The World Book Illustrated

Home
Medical
Encyclopedia

The World Book Illustrated

Home Medical Encyclopedia

Volume One
Medical Reference Guide, A - H

Published by

World Book Encyclopedia, Inc.

a Scott Fetzer company

Chicago

**The World Book Illustrated
Home Medical Encyclopedia**

1984 Revised Printing
Copyright © 1980 by
World Book-Childcraft International, Inc.
Merchandise Mart Plaza, Chicago, Illinois 60654
and Mitchell Beazley Publishers Limited
London, Great Britain

For text only on pages 24-45, 55-502, 504-509,
514-518, 566-567, 594-595, 800-919, 927-955,
964-965, 998-1005: Copyright © 1980 by Fennlevel
Limited, London, Great Britain

Printed in the United States of America
ISBN 0-7166-2060-X
Library of Congress Catalog Card No. 79-56907
d/hd

Introduction

For most individuals and families, health care is a major concern and significant expenditure. People are becoming increasingly concerned about achieving and maintaining good health and getting the most out of the money spent for medical care. Key to obtaining these objectives is a basic understanding of how the body works, diseases and disorders that can affect the body, and ways to achieve and maintain a healthy body. The layman also needs to understand basic medical terms and procedures in order to communicate effectively with health professionals.

It is for these reasons that the editors of THE WORLD BOOK ENCYCLOPEDIA decided to produce a publication that would present the current state of medical and health care in a way that was easy for the average reader to understand. The result of this effort is *The World Book Illustrated Home Medical Encyclopedia*.

Designed to provide the average family with accurate and up–to–date information, *The World Book Illustrated Home Medical Encyclopedia* has been organized and written in such a way that is both easy–to–use and easy–to–read. The information is presented with the intent that, should the need arise, clear, correct, and current data will be within easy access for quick reference.

The World Book Illustrated Home Medical Encyclopedia has been prepared by and with the advice of leading medical professionals in both the United States and Great Britain. Each key entry and important subject area has been reviewed by medical specialists. Illustrations have been thoroughly researched and reviewed to ensure the factual correctness of the procedures being shown. And experienced medical illustrators and photographers have been used throughout.

This group has been supported by a large staff of skilled editors and medical writers. The staff has been dedicated to the goal of maintaining the highest level of factual accuracy while at the same time preparing materials that are easy–to–read, easy–to–use, and easy–to–understand.

The World Book Illustrated Home Medical Encyclopedia is divided into several major sections. The first section, illustrated in full–color, details the structure and workings of the human body. An "Index of symptoms" and "Charts of related symptoms" enable a user to locate quickly and easily the various diseases and disorders discussed in the text. A thorough glossary helps a user to find the meaning of most of the medical terms he or she is likely to encounter. And thousands of entries in the A to Z portion of the set give vital background about diseases and

disorders currently of concern, and about the drugs and procedures used to combat them. A question–and–answer technique is
used to spotlight key information.

First-aid materials, featuring step–by–step illustrations for all
important procedures, help prepare a user to deal sensibly with
emergency situations. Safety–related materials provide valuable
information designed to help a reader avoid various kinds of life
threatening situations. An illustrated section on "Care of the sick
in the home" presents in a careful, step–by–step way, dozens of
recommended procedures to aid in the accomplishment of this
most difficult of responsibilities. And "Professional care for the
sick" discusses the current structure of medical care so that the
reader can become a more intelligent medical consumer.

Finally, extensive and detailed coverage has been given to a
variety of topics that should be of major concern to every family.
The World Book Illustrated Home Medical Encyclopedia devotes
a great deal of attention to such important topics as child care,
health maintenance at various age levels, nutrition, and physical
fitness.

All of the information in *The World Book Illustrated Home
Medical Encyclopedia* has been organized in such a way as to
enhance its usefulness. The material is divided into four handy–
sized volumes. Volumes 1 and 2 are devoted primarily to the A-
to-Z guide to medicine and current medical practice. Volume 3
contains sections on first aid, safety, and care of the sick. Volume
4 features coverage of child care, health maintenance, and
physical fitness.

Each major section within a volume is prefaced by an introduction describing the section's subject and by a table of contents.
The content itself has been thoroughly cross–referenced. Within
an entry in the A to Z portion of the set, the title of other entries
in which additional or related information may be found is
printed in SMALL CAPS. Articles in Volumes 3 and 4 refer the
reader to related information through the use of **boldface titles**
with **page numbers.** The entire presentation is completed by an
extensive and thorough index.

Of course, the information contained in *The World Book
Illustrated Home Medical Encyclopedia* **is not intended to take the
place of the care and attention of a physician or other medical or
health care professional.** Trained professionals must always be
consulted over matters as important as those involving a person's
health or well–being. The years of training and experience to
which such people have been subjected can never be replaced by
a single publication. What *The World Book Illustrated Home
Medical Encyclopedia* is intended to do is to provide today's
family with accurate, authoritative, up–to–date, and easy–to–use
information about medicine, its practice and procedures, and
about health care.

Contents,
Volume One

How your body works

Section contents

Introduction

This section is designed to tell a reader exactly how the body works, in words and pictures, with diagrams and captions. Every part of the body is examined and explained, either as part of one of the systems of the body or as a specific organ. The composition of each is clearly shown and the function described in detail.

The body is made up primarily of cells, of which there are many kinds. There are as many as 10 million million cells in the adult human body. The first pages of the section describe these "building blocks of life", and include information on structure and function, and on heredity, which is governed by the contents of most human cells.

The bones and joints make up the framework of the entire human body. There are about 206 bones in an adult, 22 of which alone form the skull. The joints are commonly thought only to exist to enable movement, but in fact many of them permit no movement whatever. The body has evolved clever systems of avoiding friction in those joints that do not move.

Movement, digestion, respiration, blood circulation, and other internal systems, are all made possible by the muscles. To enable movement, even in the heart, layers of muscle tissue lie across one another in an intricate crisscrossed pattern.

The heart is the body's engine, and pumps blood around the circulation system through the arteries and veins. It is the blood that exchanges carbon dioxide for life-giving oxygen in the lungs, during the process of respiration. That same process is made use of in a different way in order to talk, although speech also involves other organs in the throat and mouth.

The mouth is also the beginning of the digestive system, which consists of a tube about 30 feet long, all the way to the anus. On the way, many processes, including those within the stomach, absorb and make use of substances in the food swallowed.

The brain interprets anything felt, smelled, heard, tasted, or seen, through the nervous system. The association centers and motor areas of the brain coordinate the mechanisms and chemical reactions of the body, including the hormones secreted by the endocrine glands.

Finally, in this section the process of reproduction is fully explained.

1

A collection of cells

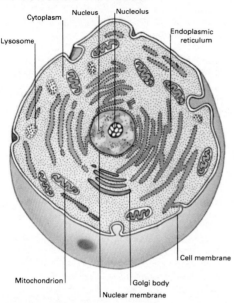

All body cells have the same basic constituents. The cell is enclosed in a membrane and comprises the cytoplasm and nucleus. The cytoplasm contains organelles vital to cell activity, such as mitochondria, for energy production, and the endoplasmic reticulum, running from membrane to nucleus, that bears ribosomes essential to protein building. Instructions for protein manufacture are given by the DNA of the nucleus.

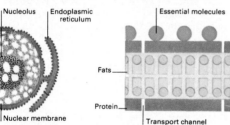

In the nucleus, information is housed in the chromosomes. The nucleolus aids protein synthesis. Substances pass in and out of pores in the membrane.

The cell membrane consists of two layers of protein enclosing a layer of fats. Special areas in the membrane allow molecules to enter and leave the cell.

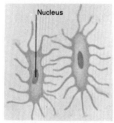

Cells called osteoblasts make the hard substances in bone. The minerals are molded by the cells' long cytoplasm-filled arms.

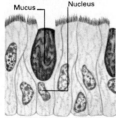

Goblet cells form part of a mucous membrane. They secrete mucin, which combines with water to form slippery mucus.

All plants and animals are composed of microscopic "building blocks" called cells. Most cells measure only a few thousandths of a millimeter across. An adult human's body contains about 10 million million cells. Each human being starts life as a single cell, a fertilized egg, which divides during embryonic development. In the course of this duplication, specialized cells do various jobs.

Cells group together to form tissues; tissues combine to compose body organs; and collections of organs make up the body systems. For example, the lining of the stomach is a tissue, and the stomach an organ that is part of the digestive system.

The cells in the body's tissues and organs vary greatly in size, shape, and appearance, but all cells are built to the same basic plan. Every cell has an outer membrane enclosing a jelly like substance, the cytoplasm, in which are found substances that provide food, energy, building materials, and waste products for removal, plus many tiny bodies (organelles). The membrane is also involved in cell operations by assisting the minute-by-minute passage of selected materials in and out of the cell. The close positioning of membranes of adjacent cells helps to ensure communication of chemical information between cells.

Of all the bodies within the cytoplasm the most prominent is the nucleus, a spherical structure vital to life. The nucleus directs all the activities of the cell because it is the store of cell information. This information is housed in strands called chromosomes, within the nucleus. Nearly all human cells contain forty-six chromosomes arranged in twenty-three pairs. Onto the chromosomes are "threaded" the genes, units made of deoxyribonucleic acid (DNA), a remarkable substance that has the ability to duplicate itself. This duplication ensures human reproduction and cell replacement processes, which continue throughout life.

The DNA in the genes works by directing the production of proteins, molecules essential for cell survival. The manufacture of proteins is assisted by the nucleolus, a center inside the nucleus, and by minute structures called ribosomes. The ribosomes lie outside the nucleus on the endoplasmic reticulum, a network of tubes running through the cytoplasm from the wall of the nucleus to the cell membrane. Both nucleolus and ribosomes contain a different nucleic acid, ribonucleic acid (RNA), which helps to control the build-up of raw materials into proteins. Once made, the proteins act as building materials, as chemical messengers (hormones), and as enzymes, the biological catalysts that direct chemical reactions within all cells. Proteins are "packaged" for removal from the cell in collections of minute tubes, the Golgi bodies.

Cells contain other vital organelles. The sausage-shaped mitochondria provide the cell with energy by breaking down substances passed to the cell in the blood. In round structures called lysosomes, large molecules are fragmented for use in the cell.

The variations between cells reflect the tasks of different cells. Some of the cells nearest to the "basic" design include the hexagonal liver cells, which perform many complex chemical reactions. Other simple cells are those that provide support and lining in many tissues. Often these column-shaped cells produce the sticky substance mucus and are edged with minute hairlike projections (cilia), which can move substances along. The fat cells found beneath the skin and around many organs are simple cells whose cytoplasm is packed with globules of fat. The fat is used to provide insulation and energy. Red blood cells, which carry oxygen and carbon dioxide round the circulation, are

unusual in having no nuclei in their mature form. In contrast, many of the white blood cells, part of the body's defense system against disease, have very large nuclei.

Three of the most specialized sorts of cells are muscle cells, nerve cells, and reproductive cells. Muscle cells are greatly elongated and have the power of contraction made possible by special proteins that can slide over one another. Because muscle contraction is energy-intensive, muscle cells have huge numbers of mitochondria.

Nerve cells are also elongated but have membranes specialized for transmitting the electrical impulses of nerve messages. Each nerve cell ends in a cell body bearing projections that lie close to similar projections on adjacent nerve cells. Messages "jump the gaps" with the aid of chemicals made in the nerve cells.

Reproductive cells, sperm from the male and eggs from the female, are unique in containing only half the usual number of chromosomes. This is necessary so that the number can be restored to forty-six when sperm and egg combine at fertilization.

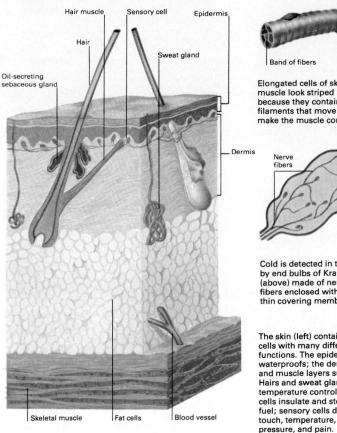

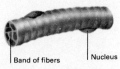

Elongated cells of skeletal muscle look striped because they contain filaments that move to make the muscle contract.

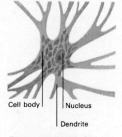

The transmission of impulses between nerve cells is achieved with the help of outgrowths (dendrites) from each cell body.

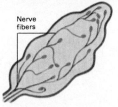

Cold is detected in the skin by end bulbs of Krause (above) made of nerve fibers enclosed within a thin covering membrane.

The skin (left) contains cells with many different functions. The epidermis waterproofs; the dermis and muscle layers support. Hairs and sweat glands aid temperature control; fat cells insulate and store fuel; sensory cells detect touch, temperature, pressure, and pain.

Spherical fat cells can expand to accommodate large stores of energy-rich fats. They have small nuclei.

Mature red blood cells, flattened concave disks that have no nuclei, carry oxygen and carbon dioxide.

3

Bones and joints

The body's skeleton is its internal support system. Its bones also surround and protect vital organs and, together with the muscles, make movement possible. Some bones have the additional job of making blood cells.

Bone is a living tissue that is both rigid and resilient. Most bones are first formed as cartilage, a gristle-like elastic substance. The cartilage is then invaded by bone-building cells, which harden it by depositing calcium salts. Even when fully formed, many bones retain some cartilage at their ends to aid binding between bones or joint articulation.

In a mature bone the cells at the center are arranged in a lattice to give lightness, whereas those toward the outside are densely packed for strength. The bone cells in the outer area are grouped in rod-shaped units, each penetrated by blood vessels that supply nutrients. Meshed between the rods are supple fibers that give bone its elasticity.

There is an average of 206 bones in the human skeleton, divided into two groups. The skull, spine, and ribcage make up the axial skeleton. The limbs, shoulder (pectoral) girdle, and hip (pelvic) girdle compose the appendicular skeleton. The twenty-two skull bones form a protective vault for the brain and sockets for the eyes, ears, and organs of smell. The only skull bone that can move is the lower jaw. Teeth are embedded in this bone, and in the upper jaw.

Beneath the skull is a total of thirty-four vertebrae, which make up the spine (backbone) and encase the spinal cord. Toward the base of the spine, five vertebrae are fused together to form the sacrum, with the fused bones of the coccyx beneath them. The twenty-four curved rib bones are attached to the spine. At the front of the body the top ten rib pairs are attached to the breastbone (sternum). The ribcage protects the heart, lungs, and large blood vessels; it can move in and out during breathing.

Lying over the upper part of the ribcage at the back of the body are the shoulder blades (scapulae). The collarbones (clavicles) link the shoulder blades with the breastbone and give support to the shoulders. The upper arm bone (humerus) fits into a socket in the shoulder blade.

The bones of the arms and shoulder girdle are designed for dexterity. In contrast, those of the hip girdle and legs are constructed for

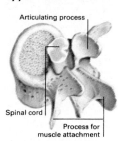

Articulating process

Spinal cord

Process for muscle attachment

A lower back spine bone (above), turned side-on shows the processes designed for articulation and muscle attachment.

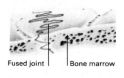

Fused joint | Bone marrow

The flat bones of the skull (above) are connected by fused unmovable joints. Red blood cells are made in the marrow of skull bones, long bones, and vertebrae.

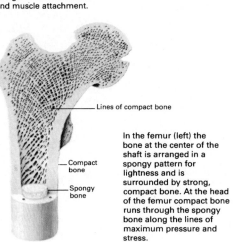

Lines of compact bone

Compact bone

Spongy bone

In the femur (left) the bone at the center of the shaft is arranged in a spongy pattern for lightness and is surrounded by strong, compact bone. At the head of the femur compact bone runs through the spongy bone along the lines of maximum pressure and stress.

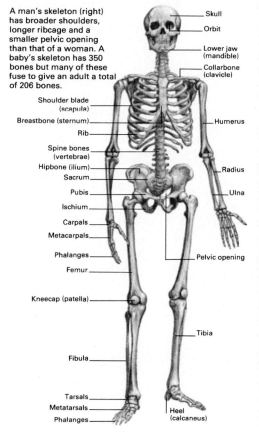

A man's skeleton (right) has broader shoulders, longer ribcage and a smaller pelvic opening than that of a woman. A baby's skeleton has 350 bones but many of these fuse to give an adult a total of 206 bones.

Skull
Orbit
Lower jaw (mandible)
Collarbone (clavicle)
Shoulder blade (scapula)
Breastbone (sternum)
Rib
Humerus
Spine bones (vertebrae)
Hipbone (ilium)
Sacrum
Radius
Pubis
Ischium
Ulna
Carpals
Metacarpals
Phalanges
Pelvic opening
Femur
Kneecap (patella)
Tibia
Fibula
Tarsals
Metatarsals
Phalanges
Heel (calcaneus)

weight-bearing and walking. The pelvic girdle also houses and supports the organs of the lower abdomen. It is made up of three fused bones on each side of the body. Each hip-bone (ilium) is bound to the sacrum of the spine, and the two pubic bones are united at the front of the body. Each ischial bone of the girdle joins with the base of the hipbone and the pubic bone. The upper leg bone (femur) is socketed into a cavity at the junction of the three bones.

Joined to the strong upper bones of each limb are paired parallel bones – the radius and ulna in the forearm, the tibia and fibula in the lower leg. The wrist and the ankle are composed of a number of small bones. The framework of the hand is made up of meta-carpals; the foot is composed of metatarsals. The fingers and toes are constructed of bones called phalanges, those of the fingers being much longer than those of the toes.

Movements of the skeleton are made possible by the joints formed wherever two bones meet. The joints that allow most freedom of action are those at the shoulder and hip. Here a ball at the end of the limb bone fits into a socket on the girdle. At knee

and elbow, hinge joints permit the limbs to bend in one direction only. The elbow also has a pivot joint enabling the arm to twist.

Other mobile joints include the ellipsoid joints between the hand's phalanges and metacarpals, which permit circular movement. The saddle joint of the thumb enables the thumb to touch each finger in turn.

Some joints are designed for only restricted motion or none at all. Disks of cartilage between the vertebrae permit only slight movement of the spine. The fused jigsaw-like joints between the skull bones eliminate all movement; their purpose is protection rather than mobility.

The detailed structure of each joint depends on the job it has to do. Wherever freedom of action is possible, the ends of each bone are capped with cartilage to cut down friction. A freely movable joint is lubricated with liquid produced by the capsule surrounding it. A large joint, such as the knee, also has a fluid-filled cavity (bursa) to the front that acts as a shock absorber. Joint strength is enhanced by ligaments and by tendons, which are extensions of the muscles whose action makes joints move.

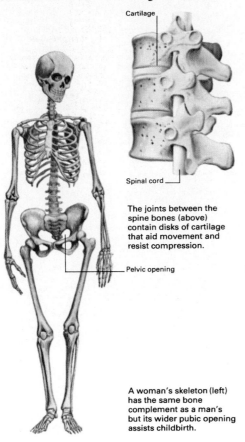

The joints between the spine bones (above) contain disks of cartilage that aid movement and resist compression.

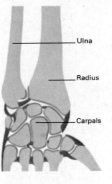

At the gliding joints between the carpal bones of the wrist (above) the surfaces of the bones slide over one another.

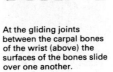

The hinge joints between the bones of the fingers (above) allow movement in one plane only. The joints are bound with ligaments and connected by tendons to muscles of the hand and arm.

A woman's skeleton (left) has the same bone complement as a man's but its wider pubic opening assists childbirth.

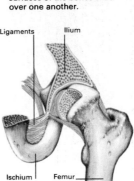

The ligaments that bond the ball-and-socket joint of the hip (left) also carry nerves and blood vessels to the joint.

Muscles

Muscles are the motive force that makes possible the wide range of human movements. The activities of muscles are also essential for digestion, respiration, blood circulation, and other vital internal mechanisms. All muscles operate by shortening in length (contracting), and all muscle contraction is controlled by messages received from the nervous system.

There are three types of muscles: skeletal muscles, smooth muscles, and cardiac muscle. Skeletal muscles are those that allow body movement. They are also called voluntary muscles because their actions can be consciously controlled by the brain. Smooth muscles are found in the intestines, arteries, bladder, and other internal organs. Cardiac muscle, found only in the heart, is the driving force of the heartbeat. Both smooth and cardiac muscles act involuntarily, under the influence of the automatic (autonomic) section of the nervous system.

More than 600 skeletal muscles, arranged in layers, cover the bones. Many of these muscles are attached directly to bones by fibrous extensions known as tendons. Other skeletal muscles are linked to neighboring muscles or to the skin. At the joints between bones, skeletal muscles can produce bending, straightening, and turning movements; or they can move the limbs to and from the side of the body. In the face, skeletal muscles attached to the skin control facial expressions such as smiling and frowning.

Most skeletal muscles are positioned and operate in pairs. In the arm, for example, the biceps muscle at the front of the upper arm links the radius bone of the forearm with the bones of the shoulder and upper arm. The triceps muscle at the back of the upper arm links the ulna of the forearm with the shoulder and upper arm bones. When the forearm is raised, operating the elbow joint, the biceps contracts and the triceps relaxes. When the arm is straightened at the elbow, the biceps relaxes and the triceps contracts.

A skeletal muscle is made up of many bundles of long, straight fibers up to 12 inches (30cm) long. Every fiber is composed of smaller units known as myofibrils. If viewed under a microscope, the fibers and myofibrils appear to have crosswise stripes. For this reason, skeletal muscle is often called striped or striated muscle. The stripes

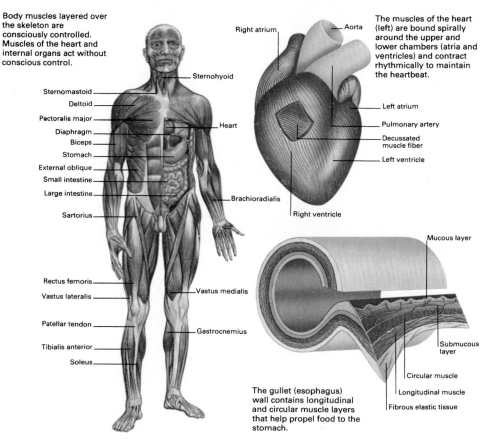

Body muscles layered over the skeleton are consciously controlled. Muscles of the heart and internal organs act without conscious control.

Sternomastoid
Deltoid
Pectoralis major
Diaphragm
Biceps
Stomach
External oblique
Small intestine
Large intestine
Sartorius

Sternohyoid
Heart

Brachioradialis

Rectus femoris
Vastus lateralis
Vastus medialis

Patellar tendon
Gastrocnemius
Tibialis anterior
Soleus

Right atrium
Aorta

The muscles of the heart (left) are bound spirally around the upper and lower chambers (atria and ventricles) and contract rhythmically to maintain the heartbeat.

Left atrium
Pulmonary artery
Decussated muscle fiber
Left ventricle

Right ventricle

Mucous layer

Submucous layer
Circular muscle
Longitudinal muscle
Fibrous elastic tissue

The gullet (esophagus) wall contains longitudinal and circular muscle layers that help propel food to the stomach.

are created by overlapping strands of protein inside the myofibrils. To make a skeletal muscle contract, nerve messages are sent to the muscle fibers. When a message reaches a fiber a chemical is released that makes the protein strands in the myofibrils slide over each other, so reducing the fiber's length.

The cardiac muscle of the heart has cross-striations like those of skeletal muscle, but its fibers are branched and its actions cannot be voluntarily controlled. Cardiac muscle is exceptional because it has a built-in rhythm of contraction. In the body this rhythm is regulated by the involuntary nervous system to produce a regular, coordinated pumping action. During a heartbeat, the muscle relaxes as the heart fills with blood, then contracts to pump blood out of the heart.

The muscle of the internal organs is called smooth muscle because its unbranched fibers are not striped like those of voluntary and cardiac muscle. Smooth muscles are composed of fibers rarely more than 0.02 inches (0.5mm) long. These fibers are generally grouped in bundles or sheets. The body's largest concentration of smooth muscle is in the tube that forms the intestine.

Here smooth muscles are arranged and work in a paired way comparable to the action of skeletal muscles. Circular muscles lie around the intestinal tube, and longitudinal muscles run along its length. By alternate contraction and relaxation of the two sets of muscles, a wavelike motion called peristalsis is created that pushes food along the tube.

Elsewhere in the body, groups of smooth muscle fibers act without the need for pairing. In the skin, a bundle of smooth muscle fibers is attached to the tissues that surround the base of each hair. When the body is cold the fibers contract, making the hair stand up.

It is sometimes possible for the brain to override the instructions of the involuntary nervous system in the control of smooth muscle activity. The smooth muscle surrounding the exit to the bladder, for example, is normally kept contracted, closing the outlet. When the bladder is full, involuntary nerve messages instruct the muscle to relax so that urine can be passed. With training, nerve signals from the brain can cancel this command until urination is convenient.

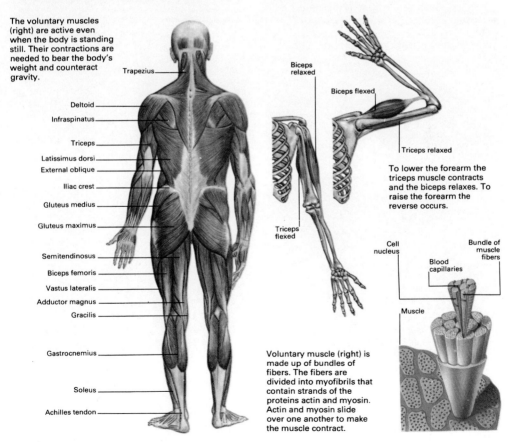

The voluntary muscles (right) are active even when the body is standing still. Their contractions are needed to bear the body's weight and counteract gravity.

Trapezius

Deltoid
Infraspinatus
Triceps
Latissimus dorsi
External oblique
Iliac crest
Gluteus medius
Gluteus maximus
Semitendinosus
Biceps femoris
Vastus lateralis
Adductor magnus
Gracilis
Gastrocnemius
Soleus
Achilles tendon

Biceps relaxed

Biceps flexed

Triceps relaxed

To lower the forearm the triceps muscle contracts and the biceps relaxes. To raise the forearm the reverse occurs.

Triceps flexed

Cell nucleus

Blood capillaries

Bundle of muscle fibers

Muscle

Voluntary muscle (right) is made up of bundles of fibers. The fibers are divided into myofibrils that contain strands of the proteins actin and myosin. Actin and myosin slide over one another to make the muscle contract.

The heart

The blood circulation is the body system that carries essential supplies of food and fuel to every living cell and exchanges them for potentially harmful waste products. The adult circulation consists of thousands of miles of tubing containing about 10 pints (4.7 liters) of blood. The blood is kept flowing round the body by the pumping action of the heart.

Blood is made up of a pale yellow liquid (plasma) containing dissolved nutrients and wastes, plus blood cells, hormones, and other substances. Most numerous of these cells are the disk-shaped red blood cells (corpuscles). Their color comes from the presence of the substance hemoglobin, which combines with oxygen. When red corpuscles charged with oxygen approach body cells, the oxygen is delivered in exchange for the waste product carbon dioxide. Other two-way transportation of materials takes place between the body cells and the plasma, and all unwanted substances are carried away in the blood for excretion by the kidneys, lungs, and liver. Plasma also contains white blood corpuscles, which help to fight infection, and platelets, which are involved in blood clotting.

In its passage through the body, blood is carried in tubes known as arteries and veins. Most arteries transport oxygen-rich (oxygenated) blood, whereas most veins transport carbon dioxide-rich (deoxygenated) blood. The largest artery is the aorta, which stems directly from the heart. The aorta and other large arteries have thick walls lined with muscle. Blood flow is assisted by the contraction of this muscle and the impetus given by the heartbeat. The "push" from the heart can be felt as the pulse where large arteries run near the body surface.

As they penetrate the tissues, arteries split into narrow branches called arterioles, which in turn divide into capillaries. It is across the very thin capillary walls that the blood gives

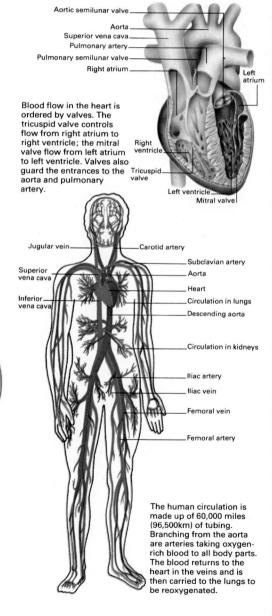

Aortic semilunar valve
Aorta
Superior vena cava
Pulmonary artery
Pulmonary semilunar valve
Right atrium
Left atrium
Right ventricle
Tricuspid valve
Left ventricle
Mitral valve

Blood flow in the heart is ordered by valves. The tricuspid valve controls flow from right atrium to right ventricle; the mitral valve flow from left atrium to left ventricle. Valves also guard the entrances to the aorta and pulmonary artery.

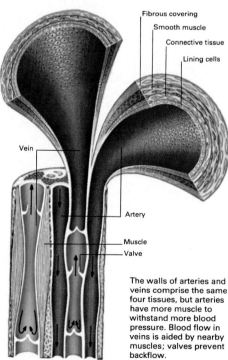

Fibrous covering
Smooth muscle
Connective tissue
Lining cells
Vein
Artery
Muscle
Valve

The walls of arteries and veins comprise the same four tissues, but arteries have more muscle to withstand more blood pressure. Blood flow in veins is aided by nearby muscles; valves prevent backflow.

Jugular vein
Carotid artery
Subclavian artery
Superior vena cava
Aorta
Heart
Inferior vena cava
Circulation in lungs
Descending aorta
Circulation in kidneys
Iliac artery
Iliac vein
Femoral vein
Femoral artery

The human circulation is made up of 60,000 miles (96,500km) of tubing. Branching from the aorta are arteries taking oxygen-rich blood to all body parts. The blood returns to the heart in the veins and is then carried to the lungs to be reoxygenated.

up its oxygen and nutrients and receives carbon dioxide and wastes. Deoxygenated blood in the capillaries flows into narrow veins (venules) and then into veins. The two largest veins, the venae cavae, return this blood to the heart. Veins have thin walls compared with those of arteries, and blood moves through the veins much more slowly. Blood flow in the veins is assisted by the action of muscles in surrounding tissues, and backflow is prevented by one-way valves.

The deoxygenated blood delivered to the heart along the veins is no use to body cells until it has been recharged with oxygen. To ensure reoxygenation, the circulation has a second "loop." In this part of the system, blood rich in carbon dioxide travels from the heart along the pulmonary artery to the lungs, where carbon dioxide is exchanged for oxygen breathed in. The pulmonary artery is the only artery to carry deoxygenated blood. The newly oxygenated blood is carried back to the heart along the pulmonary vein, the only vein to transport oxygenated blood.

The heart is a muscular organ about the size of a clenched fist. The structure and action of the heart are designed to serve the two loops of the circulation. Inside, the heart is divided vertically by a muscular wall. On each side of this wall is an upper chamber (atrium) and a thicker, lower chamber (ventricle). Blood moves through each side of the heart systematically. Deoxygenated blood is delivered into the right atrium. It then enters the right ventricle, from where it is pumped out into the pulmonary artery and to the lungs. Oxygenated blood returning in the pulmonary vein flows into the left atrium. This blood enters the left ventricle and is then pumped into the aorta for circulation.

The flow of blood in each side of the heart is controlled by a series of valves. The pumping action of the heart is achieved by the contraction of the cardiac muscle of which the heart is largely composed. The rhythm of the heartbeat is regulated by bursts of electrical impulses sent out by a concentration of specialized heart tissue called the pacemaker.

Under the influence of the pacemaker, the heart of an adult at rest beats at a rate of 70 to 80 beats a minute. The pacemaker also helps to ensure the correct sequence of activities during each heartbeat; first the two atria contract, followed rapidly by the ventricles. The powerful contraction of the ventricles pushes blood into the aorta and pulmonary artery. This period of contraction (systole) is followed by a period of relaxation (diastole), during which the heart refills. The complete sequence is accompanied by electrical activity of the muscle, which can be monitored as an electrocardiogram (EKG).

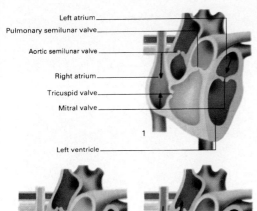

Left atrium
Pulmonary semilunar valve
Aortic semilunar valve
Right atrium
Tricuspid valve
Mitral valve
1
Left ventricle

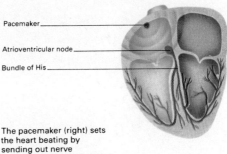

Pacemaker
Atrioventricular node
Bundle of His

The pacemaker (right) sets the heart beating by sending out nerve impulses which pass to the atria, then to the ventricles via other special nerve tissues.

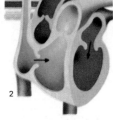
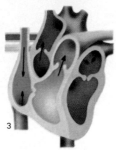

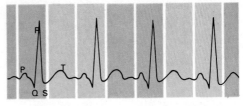

2   3

As a heartbeat begins (1) right and left atria fill with blood. The atria contract (2) forcing blood into the right and left ventricles.

The ventricles then contract strongly (3) so that blood is pushed into the aorta and pulmonary artery.

An electrocardiogram (EKG) records the waves of nerve impulses of each heartbeat. The P wave starts just before the atria

contract, the QRS wave indicates the contraction of the ventricles, and the T wave the recovery period before the next contraction.

Respiration

Respiration is the process of breathing and the mechanism by which all cells in the body release energy from the materials they consume. The two sorts of respiration are closely linked. To produce energy, cells use oxygen and generate carbon dioxide and water. The movement of air in and out of the lungs makes oxygen available to the body and removes carbon dioxide and water.

Air enters the respiratory system through the mouth and nose, where it is warmed and moistened. Air breathed in through the nose is filtered by the coarse hairs that line the nostrils, which trap large dust particles. Smaller particles are trapped in a sticky fluid (mucus) produced by the cells lining the passage between nose and mouth. This mucus is continuously moved away by the beating of minute hairlike projections (cilia).

From the mouth, air travels through the throat (pharynx), voicebox (larynx), and windpipe (trachea). At the entry to the windpipe is a flap, the epiglottis, which closes to prevent choking when food is swallowed. At its base the windpipe divides into two

tubes or bronchi, and one bronchus enters each lung. Both windpipe and bronchi are stiffened by rings of cartilage. As in the nose, the windpipe and bronchi produce dust-trapping mucus and have cilia to move this mucus up to the mouth.

Within each lung the bronchi split successively into smaller bronchi and then into many thousands of even narrower tubes called bronchioles. The bronchioles branch through the lungs and lead into millions of air sacs (alveoli) of the lung tissue. It is in the air sacs that gases are exchanged. Each air sac is meshed with small blood vessels (capillaries) carrying blood from the heart containing carbon dioxide and water. Oxygen from the air breathed in passes into the blood and, in return, carbon dioxide and water vapor are

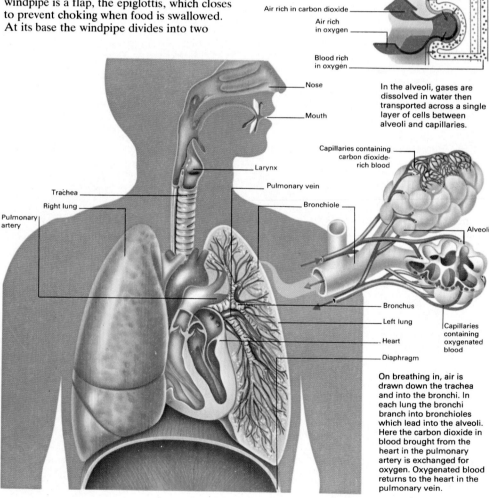

Blood rich in carbon dioxide

Layer of cells

Film of water

Air rich in carbon dioxide

Air rich in oxygen

Blood rich in oxygen

In the alveoli, gases are dissolved in water then transported across a single layer of cells between alveoli and capillaries.

Nose

Mouth

Capillaries containing carbon dioxide-rich blood

Larynx

Pulmonary vein

Trachea

Right lung

Bronchiole

Pulmonary artery

Alveoli

Bronchus

Left lung

Heart

Capillaries containing oxygenated blood

Diaphragm

On breathing in, air is drawn down the trachea and into the bronchi. In each lung the bronchi branch into bronchioles which lead into the alveoli. Here the carbon dioxide in blood brought from the heart in the pulmonary artery is exchanged for oxygen. Oxygenated blood returns to the heart in the pulmonary vein.

released into the air sacs of the lungs to be breathed out. The blood in the capillaries, now rich in oxygen, flows into the pulmonary vein and back to the heart for redistribution.

The lungs are housed in a bony cage made up of the ribs, breastbone, and backbone. The floor of the cage is formed by a sheet of muscle called the diaphragm. When a person breathes in, the muscles of the diaphragm contract, pulling the diaphragm downward. At the same time the ribcage is pulled up and out, by the contraction of the muscles between the ribs, and air rushes in. When a person breathes out, the diaphragm and rib muscles relax and the chest subsides.

Respiration takes place ten to fifteen times a minute and is normally controlled unconsciously by a collection of cells in the brain called the respiratory center. After air has been breathed out, carbon dioxide builds up again in the bloodstream. The cells in the respiratory center are extremely sensitive to carbon dioxide concentrations. When the carbon dioxide in the blood reaches a certain level, messages are sent from the respiratory center to the diaphragm and rib muscles telling them to contract. This once more initiates breathing in. As the lungs expand during inspiration, cells (stretch receptors) in the lung walls send signals back to the respiratory center. The center responds by instructing the muscles of ribs and diaphragm to relax so that breathing out takes place.

Respiration is not always a quiet process. The presence of many dust particles in the nose can trigger off sneezing. Irritants or too much mucus in the windpipe and bronchi cause coughing. Speech is also a special sort of "noisy" breathing. The sounds of speech are produced in the voicebox (larynx) and molded into words in the mouth.

The larynx consists of a box of cartilage. Across the inside of the box are flaplike structures, the vocal cords. The cords are made to move by the action of muscles attached to the cartilages of the larynx. During normal breathing, the vocal cords are held apart. For speech the cords are pulled together after a breath in, so that during breathing out the air is forced between the cords, making them vibrate. The tighter the cords are pulled together, the higher is the pitch of the sound produced. For loud sounds the air is forced through the cords faster than it is for soft sounds. The movements of the lips and of the tongue against the teeth and roof of the mouth achieve articulation. The resonance of spoken sounds and the characteristics of every individual voice are created by the cavities of the sinuses, nose, throat, and chest.

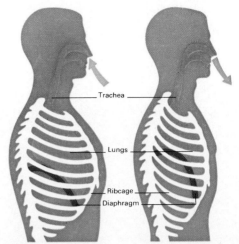

Trachea

Lungs

Ribcage
Diaphragm

Breathing in is an active process. Air is drawn in as the ribcage expands and the diaphragm contracts.

Breathing out is passive: the lungs recoil, the diaphragm relaxes, and the ribcage subsides.

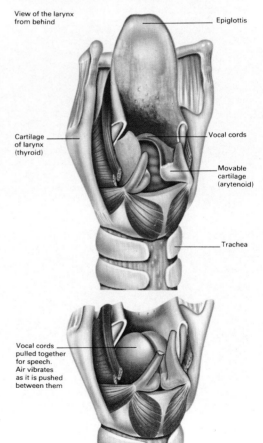

View of the larynx from behind

Epiglottis

Cartilage of larynx (thyroid)

Vocal cords

Movable cartilage (arytenoid)

Trachea

Vocal cords pulled together for speech. Air vibrates as it is pushed between them

In normal breathing, the epiglottis is held upward and the vocal cords, joined to movable cartilages, are

wide apart. In swallowing, the epiglottis is lowered. For speech the vocal cords are drawn close together.

11

The digestive system

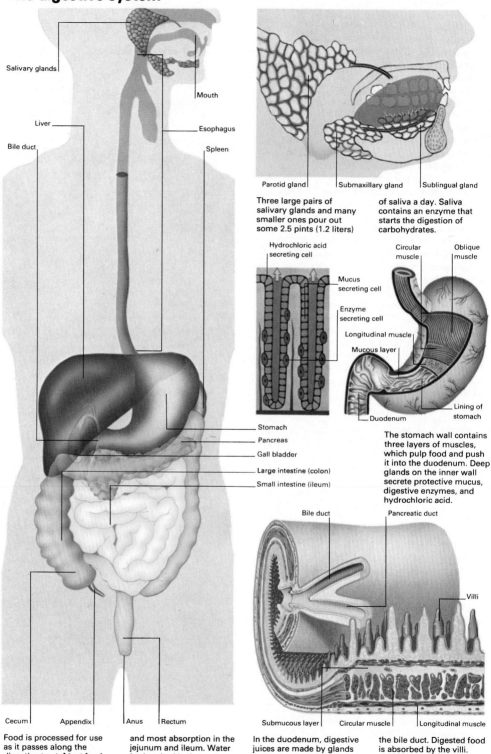

Salivary glands

Mouth

Liver

Esophagus

Bile duct

Spleen

Parotid gland | Submaxillary gland | Sublingual gland

Three large pairs of salivary glands and many smaller ones pour out some 2.5 pints (1.2 liters) of saliva a day. Saliva contains an enzyme that starts the digestion of carbohydrates.

Hydrochloric acid secreting cell

Mucus secreting cell

Enzyme secreting cell

Circular muscle

Oblique muscle

Longitudinal muscle

Mucous layer

Lining of stomach

Duodenum

Stomach

Pancreas

Gall bladder

Large intestine (colon)

Small intestine (ileum)

The stomach wall contains three layers of muscles, which pulp food and push it into the duodenum. Deep glands on the inner wall secrete protective mucus, digestive enzymes, and hydrochloric acid.

Bile duct

Pancreatic duct

Villi

Cecum | Appendix | Anus | Rectum

Submucous layer | Circular muscle | Longitudinal muscle

Food is processed for use as it passes along the digestive tract. Most food breakdown occurs in the stomach and duodenum, and most absorption in the jejunum and ileum. Water is absorbed in the cecum and colon, while wastes are passed at the anus.

In the duodenum, digestive juices are made by glands on the inner wall. More juices enter from the gall bladder and pancreas via the bile duct. Digested food is absorbed by the villi. Amino acids and sugars enter the blood, fats the lymph vessels.

Proteins, carbohydrates, fats, and liquids supply the body with energy and building materials. But these foods are of no use until they have been broken down into substances that can be absorbed into the blood circulation and transported via the liver to all body cells. This breakdown and absorption are the functions of the digestive system.

The digestive system consists of a tube about 33 feet (10 meters) in length that runs from the mouth to the anus. Within the tube many secretions are produced to aid the digestive process. These secretions include enzymes, which are biological catalysts that help to speed essential chemical reactions.

Food starts its journey through the digestive system in the mouth. There it is broken up by the teeth and moistened by secretions released from the salivary glands. Saliva also starts digestion, because it contains an enzyme that begins breaking down carbohydrates. The tongue and the teeth form each mouthful of food into a ball (bolus) and the tongue pushes it to the back of the mouth to be swallowed.

After leaving the mouth, food passes down the esophagus (gullet) and into the stomach. Most food stays in the stomach for up to four hours. During this time it is churned and mixed with secretions produced by the cells of the stomach lining. These secretions include the enzyme pepsin, which begins breaking down proteins; hydrochloric acid sterilizes food and provides the right environment for stomach enzymes to work; and the sticky fluid (mucus) that protects the stomach cells from digesting themselves.

Digestion in the stomach converts food into a thick sludge called chyme. The chyme passes into the duodenum, the first part of the small intestine. The small intestine is a tube about 21 feet (6.4 meters) long, named for its width rather than its length. In passing down the small intestine – and the large intestine that follows it – food is moved along by peristalsis, rhythmic, wavelike contractions of the muscles in the intestine wall.

In the 10-inch (25cm) duodenum, many digestive juices are poured onto the chyme. The duodenum wall secretes alkaline juices that neutralize the acid from the stomach and contain enzymes and protective mucus. Further enzyme-containing juices enter the duodenum from the pancreas. The two sets of enzymes digest proteins, carbohydrates, and fats. Fat digestion is assisted by bile, which is made in the liver. Bile contains no enzymes but breaks fats into small globules that are easier for the enzymes to work on.

By the time it leaves the duodenum, most food has been broken down into absorbable fragments. Proteins have become amino acids; carbohydrates are now glucose; and other simple sugars and fats have been converted to glycerol and fatty acids. Some of these substances are absorbed in the duodenum, but most are taken up in the 8-foot (2.5m) jejunum and 12-foot (3.6m) ileum.

The inner wall of the small intestine is folded into millions of finger-like projections called villi, which provide a large surface area for absorption. Within each villus are small blood vessels (capillaries) and narrow branches of the lymphatic system. Amino acids and sugars are absorbed into the capillaries, while glycerol and fatty acids enter the lymphatic vessels, which drain into the bloodstream. Nutrients from digested food are then transported in the blood to the liver for storage until required by body cells.

Digestion in the small intestine takes four to five hours. The liquid remaining after absorption passes into the large intestine (colon), hanging from which is the appendix, an organ with no apparent useful function. Movement of the remnants of digestion through the large intestine takes fifteen hours or more. In this time more than half the water contained is absorbed into the blood. The colon is also filled with bacteria. Some of these can break down the plant carbohydrate cellulose into usable sugars whereas others make vitamin B.

The feces (stools), the final products of digestion, leave the large intestine via the anus. Water makes up 75 percent of the stools. The remaining 25 percent consists of worn-out digestive cells, dead bacteria, and undigested plant fibers. The urge to defecate occurs when the rectum fills with feces.

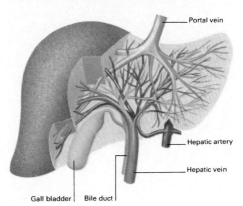

Portal vein

Hepatic artery

Hepatic vein

Gall bladder   Bile duct

Digested food reaches the liver in the portal vein and oxygen in the hepatic artery. Essential substances such as sugars, vitamins, and minerals are extracted for storage and spent blood leaves in the hepatic vein. Bile formed in the liver is stored in the gall bladder until needed for digestion.

The urinary system

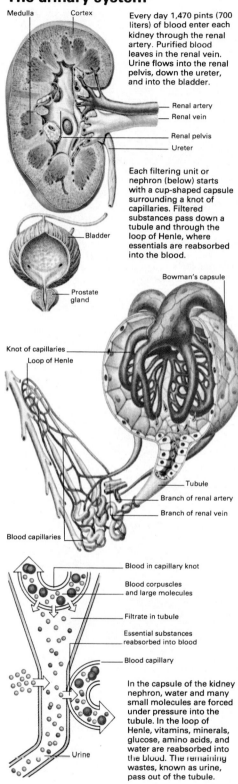

Medulla   Cortex

Every day 1,470 pints (700 liters) of blood enter each kidney through the renal artery. Purified blood leaves in the renal vein. Urine flows into the renal pelvis, down the ureter, and into the bladder.

Renal artery
Renal vein

Renal pelvis
Ureter

Each filtering unit or nephron (below) starts with a cup-shaped capsule surrounding a knot of capillaries. Filtered substances pass down a tubule and through the loop of Henle, where essentials are reabsorbed into the blood.

Bladder

Prostate gland

Bowman's capsule

Knot of capillaries
Loop of Henle

Tubule
Branch of renal artery
Branch of renal vein

Blood capillaries

Blood in capillary knot

Blood corpuscles and large molecules

Filtrate in tubule

Essential substances reabsorbed into blood

Blood capillary

In the capsule of the kidney nephron, water and many small molecules are forced under pressure into the tubule. In the loop of Henle, vitamins, minerals, glucose, amino acids, and water are reabsorbed into the blood. The remaining wastes, known as urine, pass out of the tubule.

Urine

The urinary system filters soluble waste products from the blood. It consists of two kidneys, two ureters, the urinary bladder, and the urethra. The kidneys are about 4½ inches (11cm) long and about 2½ inches (6cm) wide. They lie in the upper part of the abdomen at the back. The ureters are tubes about 10 inches (25cm) long that drain urine from the core of the kidneys, the renal pelvis, to the bladder. The bladder lies in the lower abdomen at the front of the body. The urethra is the tube through which urine is passed to the outside.

The renal pelvis is funnel-shaped; its widest part is in the center of the kidney. As the renal pelvis narrows, it projects from the kidney and becomes the top of the ureter. The widest part of the renal pelvis is surrounded by the renal medulla, which is in turn surrounded by the renal cortex. The renal cortex is covered by tough fibrous tissue that forms the protective outer layer of each kidney.

Blood is brought to the kidneys by the renal arteries and, after filtration, is returned to the circulation through the renal veins. The blood vessels join the kidneys close to each renal pelvis.

The functional units of the kidney are microscopic filters. The renal cortex contains about one million of these filters. Each consists of a cup-shaped capsule (Bowman's capsule) that encloses a knot (glomerulus) of blood capillaries. Blood from the renal artery is pumped into the glomerulus by blood pressure. Water, sugar, salts, urea (a waste product of the breakdown of proteins), and other small molecules pass through the capillary walls into the Bowman's capsule. Blood cells and large molecules, such as whole proteins and fats, remain in the blood.

Filtered fluids pass from the Bowman's capsule into a coiled tube, the nephron, that leads through the renal medulla to the renal pelvis. Each nephron has a U-shaped loop, the loop of Henle, half-way along its length. The whole tube is closely surrounded by blood capillaries. As the filtered fluid passes through the tube, substances that the body needs, especially water, essential salts, and sugar, are reabsorbed from the fluid in the tube into the surrounding blood capillaries.

The concentrated fluid (urine) that results from the filtration and reabsorption processes collects in the renal pelvis before passing through the ureter to the bladder. A circular ring of muscle at the top of the urethra keeps urine in the bladder until voluntarily relaxed.

The nose, mouth, and throat

The nose has two primary functions: (1) to filter, warm, and humidify air before it reaches the lungs; and (2) to smell.

The internal surface of the nose is covered with tiny hairs (cilia) that are surrounded by sticky, fluid mucus. Both cilia and mucus remove dust particles and water droplets from the air that is breathed through the nostrils. At the top of the nasal cavity there are two areas of tissue in which the cells are sensitive to smell. When a substance is trapped in the mucus by the cilia, it causes a chemical change to affect the sensitive cells. The cells react by sending a nerve impulse to the brain that is interpreted there as a smell.

The mouth is the beginning of the digestive tract. The teeth, the tongue, and the salivary glands prepare food for digestion. The saliva contains enzymes that start the process of digestion. The organs of taste (taste buds) are located in tiny projections (papillae) on the surface of the tongue. Each taste bud consists of a cluster of receptor cells that react to a chemical change by sending a nerve impulse to the brain, where it is interpreted as a taste.

When food is swallowed, a flap of cartilage (the epiglottis) folds down to cover the opening to the trachea (windpipe). This action prevents food from going on down into the lungs.

The vocal cords are located in the trachea, just below the epiglottis. Sound is produced when air from the lungs passes between vocal cords that have been voluntarily tensed. The sounds of the human voice are controlled by the movements of the vocal cords in combination with movements of the tongue and lips.

The back of the nose and mouth is lined with pads of spongy tissue containing many lymph vessels. These pads include the adenoids in the nose, the tonsils at the back of the mouth, and a similar pad of lymphoid tissue on the back of the tongue. Invading bacteria are collected and destroyed by the cells (lymphocytes) that are concentrated in lymphoid tissue. A large number of lymph nodes in the tissues at the top of the throat and below, in the neck, support this defense mechanism.

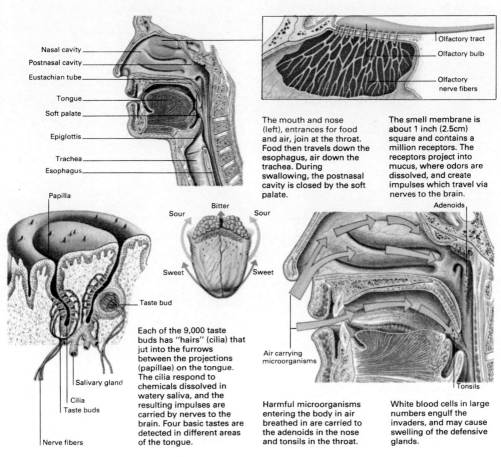

Nasal cavity
Postnasal cavity
Eustachian tube
Tongue
Soft palate
Epiglottis
Trachea
Esophagus
Papilla

Olfactory tract
Olfactory bulb
Olfactory nerve fibers

The mouth and nose (left), entrances for food and air, join at the throat. Food then travels down the esophagus, air down the trachea. During swallowing, the postnasal cavity is closed by the soft palate.

The smell membrane is about 1 inch (2.5cm) square and contains a million receptors. The receptors project into mucus, where odors are dissolved, and create impulses which travel via nerves to the brain.

Sour   Bitter   Sour
Sweet   Sweet
Adenoids

Taste bud

Salivary gland
Cilia
Taste buds
Nerve fibers

Air carrying microorganisms

Tonsils

Each of the 9,000 taste buds has "hairs" (cilia) that jut into the furrows between the projections (papillae) on the tongue. The cilia respond to chemicals dissolved in watery saliva, and the resulting impulses are carried by nerves to the brain. Four basic tastes are detected in different areas of the tongue.

Harmful microorganisms entering the body in air breathed in are carried to the adenoids in the nose and tonsils in the throat.

White blood cells in large numbers engulf the invaders, and may cause swelling of the defensive glands.

The eye and ear

The eyes and ears are organs vital to the body's interpretation of its environment. The eyes detect light rays; the ears pick up sound waves. The ears also contain the organs of balance.

Each eye is a spherical structure protected at its back and sides by the bones of the skull and at the front by two lashed eyelids. The outer covering of the eye, the sclera or "white," is both protective and structural. Light penetrates the sclera only at the front of the eye, where the outer surface bulges into the transparent cornea, a delicate structure overlaid with a thin defensive membrane, the conjunctiva. Under each upper eyelid is a tear-secreting lacrimal gland whose constant activity keeps the conjuctiva moist and free from germs.

Light entering the eye passes through the cornea and then through a watery fluid, the aqueous humor, in the front of the eye. Behind the fluid is the iris, a ring of muscle with a central hole, the pupil. The cornea focuses light rays so that they pass through the pupil. The iris determines how much light enters the eye. In dim light its muscles relax to let in more light; in bright light its muscles

contract to reduce pupil size and restrict light entry.

The fine focusing of light is achieved by the lens, a soft, transparent structure lying behind the iris. The lens is held in place by ligaments attached to internal eye muscles. The actions of these muscles bring about changes in the shape of the lens so that close and distant objects can be focused upon. For viewing near objects the muscles make the lens shorter and fatter; for viewing distant objects the lens becomes longer and thinner. This process is known as accommodation.

From the lens, light passes through the thick jelly (vitreous humor) that fills the center of the eye. The light is projected onto the retina, a light-sensitive layer inside the sclera from which it is separated by the choroid, a dark layer of tissue rich in blood vessels. The retina contains two sorts of light-receptor cells: rods, which detect shades of black and white; and cones, which are sensitive to color. In response to light, the rods and cones generate nerve impulses that pass along the optic nerve to the brain to be interpreted as vision. The concentration of cones is densest at a single spot called the

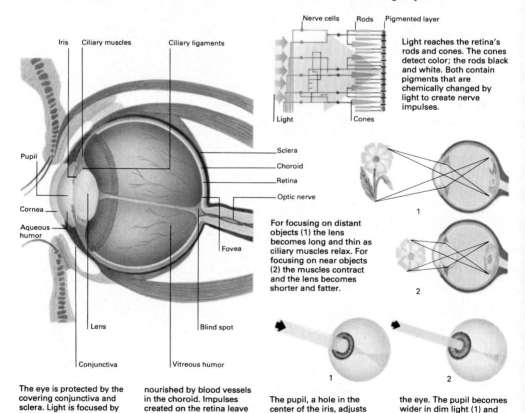

Nerve cells   Rods   Pigmented layer

Light reaches the retina's rods and cones. The cones detect color; the rods black and white. Both contain pigments that are chemically changed by light to create nerve impulses.

Light   Cones

Iris   Ciliary muscles   Ciliary ligaments

Pupil

Cornea

Aqueous humor

Lens   Blind spot

Conjunctiva   Vitreous humor

Sclera
Choroid
Retina
Optic nerve

Fovea

For focusing on distant objects (1) the lens becomes long and thin as ciliary muscles relax. For focusing on near objects (2) the muscles contract and the lens becomes shorter and fatter.

1

2

1

2

The eye is protected by the covering conjunctiva and sclera. Light is focused by the cornea and lens onto the retina, which is

nourished by blood vessels in the choroid. Impulses created on the retina leave the eye along the optic nerve.

The pupil, a hole in the center of the iris, adjusts by reflex to control the amount of light entering

the eye. The pupil becomes wider in dim light (1) and becomes smaller in bright (2).

fovea. Where the optic nerve leaves the back of the eye there are no rods or cones; this is called the blind spot.

The ears, like the eyes, are housed mostly deep in the bone structure of the skull. Each ear is divided into outer, middle, and inner sections. The only visible part is the flap of cartilage (pinna) of the outer ear, which helps to collect sounds and concentrates them into a tube, the auditory canal. At the end of the canal is a thin membrane, the eardrum (tympanic membrane). When sounds reach the eardrum, they make it vibrate. These vibrations are transmitted and amplified through the middle ear by a chain of three small bones, the hammer (malleus), anvil (incus), and stirrup (stapes). The cavity of the middle ear, in which the bones are contained, is joined to the throat by the Eustachian tube. The tube ensures that the air pressure in the middle ear remains the same as that on the outer side of the eardrum. The middle ear also connects with the air cells in the mastoid bone behind the ear.

The stirrup, the last of the middle ear bones, rests against a membrane, the oval window, that leads to the cochlea, the part of the inner ear concerned with hearing. The cochlea is a spiral, fluid-filled tube divided internally along its length by a strip of tissue, the basilar membrane. The vibrations carried by the middle ear bones are transported in the fluid as pressure waves. These waves make special hair-bearing cells on the basilar membrane vibrate according to the loudness and pitch of sound. Their vibration sets up nerve impulses that are then carried to the brain along the auditory nerve, to be interpreted there as hearing. The hair-bearing cells and the membrane on which they are found are known as the organ of Corti.

The inner ear also contains the organs of balance which, like the cochlea, consist of fluid-filled chambers. Three of these, the semicircular canals, are set in planes at right angles to one another. At the ends of the chambers are collections of fine hairs. As the head moves, the fluid in each canal starts to move accordingly, and stimulates the hairs to generate nerve messages. Even when the head is still, body posture is detected by two further chambers, the utricle and saccule. Impulses from these chambers travel to the area of the brain responsible for balance.

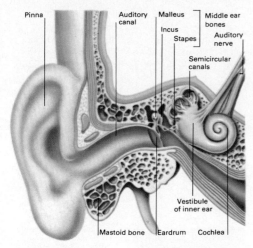

Sounds received by the ear's pinna pass along the auditory canal to the eardrum. Vibrations are carried by three bones to the cochlea, from which nerve impulses are sent to the brain.

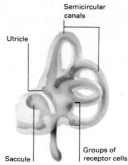

The spiral cochlea is divided internally into three compartments. Within the central one lies the organ of Corti. This has hairs that vibrate in response to sounds and create nerve impulses that travel via the auditory nerve to the brain for analysis.

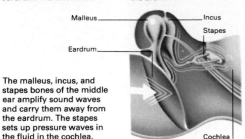

The malleus, incus, and stapes bones of the middle ear amplify sound waves and carry them away from the eardrum. The stapes sets up pressure waves in the fluid in the cochlea.

The semicircular canals detect body movement in three planes as the fluid they contain stimulates hairlike receptors. Utricle and saccule register the position of the head.

17

The brain

The brain is an organ constructed to receive, process, and store the information that floods into it from inside and outside the body, and to issue "instructions" for body action. It is the seat of human consciousness, intellect, memory, emotions, and personality. The brain is a delicate structure weighing about 3lb (1,380gm) in a man, and 2lb 12oz (1,250gm) in a woman; it is protected by a covering membrane (meninges) and by the bones of the skull.

More than 30,000 million nerve cells (neurons) make up the brain. To accommodate these cells the surface of the brain is much folded. Most of the brain is symmetrically divided into right and left halves, linked by nerve tissue. Each half is made up of three main areas: the hind-, mid-, and forebrain. Different parts of each area have distinct functions that are carried out by the nerve cells that compose them. Lying deep within the brain are cavities (ventricles) filled with fluid.

The hindbrain, at the brain's base and joined to the spinal cord, is composed of two parts: the brainstem and the cerebellum. The brainstem controls essential life-supporting functions, such as respiration and heartbeat, and acts on the huge inflow of information it receives about the state of the body. Running through the brainstem is the reticular formation that helps to determine the whole level of brain activity and, for example,

whether a person is asleep or awake. The reticular formation also has an influence on the emotions. The cerebellum, just behind and above the brainstem, controls the coordination of body movements, posture, and balance, although it has no power to initiate movements.

Composing the midbrain are the hypothalamus, thalamus, pituitary gland, and limbic system. The hypothalamus is responsible for controlling the basic drives that ensure human survival: hunger, thirst, and sex. In addition, the hypothalamus helps to regulate body temperature and governs the activity of the pituitary gland, the gland that produces many hormones which control other glands in the endocrine system. Encircling the hypothalamus is the limbic system, which is involved in the expression of emotions such as anger and fear, in mood changes, and in the power of human memory. The limbic system also serves to integrate messages from the higher centers of the forebrain, while the thalamus acts as a relay station for information transfer between sense organs and the forebrain.

The forebrain, or cerebrum, making up 70 percent of the brain, is composed of two cerebral hemispheres linked by a bundle of nerve fibers, the corpus callosum. Each hemisphere is composed of an outer cortex (gray matter), containing millions of nerve cells, and an inner layer (white matter),

Corpus callosum

Limbic system

Thalamus

Cerebellum

Brainstem

Hypothalamus

Pituitary gland

Cerebral hemisphere

The brain's three main areas reflect its evolution. The hindbrain (brainstem and cerebellum) is less advanced than the midbrain (consisting of thalamus, hypothalamus, pituitary, and limbic system). Most advanced are the cerebral hemispheres of the forebrain.

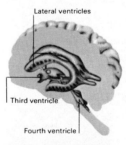

Lateral ventricles

Third ventricle

Fourth ventricle

Four cavities (ventricles) in the brain contain a clear fluid that flows out of the fourth ventricle in the brainstem to lubricate the surfaces of brain and spinal cord. This cerebrospinal fluid is made by cells in the brain and acts to cushion the brain against injury.

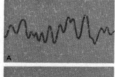
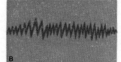
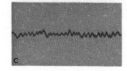

An electroencephalogram (EEG) is a trace of the electrical activity of the cells in the brain's cortex. The trace is obtained by placing electrodes on the scalp. In deep sleep (A), the waves are large and well spaced. When the body is awake but relaxed (B), the waves become sharper and more frequent; and are very fast and close together in physical exertion (C).

consisting largely of nerve fibers that carry messages in and out of the cortex. The cortex is the brain's chief receiver, processor, and storer of information, and the main issuer of instructions for action.

The nerve fibers entering and leaving the cerebral hemispheres from all parts of the body cross over in the brainstem. This means that the left hemisphere serves the right side of the body, and the right hemisphere the body's left side. The two hemispheres do not, however, work completely equally. In most people the left hemisphere is the "logical" brain, the right hemisphere usually acts as the "artistic" brain, directing visio-spatial and musical skills.

Each cerebral hemisphere is divided into four lobes, which are known to perform specific tasks. Largest of these lobes are the frontal lobes at the front of the hemispheres. One area toward the back of each lobe (the

motor cortex) is responsible for directing voluntary movements. The rest of each frontal lobe is involved in personality development and the ability to form abstract concepts.

Behind the frontal lobes are the parietal lobes, which are primarily responsible for receiving sensations of touch and body position. The occipital lobes at the back of the hemispheres are the receivers and analyzers of visual information. And the senses of hearing and smell are made possible by the temporal lobes that form the sides of each hemisphere.

To ensure that information reaching the four lobes of each hemisphere is properly integrated, the cerebral cortex contains groups of nerve cells which make up association areas. These areas allow the brain to create a total "picture" of the body's state and environment.

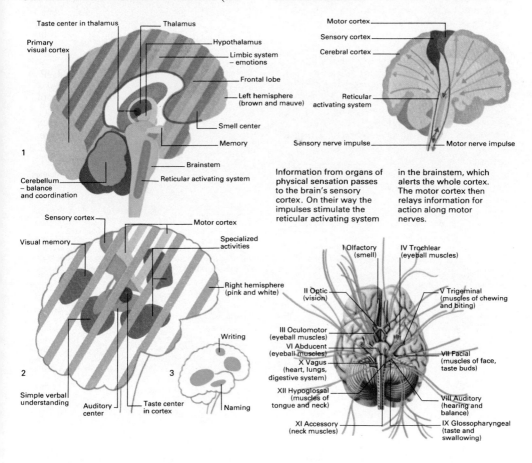

Information from organs of physical sensation passes to the brain's sensory cortex. On their way the impulses stimulate the reticular activating system in the brainstem, which alerts the whole cortex. The motor cortex then relays information for action along motor nerves.

Many of the brain's functions have been "mapped." Indicated here are the major activities governed by the left hemisphere, shown from inside (1) and outside (3), and of the right hemisphere (2) shown from the outer aspect.

Arising from the underside of the brain are 12 pairs of cranial nerves that receive and relay information to and from many organs.

Nerves carrying incoming messages are shown in green; those sending out instructions in orange.

19

The nervous system

The function of the nervous system is to receive and respond to information from the body's environment. The system also coordinates and controls body activities. It is made up of millions of nerve cells, or neurons, each consisting of a cell body with an extension called an axon. In some cells, the axon may be lengthy. Nerve fibers are formed when the axons of many neurons group together.

The nervous system is in two parts. The central nervous system (CNS) comprises the brain and spinal cord. The peripheral nervous system spreads out from both brain and spinal cord, all over the body, carrying information to and from the central nervous system.

In the peripheral system, 31 pairs of spinal nerves branch from the spinal cord, and 12 pairs of cranial nerves arise from underneath the brain. There are also autonomic nerves, located outside the spinal cord.

Most of the spinal and cranial nerves have sensory and motor components. Sensory nerves convey information from the sense organs to the central nervous system. They also monitor such internal conditions as muscle tension, and the oxygen content of the blood. Some of them, such as the optic and auditory nerves, are partly under conscious control. Motor nerves transmit instructions to the muscles to carry out the movements desired, and are thus totally under conscious control.

The autonomic nerves work unconsciously to regulate such functions as heartbeat, respiration, and digestion. There are two kinds: sympathetic and parasympathetic. The sympathetic nerves prepare the body for immediate action; the parasympathetic nerves relax the body after exertion and keep the body functioning at a reduced level during sleep.

The messages that move along the nerves depend on electrically charged particles (ions) of sodium and potassium, which pass through the covering membrane and cause an electric charge to pass through the nerve fiber. The charge is then transmitted to the adjacent nerve cell body, and so on to its destination.

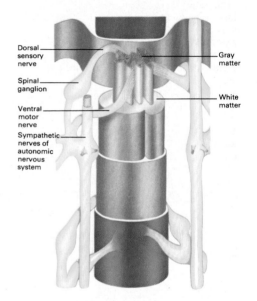

Dorsal sensory nerve

Spinal ganglion

Ventral motor nerve

Sympathetic nerves of autonomic nervous system

Gray matter

White matter

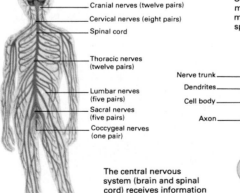

Cerebrum
Cerebellum
Cranial nerves (twelve pairs)
Cervical nerves (eight pairs)
Spinal cord

Thoracic nerves (twelve pairs)

Lumbar nerves (five pairs)
Sacral nerves (five pairs)
Coccygeal nerves (one pair)

The central nervous system (brain and spinal cord) receives information via the peripheral nervous system that branches from it and runs throughout the body. The information is used for making conscious and unconscious decisions, resulting if necessary in orders for body actions.

Sensory nerves bring messages to the gray matter in the center of the spinal cord; motor nerves take away instructions for action. Messages are relayed to and from the brain in the white matter.

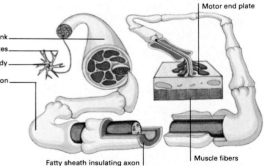

Nerve trunk
Dendrites
Cell body
Axon

Motor end plate

Fatty sheath insulating axon

Muscle fibers

A nerve cell consists of a cell body and a long axon. Impulses are transmitted as electrical charges created when sodium ions enter and potassium ions leave the axon. An impulse is transmitted to a muscle by a chemical transmitter substance that stimulates the muscle fibers to contract.

Endocrine glands

Endocrine glands are collections of tissue that control body functions by producing hormones. The endocrine glands release hormones directly into the blood.

The chief endocrine gland is the pituitary, situated beneath the brain and divided into two lobes. The front (anterior) lobe produces a group of stimulating (tropic) hormones that are carried to other endocrine glands - the thyroid, adrenals, and sex glands - to trigger hormone production.

Other anterior pituitary hormones exert their influence directly. They include prolactin, which maintains milk production from the breasts, and growth hormone. The back (posterior) lobe of the pituitary produces two hormones: ADH (vasopressin), which is carried to the kidneys to help control body water content, and oxytocin, which assists the contraction of the womb during labor and encourages the flow of milk into the breasts after the birth of a baby.

Each of the adrenal glands, sited over the kidneys, is divided into an outer (cortex) and inner (medulla) region. The medulla makes the hormones adrenaline (epinephrine) and noradrenaline (norepinephrine), which help to prepare the body for "fight or flight" in response to danger. The hormones of the cortex include steroids involved in the body's metabolism of sugars and proteins, and in balancing body water content.

The thyroid gland lies below the voicebox or upper part of the windpipe. It secretes hormones that control the rate at which cells use nutrients. Attached to the back of the thyroid are the four small parathyroid glands whose hormones regulate the amounts of calcium and phosphate in the blood, an activity vital to bone building.

The amount of glucose in the blood is governed by cells in the pancreas, situated beside the duodenum. The endocrine cells of the gland are clustered in small masses and make two hormones: glucagon, which raises blood glucose levels; and insulin, which decreases them. The sex glands - ovaries in a female and testes in a male - produce hormones that control the production of mature sex cells and help to determine a person's total sexual makeup.

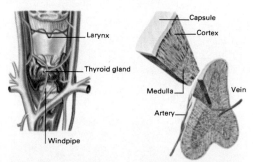

Hormones of the thyroid gland contain the mineral iodine. They help to control the rate at which the body burns and stores sugars.

The adrenal gland's cortex makes steroid hormones. The medulla's hormones prepare the body for "fight or flight."

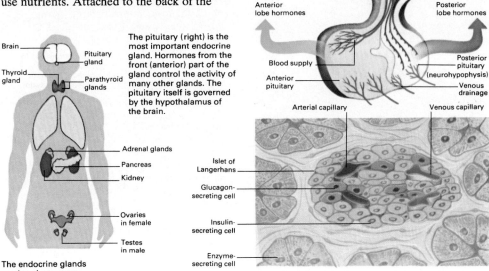

The pituitary (right) is the most important endocrine gland. Hormones from the front (anterior) part of the gland control the activity of many other glands. The pituitary itself is governed by the hypothalamus of the brain.

The endocrine glands produce hormones, chemical messengers that travel in the blood and influence a wide variety of body activities over long periods.

Groups of cells in the islets of Langerhans in the pancreas make two hormones that regulate body sugars. Insulin decreases the amount of sugar in the blood; glucagon increases it. The remainder of the gland secretes digestive enzymes.

Reproduction

The biological purpose of the sex organs is the reproduction of the human race. To make this possible, a male's reproductive system must be able to make sex cells (sperm) and place them inside the female. The female's system must be able to release mature female sex cells (eggs or ova). The sperm enter and fertilize the eggs, and the developing baby (fetus) is nurtured within the female until it is born.

In a mature man sperm are made in the two testes (testicles), organs filled with many coiled tubes. The testes are suspended in a sac, the scrotum, outside the body. The

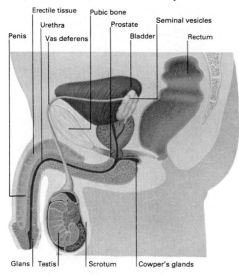

Erectile tissue Pubic bone
Urethra Prostate Seminal vesicles
Penis Vas deferens Bladder Rectum

Glans | Testis | Scrotum | Cowper's glands

In the male, sperm are made in the testes. During intercourse they pass along the vas deferens and the urethra in the penis. Seminal vesicles, prostate, and Cowper's glands make fluids that compose semen.

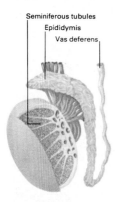

Seminiferous tubules
Epididymis
Vas deferens

Sperm are made in the coiled seminiferous tubules of the testis, then stored in the adjoining epididymis until coitus.

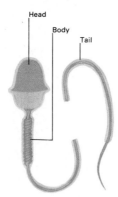

Head
Body
Tail

The miscroscopic sperm has a head containing genetic material, a "body" that provides energy, and a whiplash tail for movement.

scrotum lies behind the penis, the organ sensitive to sexual arousal through which the sperm are transmitted to the female. Sperm are made continuously in the testes and stored in the seminal vesicles, two small structures next to the prostate gland. During sexual intercourse, some 250 million tadpole-like sperm are released (ejaculated) from the penis, together with secretions from several sex glands, including the prostate and the seminal vesicles. The mixture of sperm and fluids is known as semen.

All the reproductive organs of the female body are internal. Eggs are produced in a pair of organs, the ovaries. The ovaries are connected to the womb (uterus), the site of fetus development, by the fallopian tubes. The womb leads, through a narrow opening (the cervix), into the vagina, the cavity into which the penis is placed during intercourse. Surrounding the entrance to the vagina, on the outside of the body, are two pairs of skin folds. The larger pair (labia majora) lie outside the smaller (labia minora). Behind these folds is the clitoris, an organ of sexual arousal equivalent to the penis.

Puberty, the start of sexual development, begins in boys at the age of twelve or thirteen. The hypothalamus in the base of the brain stimulates the pituitary gland to secrete two hormones. These hormones act on the testes, to make them release male hormones (androgens), the most important of which is testosterone. This hormone brings about the enlargement of the sex organs, the start of sperm production, and the appearance of secondary sexual characteristics. Among these characteristics are the growth of hair on the body and face, the deepening of the voice, and increased development of bones and muscles. Maturation to manhood is not usually complete until about age twenty.

Girls start to mature sexually about two years earlier than boys. The pituitary, under the influence of the hypothalamus, secretes the identical hormones, which act on the ovaries and stimulate them to produce the two hormones estrogen and progesterone. Estrogen brings about enlargement of the sex organs, and controls the development of the female secondary sexual characteristics. These include the growth of the breasts, the widening of the hips, and the appearance of hair in the armpits and pubic region. The whole body grows rapidly and maturity is usually reached by the age of sixteen.

A girl experiences her first menstrual period at about the same time as ovulation begins. Menstruation, a bleeding from the womb, takes place about every 28 days and lasts for four or five days. It is closely controlled by hormones. In the ovary, each egg develops in a sac called a follicle. As the egg is prepared for release, the follicle produces the hormone estrogen, which starts the build-up of the lining of the womb in preparation for receiving a fertilized egg. Once the egg has left the ovary the empty follicle secretes more estrogen, plus a second hormone, progesterone. Together estrogen and progesterone aid further thickening of the womb lining. If the egg is not fertilized, the follicle degenerates, hormone output ceases, and the womb lining is shed as the menstrual period. If the egg is fertilized, it

makes yet another hormone that keeps the womb lining going to nurture the embryo until birth.

In a man, the production of sex hormones and sperm continues from maturity for the rest of life, although there is a gradual decline from the 40s and 50s onward. In a woman, however, ovulation becomes less frequent as she becomes older, and the ovaries less responsive to the pituitary hormones. Eventually, the ovaries do not respond at all and menstruation ceases (the menopause). This commonly occurs during the mid-40's.

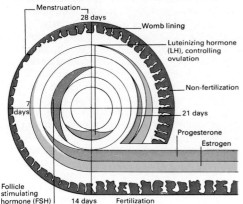

In the female, eggs are made in the ovaries and move through the fallopian tubes to the womb, where they will develop if fertilized. During intercourse the male penis is placed in the vagina.

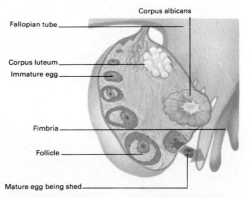

The ovaries of a baby girl contain thousands of immature eggs. After puberty, one egg ripens and is shed each month, leaving a corpus luteum, which makes hormones essential to the early stages of pregnancy. Fertilization usually occurs in the fimbria of the fallopian tubes.

Hormones regulate the menstrual cycle. The egg matures under FSH influence, estrogen starts the build-up of the womb lining, and LH controls egg release. Progesterone completes the womb lining. If the egg is not fertilized, hormone production stops and menstruation occurs.

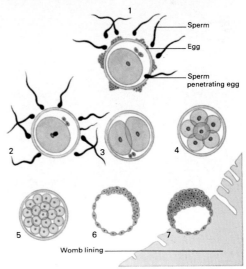

After fertilization (1), the egg divides (2-5) to form a ball of cells. A fluid-filled cavity then develops inside the structure (6), which enters the womb lining (7) a week after fertilization. When implanted in the womb lining, the structure develops into the embryo.

Index of symptoms

Section contents

Introduction

The Index of symptoms has been designed to be an easy-to-use reference guide to the A-Z section that follows it. Organization of this index enables a user to quickly relate a given set of symptoms to the various conditions and disorders described in the A-Z section.

The index is divided into two parts: the first part is pictorial, the second part is diagrammatic.

Each page of the Pictorial index contains an illustration or illustrations of a portion of the human body. Placed around each illustration are lists of the titles of relevant articles in the A-Z section.

The first section on every page informs the user of the titles of general articles in the A-Z section that may give background information about the part of the body illustrated.

Each of the other lists on the page is headed by a specific symptom and informs the user of the title of every article related to that symptom in the A-Z section. The lists have been enclosed by boxes to enhance usefulness. Lines drawn from the boxes to specific sites on the illustration indicate where in or on the body each symptom may occur.

The diagrammatic part of the index, Charts of related symptoms, is designed to direct a user to appropriate articles in the A-Z section when two or more symptoms occur simultaneously. Information as to the best immediate course of action is included. This part of the index has its own introduction, explaining how, using these charts, the appropriate articles in the A-Z may be quickly identified.

The user should keep in mind throughout that the information contained in the Index of symptoms **is not intended to replace the knowledge or expertise of a trained physician. It is not intended to be, and should under no circumstances be used as, a means of self-diagnosis.** This is no substitute for the background, training, and experience of a physician.

However, an understanding of various disorders and their symptoms can help a patient to more accurately communicate with his or her physician when a medical problem does arise. And this is the strength of the Index of symptoms and the accompanying A-Z section.

The eye

General articles
Blindness
Eye
Eye disorders

Blurred vision
Alcoholism
Amblyopia
Astigmatism
Cataract
Conjunctivitis
Detached retina
Diabetes
Eclampsia
Farsightedness
Glioma
Glaucoma
Hyperopia
Iritis
Migraine
Multiple sclerosis
Myopia
Retinitis
Retrobulbar
  neuritis
Sarcoma

Double vision
Diplopia
Head injury
Multiple sclerosis
Strabismus

**Impaired color
  perception**
Color blindness

**Intolerance of
  light**
Conjunctivitis
Encephalitis
Hay fever
Iritis
Measles
Meningitis
Migraine

**Spots in front of
  eyes**
Detached retina
High blood
  pressure
Migraine
Retinitis

Squint
Strabismus

Blindness
Blindness
Cataract
Detached retina
Diabetes
Glaucoma
Migraine
Night blindness
Retrobulbar
  neuritis
Snow blindness
Stroke
Ulcer

Red or pink eye
Allergy
Cannabis
Chemosis
Conjunctivitis
Glaucoma
Hay fever
Iritis
Measles
Red eye

Yellow eyes
Jaundice

Conjunctivitis
Allergy
Conjunctivitis
Hay fever
Measles
Smoking

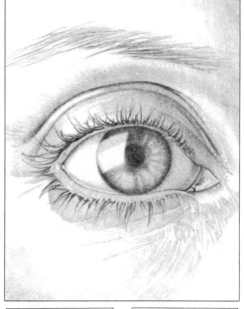

Watering eyes
Allergy
Blepharitis
Common cold
Conjunctivitis
Dacryocystitis
Ectropion
Entropion
Hay fever
Stye
Tears

Lump on lid
Chalazion
Melanoma
Mole
Papilloma
Rodent ulcer
Stye
Wart
Xanthelasma

Cysts on lid
Chalazion
Stye

Gritty feeling
Allergy
Blepharitis
Chalazion
Chemosis
Conjunctivitis
Hay fever
Iritis
Stye
Ulcer
Xerophthalmia

Protruding eyes
Edema
Iritis
Proptosis
Thyrotoxicosis

Black eye
Bruise

Lids, drooping
Bell's palsy
Horner's
  syndrome
Myasthenia gravis
Ptosis
Stroke

Lids, sore
Allergy
Blepharitis
Chalazion
Ectropion
Entropion
Hay fever
Stye

Lids, swollen
Allergy
Angioneurotic
  edema
Blepharitis
Ectropion
Edema
Entropion
Hay fever
Nephritis
Stye

Lids, twitching
Anxiety

The neck and throat

General articles
Larynx
Lymph gland
Neck
Parathyroid gland
Pharynx
Swallowing
Throat
Thyroid gland
Tonsil

Adenoids
Adenoids
Adenoidectomy
Mucus
Snoring
Tonsil

Wryneck
Stiff neck

Boils
Abscess
Boils

Lump on neck, stiff
Boils
Sebaceous cyst
Stiff neck
Whiplash injury

Swallowing, difficult
Achalasia
Bulbar paralysis
Dysphagia
Esophagus

Swallowing, painful
Pharyngitis
Peritonsillar abcess
Sore throat
Tonsillitis

Altered voice
Laryngitis
Larynx
Muscular disorders
Neurological disorders

Cough
Cough
Laryngitis
Mucus
Pharyngitis
Sinusitis

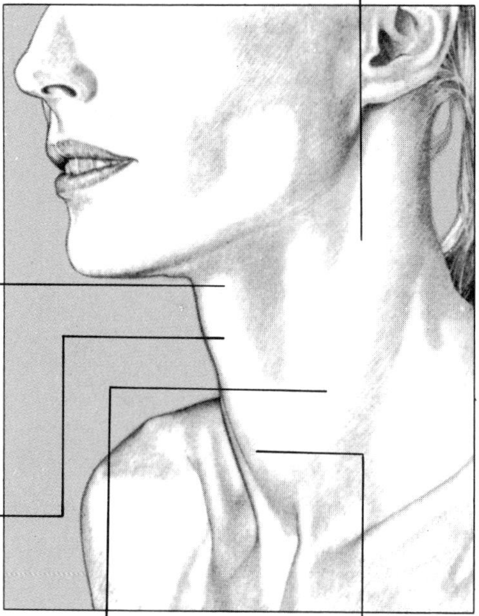

"Lump in throat"
Globus hystericus
Goiter
Laryngitis
Lymph gland
Pharyngitis

Hoarseness
Laryngitis
Pharyngitis
Smoking

Swollen glands
Goiter
Hodgkin's disease
Leukemia
Lymph gland
Lymphosarcoma
Mononucleosis
Tuberculosis

Goiter
Goiter
Myxedema
Thyrotoxicosis

Loss of voice
Aphasia
Aphonia
Laryngitis
Larynx
Mute

Neck, swollen
Goiter
Lymph gland

Swollen and painful glands
Lymph gland
Mononucleosis
Mumps
Tonsil

Sore throat
Mononucleosis
Pharyngitis
Quinsy
Sore throat
Tonsillitis
Vincent's angina

See also
Head and face
Mouth

The mouth

General articles
Jaw
Salivary glands
Taste
Teeth

Bad breath
Abscess
Bad breath
Gastritis
Gingivitis
Indigestion
Liver disorders
Pyorrhea
Sinusitis
Smoking
Sore throat
Stomach disorders
Stomatitis
Tonsillitis
Tooth decay
Trench mouth
Vincent's angina
Uremia

Cleft palate
Cleft palate

Dentures
Dentures

Teeth
Hutchinson's
  teeth
Teeth

Teeth, clenched
Abscess
Hysteria
Tetanus

Teeth, discolored
Fluorosis
Tetracyclines
Tooth decay

Teeth, painful
Abscess
Gingivitis
Impacted
Toothache
Tooth decay

Gums, pain in
Cancer
Gingivitis
Lead poisoning
Leukemia
Plaque
Pyorrhea
Vincent's angina

**Gums, spongy and
  ulcerated**
Diabetes
Gingivitis
Leukemia
Scurvy
Stomatitis
Tuberculosis

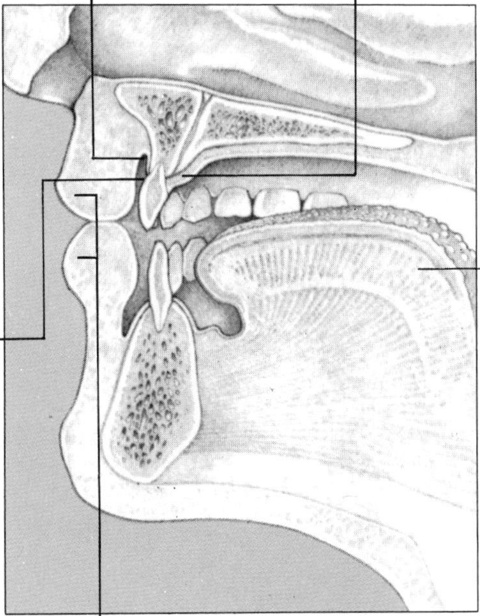

Lips
Chapping
Cold sore

Lips, blue
Cyanosis

**Lips, crack at
  corner of mouth**
Anemia
Cheilosis
Deficiency
  diseases

Teeth, loose
Abscess
Gingivitis
Plaque
Scurvy
Teeth

Inner cheek
Cancer
Leukoplakia
Lichen planus
Measles
Moniliasis
Syphilis
Thrush
Ulcer

Ulcers
Aphthous ulcer
Canker sore
Herpes simplex
Moniliasis

Gums, bleeding
Deficiency
  diseases
Hemophilia
Leukemia
Scurvy
Stomatitis
Trench mouth

Taste, bitter
Gastritis
Pyrosis
Stomatitis
Vomiting

Taste, loss of
Common cold
Head injury
Stomatitis

Tongue
Taste
Tongue

**Tongue,
  discolored**
Furred tongue
Gastritis

Tongue, red
Addison's anemia
Deficiency
  diseases
Glossitis
Scarlet fever

Tongue, sore
Glossitis
Moniliasis

Tongue, white
Furred tongue
Gastritis
Glossitis
Leukoplakia
Thrush

The head and face

General articles
Cranium
Headache
Salivary glands

Birthmarks
Birthmark
Hemangioma
Mole

Scalp, itching
Anxiety
Dandruff
Eczema
Nit
Ringworm
Seborrhea

Scurf
Dandruff
Eczema
Psoriasis
Ringworm
Seborrhea

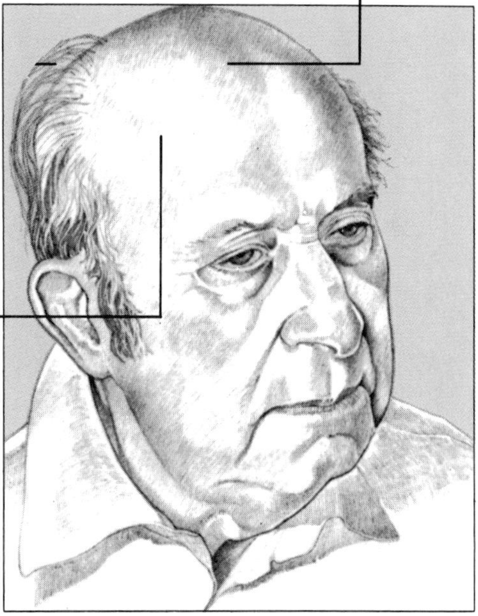

Headache
Allergy
Altitude sickness
Anxiety
Diabetes
Eye disorders
Hangover
Headache
Migraine
Sinusitis

Baldness
Alopecia
Baldness
Eczema
Ringworm
Sebaceous cyst

Pain in forehead
Headache
Herpes simplex
Migraine
Neuralgia
Shingles
Sinusitis
Tumor

Habit spasm
Anxiety
Spasm
Tic
Trigeminal
  neuralgia

**Paralysis or
  weakness**
Bell's palsy
Mastoid
Motor neuron
  disease
Muscular disorders
Myasthenia gravis
Poliomyelitis
Polyneuritis
Stroke

Fainting
Adolescence
Arteriosclerosis
Diabetes
Epilepsy
Fainting
Menstruation
Pregnancy and
  childbirth

Hangover
Alcoholism
Hangover
Headache

Concussion
Concussion
Headache
Head injury

Head, lumps
Bruise
Dermoid cyst
Head injury
Leontiasis
Osteoma
Paget's disease of
  bone
Rickets
Sebaceous cyst
Wart

Dizziness
Arteriosclerosis
Concussion
Dizziness
Ear disorders
Epilepsy
Ménière's disease
Migraine
Vertigo

See also
Neck and throat
Mouth
Ear and nose
Eye

28

Skin, pigment abnormalities
Freckles
Leprosy
Liver spot
Mole
Vitiligo

Skin, unusually brown
Addison's disease
Chloasma
Sunburn

Face, rash
Allergy
Chickenpox
Measles
Roseola
Rubella
Scarlet fever
Typhoid fever

Skin, unusually blue
Blue baby
Emphysema
Exposure
Heart disease

Face, greasy
Acne
Rosacea
Seborrhea

Skin, unusually pale
Anemia
Bleeding
Fainting
Kidney disorders
Myxedema
Pallor
Shock

Face, lumps
Abscess
Boils
Bruise
Dental disorders
Dermoid cyst
Eye disorders
Hodgkin's
  disease
Insect bite
Lymph gland
Mumps
Paget's disease of
  bone
Salivary glands
Sebaceous cyst
Sialolithiasis
Sinusitis
Tumor
Wart

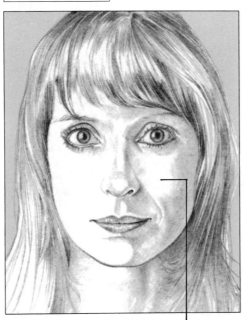

Skin, unusually red
Acne
Bruise
Erysipelas
Fever
High blood
  pressure
Hot flash
Lupus
  erythematosus
Measles
Menopause
Plethora
Polycythemia
Rosacea
Roseola
Rubella
Seborrhea

Face, spots
Acne
Adolescence
Birthmark
Blackhead
Boils
Folliculitis
Impetigo
Insect bite
Papule
Pimple
Pustule
Rodent ulcer
Shingles
Wart

Face, swollen
Acromegaly
Allergy
Angioneurotic
  edema
Cushing's
  syndrome
Dental disorders
Eye disorders
Hydrocephalus
Mumps
Myxedema
Nephrotic
  syndrome
Paget's disease of
  bone
Whooping cough

Pain in cheek
Boils
Dental disorders
Neuralgia
Shingles
Sinusitis
Tetanus
Toothache
Trigeminal
  neuralgia
Tumor

Skin, unusually yellow
Jaundice
Pernicious anemia

The ear

General articles
Deafness
Ear
Ear disorders
Mastoid

**Buzzing and
  ringing**
Labyrinthitis
Ménière's disease
Otitis
Otosclerosis
Tinnitus

Deafness
Common cold
Deafness
Influenza
Ménière's disease
Mumps
Mute
Occupational
  hazards
Otosclerosis
Otitis
Scarlet fever
Wax

Discharge
Boils
Mastoiditis
Otitis
Otorrhea
Wax

Dizziness
Concussion
Dizziness
Ménière's disease
Vertigo

Earache
Boils
Common cold
Earache
Mastoiditis
Mumps
Occupational
  hazards
Otitis
Pharyngitis
Sinusitis
Tonsillitis

Itching
Chilblains
Dermatitis
Eczema
Otitis

Lumps on ear
Pimple
Rodent ulcer
Sebaceous cyst
Tumor

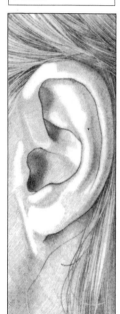

Blisters
Chilblains
Herpes zoster
Impetigo

Boil
Boils
Carbuncle
Otitis

Mastoiditis
Mastoiditis

See also
Face

The nose

General articles
Nose
Smell, sense of

Red nose
Chapping
Common cold
Influenza
Rhinophyma

Blocked
Adenoids
Common cold
Polyp
Rhinitis

Mucus
Adenoids
Allergy
Common cold
Influenza
Mucus

Snoring
Adenoids
Deviated nasal
  septum
Polyp
Snoring
Stuffy nose

Bleeding
Blood disorders
High blood
  pressure
Nosebleed
Puberty

Running nose
Allergy
Common cold
Deviated nasal
  septum
Hay fever
Measles
Mucus
Polyp
Sneezing
Vasomotor
  rhinitis

Sneezing
Allergy
Common cold
Influenza
Measles
Sneezing

Cold
Common cold
Measles

Loss of smell
Common cold
Head injury
Influenza
Mucus
Smell, sense of
Stuffy nose

Swollen
Abscess
Boils
Cellulitis
Rhinophyma

See also
Head
Face

The female breast

General articles
Breast
Breast disorders
Cancer
Nipple
Palpation

**Menstrual
  changes**
Fibroadenosis
Mastitis
Menstrual
  problems
Palpation
Pregnancy

Painful breast
Abscess
Breast disorders
Fibroadenosis
Lactation
Mastitis
Menstrual
  problems
Pregnancy and
  childbirth

Size changes
Cancer
Contraception
Fibroadenosis
Mammoplasty
Pregnancy and
  childbirth

Tenderness
Abscess
Lactation
Menstrual
  problems

Blushing, flushing
Flush
Hot flash
Menopause

Lump in breast
Abscess
Cancer
Breast disorders
Cyst
Fibroadenosis
Lipoma
Palpation

Lump under arm
Cancer
Lymph gland

**General
  lumpiness**
Abscess
Cancer
Cyst
Lactation
Lipoma
Mastitis
Menstrual
  problems

Nipple, bleeding
Breast disorders
Cancer
Nipple
Pregnancy and
  childbirth

**Nipple,
  discharging**
Breast disorders
Cancer
Colostrum
Eczema
Lactation
Nipple
Palpation
Witch's milk

Nipple, indrawn
Cancer
Nipple

Nipple, sore
Eczema
Lactation
Pregnancy and
  childbirth

Nipples, tingling
Lactation
Menstrual
  problems

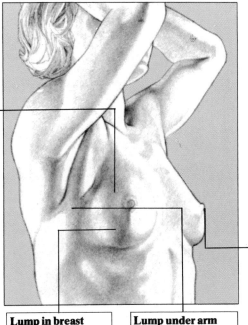

The chest

General articles
Arteriosclerosis
Heart disease
Lung disorders
Smoking
Sternum
Valvular disorders

Breathlessness
Anemia
Anxiety
Asthma
Atelectasis
Breathlessness
Emphysema
Heart failure
High blood
  pressure
Lung disorders
Myocarditis
Obesity

**Irregular
  breathing**
Asthma
Cheyne-Stokes
  breathing

Pain on breathing
Embolism
Empyema
Epidemic
  pleurodynia
Pleurisy
Pneumonia
Tietze's syndrome
Tracheitis

Tightness in chest
Angina pectoris
Asthma
Breathlessness
Coronary heart
  disease
Emphysema
Heart failure
Pneumonia

Heartburn
Hiatus hernia
Indigestion

Chest pain
Abscess
Angina pectoris
Cancer
Coronary heart
  disease
Hiatus hernia
Indigestion
Pericarditis
Pleurisy
Tietze's syndrome

Heart attack
Coronary heart
  disease
Heart attack

**Irregular
  heartbeat**
Extrasystole
Palpitations
Stokes-Adams
  syndrome

Palpitations
Fibrillation
Indigestion
Palpitation
Tachycardia

Pain, ribs
Bornholm disease
Gallstone

Pain, side
Colic
Shingles
Urinary tract
  infections

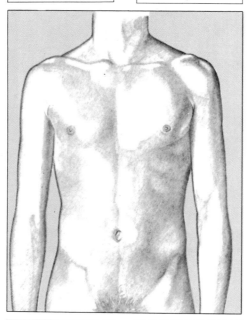

Cough
Bronchiectasis
Bronchitis
Bronchial
  pneumonia
Cough
Croup
Laryngitis
Measles
Pharyngitis
Smoking
Tracheitis
Tuberculosis
Whooping cough

Lumps
Hernia
Lipoma
Tumor
von
  Recklinghausen's
  disease

Cyst
Lipoma
Sebaceous cyst

Wheezing
Asthma
Breathlessness
Heart failure

The abdomen

General articles
Abdominal pain
Colon
Gall bladder
Liver
Stomach
Stomach disorders

Liver
Cirrhosis
Hepatitis
Jaundice
Liver

Gall bladder
Biliary colic
Gall bladder
Gallstone

**Pain, top right
and middle**
Abdominal pain
Appendicitis
Cholecystitis
Duodenal ulcer
Gall bladder
Gallstone
Gastritis
Pancreatitis
Peptic ulcer

Pain, abdominal
Aneurysm
Colic
Colitis
Crohn's disease
Food poisoning
Gastric flu
Gastroenteritis
Intestinal
  obstruction
Intussusception
Pancreatitis
Peritonitis
Pleurisy
Stomachache
Stomach disorders
Urinary tract
  infections
Volvulus
Vomiting

Gas
Belching
Flatus
Gall bladder
Gastritis
Hiatus hernia

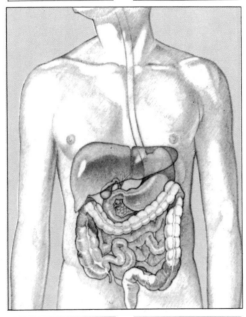

Pain, low
Appendicitis
Colitis
Diverticulitis
Diverticulosis
Dysmenorrhea
Ectopic pregnancy
False labor pains
Pregnancy and
  childbirth
Salpingitis

Hiccup
Hiatus hernia
Hiccup
Uremia

Indigestion
Cirrhosis
Dyspepsia
Gastritis
Heartburn
Hiatus hernia
Peptic ulcer

Colon
Celiac disease
Colitis
Colon
Colostomy
Digestive system
Diverticulitis
Diverticulosis
Hernia

Internal parasites
Worms

Stomach
Cancer
Diet
Digestive system
Peptic ulcer
Stomach disorders

Vomiting
Acidosis
Altitude sickness
Anxiety
Appendicitis
Cancer
Diabetes
Food poisoning
Gall bladder
Gallstone
Gastroenteritis
Hepatitis
Kidney disease
Ménière's disease
Meningitis
Migraine
Motion sickness
Peptic ulcer
Poisoning
Pregnancy and
  childbirth
Vomiting
Whooping cough

Vomiting, black
Blood, vomiting of

Vomiting, blood
Blood, vomiting of
Gastritis
Nosebleed

**Vomiting, after
food**
Anorexia nervosa
Peptic ulcer
Pyloric stenosis
Pylorospasm

Vomiting, at night
Hiatus hernia
Peptic ulcer

See also
Heart
Urinary system
Anus and rectum

The urinary system

General articles
Bladder
Bladder disorders
Cystitis
Kidney
Kidney disorders
Urinary
  abnormalities
Urine

Urine flow,
  dribble
Bladder disorders
Incontinence
Prostate problems
Urinary
  abnormalities

Urine flow,
  frequent
Alcohol
Anxiety
Bladder disorders
Cystitis
Diabetes mellitus
Kidney disorders
Nephritis
Nephrotic
  syndrome
Nocturia
Polyuria
Pregnancy and
  childbirth
Prostate problems
Pyelitis
Urinary
  abnormalities

Urine flow,
  hesitant
Anxiety
Bladder disorders
Prostate problems

Urine flow,
  incontinent
Enuresis
Epilepsy
Incontinence
Neurological
  disorders
Stress
  incontinence
Stroke

Stone
Calculus
Colic
Dysuria

Loin ache or pain
Abscess
Backache
Calculus
Kidney disorders

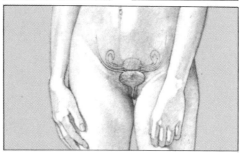

Urine flow,
  infrequent
Dehydration
Fever
Kidney disorders
Oliguria
Preeclampsia

Inability to pass
  urine
Anuria
Anxiety
Pregnancy and
  childbirth
Prolapse
Prostate problems
Retention
Strangury
Tenesmus

Urine flow, with
  pain
Bladder disorders
Calculus
Cystitis
Dysuria
Prostate problems
Pyelitis
Pyelonephritis
Strangury
Tenesmus
Venereal diseases

Urine, blood in
Bladder disorders
Calculus
Cystitis
Hematuria
Hemoglobinuria
Kidney disorders
Nephritis
Prostate problems
Schistosomiasis
Urethritis
Urinary
  abnormalities

Urine, dark
Bladder disorders
Cystitis
Hemoglobinuria
Hepatitis
Jaundice
Melanuria
Oliguria
Porphyria
Urinary
  abnormalities

Urine, smoky
Calculus
Cystitis
Hematuria
Kidney disorders
Pyelitis
Urinary
  abnormalities

See also
Reproductive
  systems

34

The anus and the rectum

General articles
Anus
Constipation
Diarrhea
Hemorrhoid
Rectum
Skin diseases

Feces
Constipation
Diarrhea
Feces

Feces, black
Cancer
Melena
Peptic ulcer

Feces, greasy
Celiac disease
Crohn's disease
Gall bladder
Hepatitis
Sprue

Feces, red
Cancer
Hemorrhoid
Diverticulitis
Diverticulosis
Dysentery
Intussusception

Feces, white
Celiac disease
Jaundice
Steatorrhea

Pain at base of back
Abscess
Bedsore
Coccyx
Ischiorectal abscess
Pilonidal sinus
Pregnancy and childbirth

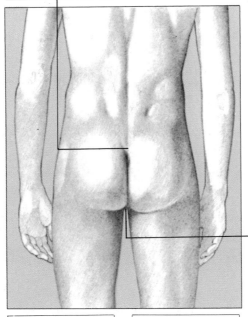

Diarrhea
Celiac disease
Cholera
Colitis
Cystic fibrosis
Diarrhea
Diverticulitis
Diverticulosis
Dysentery
Food poisoning
Gastroenteritis
Hepatitis
Ileitis
Sprue
Steatorrhea
Thyrotoxicosis
Typhoid fever

Constipation
Anxiety
Cancer
Constipation
Diverticulitis
Diverticulosis
Hemorrhoid
Hirschsprung's disease
Intestinal obstruction
Myxedema
Pregnancy and childbirth

Bleeding
Colitis
Diverticulitis
Diverticulosis
Dysentery
Fissure
Hemorrhoid
Pilonidal sinus
Polyp
Schistosomiasis

Itching
Hemorrhoid
Moniliasis
Scabies
Worms

Pain in anus
Abscess
Cancer
Fissure
Fistula
Hemorrhoid
Proctalgia
Proctitis
Tenesmus

Piles
Cirrhosis
Constipation
Hemorrhoid
Pregnancy and childbirth

Protrusion from anus
Hemorrhoid
Intussusception
Polyp
Prolapse
Wart

Lump
Hemorrhoid
Intussusception
Pilonidal sinus
Polyp
Rectum

Worms
Worms

See also
Abdomen

The female reproductive system

General articles
Gynecological
  disorders
Herpes genitalis
Menopause
Menstrual
  problems
Pregnancy and
  childbirth
Premenstrual
  tension
Sexual problems
Vagina
Vulva
Womb

Fertility
Fertility
Infertility
Pregnancy and
  childbirth
Sterility

Ovary
Corpus luteum
Fertilization
Graafian follicle
Oophoritis
Ovulation
Ovum

Venereal disease
Gonorrhea
Syphilis
Urethritis
Venereal diseases

Vulva
Clitoris
Labium
Vulva

Vulva, sore
Dyspareunia
Vulvitis

Vulva, swollen
Bartholin's cyst
Menstruation
Prolapse

Ulcer
Chancre
Chancroid
Herpes genitalis
Syphilis
Venereal diseases

Cervix
Cervical cancer
Cervical erosion
Cervical smear
Cervicitis
Contraception
Pregnancy and
  childbirth

Fallopian tube
Ectopic pregnancy
Fallopian tube
Fertilization
Ovulation
Ovum
Salpingitis
Sterilization

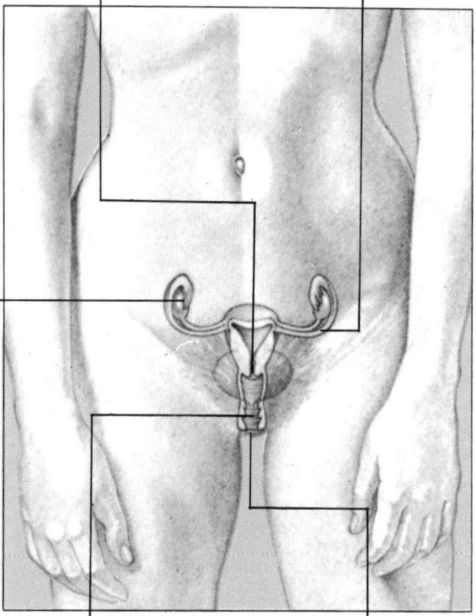

Intercourse, pain
Dyspareunia
Hymen
Sexual problems
Vaginismus

Vagina
Contraception
Pregnancy and
  childbirth

**Vaginal itching
  and irritation**
Gonorrhea
Moniliasis
Trichomonas
Urethritis
Vaginitis
Venereal diseases
Vulvitis

Vaginal discharge
Adolescence
Cervical cancer
Cervical erosion
Cervicitis
Endometritis
Gonorrhea
Lochia
Ovulation
Salpingitis
Urethritis
Vaginitis
Venereal diseases

Uterus
Contraception
Menstruation
Pregnancy and
  childbirth
Womb

**Bleeding after
  menopause**
Cervical cancer
Cervical erosion
Cervicitis
Menopause

Pain in midcycle
Menstrual
  problems
Ovulation

**Periods, flooding
  or heavy**
Adolescence
Abortion
Endometritis
Fibroid
Menorrhagia
Menstrual
  problems

Periods, irregular
Adolescence
Anxiety
Menopause
Menstrual
  problems

**Periods,
  nonexistent**
Hematocolpos
Infertility
Menarche

Periods, painful
Dysmenorrhea
Endometriosis
IUD
Salpingitis

Periods, stopped
Adolescence
Amenorrhea
Anorexia nervosa
Contraception
False pregnancy
Menopause
Pregnancy and
  childbirth

See also
Abdomen
Urinary system

The male reproductive system

General articles
Epididymis
Penis
Prostate gland
Prostate problems
Scrotum
Sexual problems
Testicle
Urinary
  abnormalities

Circumcision
Circumcision
Foreskin
Paraphimosis
Phimosis

Foreskin, tight
Paraphimosis
Phimosis

Testes, absent
Cryptorchidism
Testicle

Testes, painful
Epididymitis
Hernia
Mumps
Orchitis
Testicle
Venereal diseases

Scrotum, rash
Moniliasis
Ringworm

Scrotum, swollen
Cyst
Epididymitis
Hernia
Hydrocele
Mumps
Orchitis
Seminoma
Spermatocele
Tumor
Variocele

Sperm duct
Epididymis
Epididymitis

**Erection,
  problems with**
Alcohol
Anxiety
Depression
Diabetes
Drugs
Dyspareunia
Impotence
Priapism
Prostate problems
Sexual problems

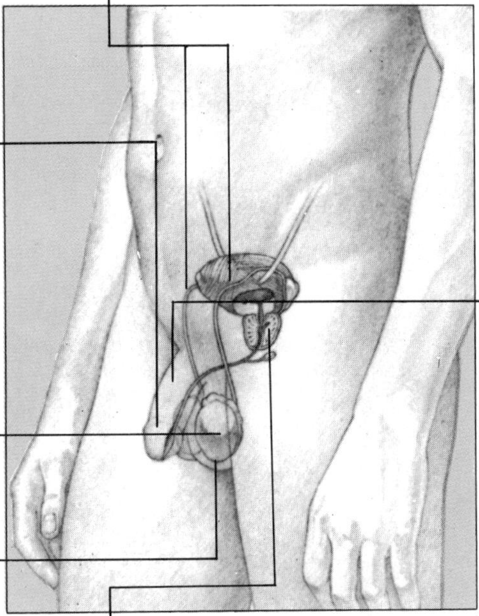

Prostate problems
Prostate problems

Venereal disease
Gonorrhea
Syphilis
Urethritis
Venereal diseases

Penis, ulcerated
Chancre
Chancroid
Herpes genitalis
Syphilis
Ulcer
Venereal diseases

Penis, warts
Venereal diseases
Wart

Impotence
Anxiety
Drugs
Depression
Impotence
Sexual problems

Infertility
Artificial
  insemination
Cryptorchidism
Fertility
Infertility
Impotence
Mumps
Prostate problems
Sterility

Penis
Erection
Foreskin
Urethra

Penis, blistered
Shingles

Penis, discharging
Balanitis
Gonorrhea
Prostatitis
Urethritis
Venereal diseases

Penis, painful
Balanitis
Cryptorchidism
Cystitis
Gonorrhea
Priapism
Prostatitis
Urethritis
Venereal diseases

**Penis, shape
  abnormalities**
Epispadias
Hypospadias
Paraphimosis
Phimosis
Priapism

See also
Abdomen
Urinary system

Back, shoulder, arm, and hand

General articles
Armpit
Arthritis
Backache
Bone disorders
Elbow
Hand
Joint disorders
Muscular disorders
Nail
Neurological
  disorders
Pulled muscle
Rheumatic
  diseases
Scabies
Shoulder
Wrist

Shoulder
Arthritis
Dislocation
Frozen shoulder

Sacrum
Coccygodynia
Myelocele
Pilonidal sinus
Sacrum
Spina bifida

Back pain
Ankylosing
  spondylitis
Backache
Depression
Dysmenorrhea
Gall bladder
Osteoporosis
Peptic ulcer
Sciatica
Slipped disk
Spondylolisthesis

Stiffness
Ankylosing
  spondylitis
Arthritis
Rheumatic
  diseases
Stiffness

Elbow
Bursitis
Capsulitis
Elbow injuries
Humerus
Osteoarthritis
Rheumatic
  diseases
Rheumatic fever

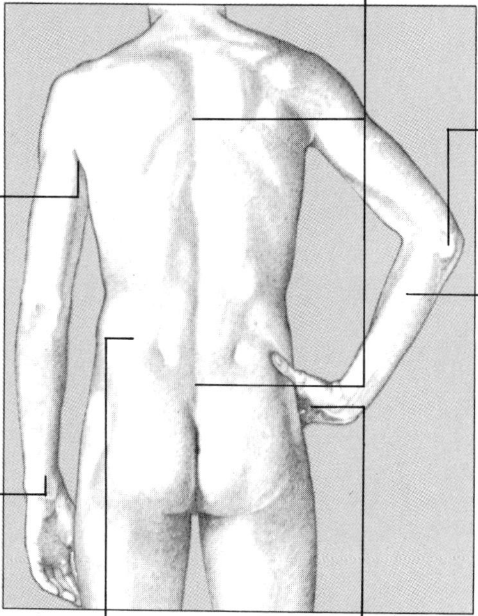

Armpit, sweating
Bromhidrosis
Hyperhidrosis

Armpit, swollen
Boils
Carbuncle
Lymph gland

Wrist
Colles' fracture
Wrist drop

Finger, blistered
Allergy
Blister
Hand-foot-and-
  mouth disease
Pompholyx

Finger, lumps
Heberden's nodes
Rheumatoid
  arthritis
Wart

Finger, painful
Arthritis
Chilblain
Polyneuritis
Raynaud's
  phenomenon
Rheumatoid
  arthritis
Whitlow

Loin pain
Kidney disorders
Pancreatitis
Pyelitis
Shingles
Strain

Nails
Clubbing
Nail

Finger, stiff
Capsulitis
Rheumatoid
  arthritis
Tenosynovitis

Hand, cramp
Carpal tunnel
  syndrome
Dupuytren's
  contracture
Scleroderma
Tetany

Hand, itching
Allergy
Dermatitis
Pompholyx
Scabies

Hand, shaking
Anxiety
Parkinson's
  disease
Thyrotoxicosis
Tremor

Arm, lumps
Bruise
Chondroma
Exostosis
Fibroma
Ganglion
Lipoma
Osteoma
von
  Recklinghausen's
  disease

Arm, painful
Causalgia
Cervical
  spondylosis
Fibrositis
Neuralgia
Osteomyelitis
Pulled muscle
Stiffness

Paralysis of the arm
Hysteria
Motor neuron
  disease
Muscular disorders
Neurological
  disorders
Poliomyelitis
Stroke

Weakness
Cerebral palsy
Muscular disorders

Leg, hip, knee, and foot

General articles
Ankle
Arthritis
Foot
Heel
Joint disorders
Knee
Muscular
 disorders
Nail
Neurological
 disorders
Pulled muscle
Rheumatic
 diseases

Paralysis
Hysteria
Neurological
 disorders
Poliomyelitis
Stroke

Weakness
Cerebral palsy
Muscular disorders
Weakness

Achilles tendon
Achilles tendon
Tendinitis

Ankle, painful
Arthritis
Gout
Joint disorders
Pott's fracture
Rheumatic
 diseases
Sprain

Ankle, swollen
Ankles, swollen
Edema
Kidney disorders
Pregnancy and
 childbirth
Thrombophlebitis
Whiteleg

Sciatica
Lumbago
Sciatica
Slipped disk

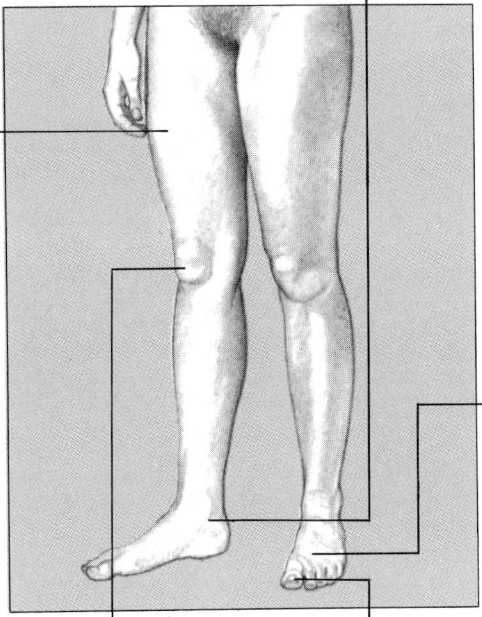

Hip, painful
Arthritis
Perthes' disease
Rheumatic
 diseases

Unsteadiness
Ataxia
Neurological
 disorders
Parkinson's
 disease

Limping
Claudication
Perthes' disease

Lumps
Bruise
Chondroma
Erythema
 nodosum
Exostosis
Fibroma
Melanoma
Osteoma
Varicose vein
von
 Recklinghausen's
 disease

Foot, blistered
Allergy
Blister
Chilblains
Hand-foot-and-
 mouth disease
Immersion foot
Pompholyx
Verruca

Foot, itching
Athlete's foot
Hyperhidrosis
Moniliasis
Pompholyx
Ringworm

**Pain in calf or
 thigh**
Buerger's disease
Causalgia
Claudication
Cramp
Osteomyelitis
Phlebitis
Sciatica
Tabes dorsalis
Tenosynovitis
Thrombophlebitis

Knee, locked
Cartilage
Chondromalacia
Osteochondritis

Knee, painful
Arthritis
Chondromalacia
Rheumatic
 diseases
Sprain

Knee, swollen
Arthritis
Bursitis
Cartilage
Chondromalacia
Gout
Sprain

Toes
Chilblains
Corn
Ingrowing nail
Pigeon toe
Ringworm

Foot, ulcerated
Diabetes
Ulcer

Foot, tingling
Chilblains
Polyneuritis
Tingling

Foot, lumps
Bunion
Corn
Hammertoe
Wart

Foot, painful
Arthritis
Buerger's disease
Callus
Chilblains
Foot disorders
Pregnancy and
 childbirth

Charts of related symptoms

Introduction
This section is most useful when two or more conditions occur at once. By beginning with a symptom that is keenly felt, and proceeding to less severe symptoms set out in parallel, a connecting line is established. When followed, this leads to brief advice on immediate action, on a time to consult a physician, and finally, the full list of relevant A–Z articles

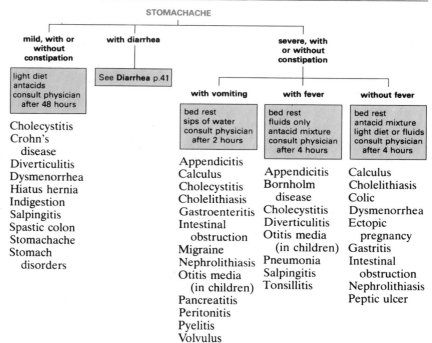

STOMACHACHE

mild, with or without constipation

light diet
antacids
consult physician
after 48 hours

Cholecystitis
Crohn's
 disease
Diverticulitis
Dysmenorrhea
Hiatus hernia
Indigestion
Salpingitis
Spastic colon
Stomachache
Stomach
 disorders

with diarrhea

See **Diarrhea** p.41

severe, with or without constipation

with vomiting

bed rest
sips of water
consult physician
after 2 hours

Appendicitis
Calculus
Cholecystitis
Cholelithiasis
Gastroenteritis
Intestinal
 obstruction
Migraine
Nephrolithiasis
Otitis media
 (in children)
Pancreatitis
Peritonitis
Pyelitis
Volvulus

with fever

bed rest
fluids only
antacid mixture
consult physician
after 4 hours

Appendicitis
Bornholm
 disease
Cholecystitis
Diverticulitis
Otitis media
 (in children)
Pneumonia
Salpingitis
Tonsillitis

without fever

bed rest
antacid mixture
light diet or fluids
consult physician
after 4 hours

Calculus
Cholelithiasis
Colic
Dysmenorrhea
Ectopic
 pregnancy
Gastritis
Intestinal
 obstruction
Nephrolithiasis
Peptic ulcer

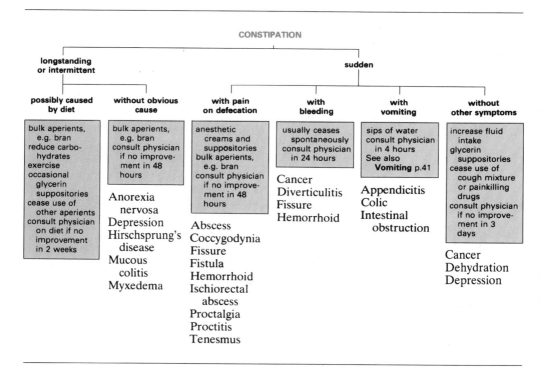

CONSTIPATION

longstanding or intermittent

possibly caused by diet

bulk aperients,
e.g. bran
reduce carbo-
hydrates
exercise
occasional
glycerin
suppositories
cease use of
other aperients
consult physician
on diet if no
improvement
in 2 weeks

without obvious cause

bulk aperients,
e.g. bran
consult physician
if no improve-
ment in 48
hours

Anorexia
 nervosa
Depression
Hirschsprung's
 disease
Mucous
 colitis
Myxedema

sudden

with pain on defecation

anesthetic
creams and
suppositories
bulk aperients,
e.g. bran
consult physician
if no improve-
ment in 48
hours

Abscess
Coccygodynia
Fissure
Fistula
Hemorrhoid
Ischiorectal
 abscess
Proctalgia
Proctitis
Tenesmus

with bleeding

usually ceases
spontaneously
consult physician
in 24 hours

Cancer
Diverticulitis
Fissure
Hemorrhoid

with vomiting

sips of water
consult physician
in 4 hours
See also
Vomiting p.41

Appendicitis
Colic
Intestinal
 obstruction

without other symptoms

increase fluid
intake
glycerin
suppositories
cease use of
cough mixture
or painkilling
drugs
consult physician
if no improve-
ment in 3
days

Cancer
Dehydration
Depression

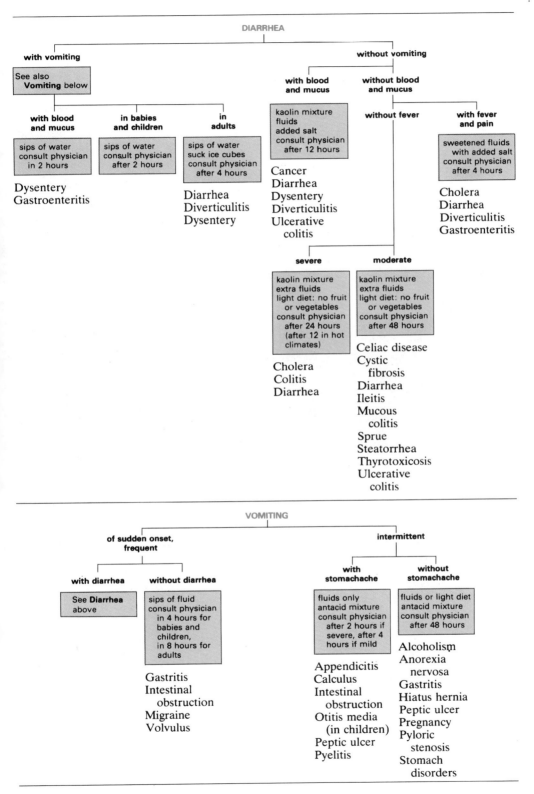

DIARRHEA

with vomiting

See also
Vomiting below

with blood and mucus

sips of water
consult physician
in 2 hours

Dysentery
Gastroenteritis

in babies and children

sips of water
consult physician
after 2 hours

Diarrhea
Diverticulitis
Dysentery

in adults

sips of water
suck ice cubes
consult physician
after 4 hours

without vomiting

with blood and mucus

kaolin mixture
fluids
added salt
consult physician
after 12 hours

Cancer
Diarrhea
Dysentery
Diverticulitis
Ulcerative
colitis

without blood and mucus

without fever

severe

kaolin mixture
extra fluids
light diet: no fruit
or vegetables
consult physician
after 24 hours
(after 12 in hot
climates)

Cholera
Colitis
Diarrhea

moderate

kaolin mixture
extra fluids
light diet: no fruit
or vegetables
consult physician
after 48 hours

Celiac disease
Cystic
fibrosis
Diarrhea
Ileitis
Mucous
colitis
Sprue
Steatorrhea
Thyrotoxicosis
Ulcerative
colitis

with fever and pain

sweetened fluids
with added salt
consult physician
after 4 hours

Cholera
Diarrhea
Diverticulitis
Gastroenteritis

VOMITING

of sudden onset, frequent

with diarrhea

See **Diarrhea**
above

without diarrhea

sips of fluid
consult physician
in 4 hours for
babies and
children,
in 8 hours for
adults

Gastritis
Intestinal
obstruction
Migraine
Volvulus

intermittent

with stomachache

fluids only
antacid mixture
consult physician
after 2 hours if
severe, after 4
hours if mild

Appendicitis
Calculus
Intestinal
obstruction
Otitis media
(in children)
Peptic ulcer
Pyelitis

without stomachache

fluids or light diet
antacid mixture
consult physician
after 48 hours

Alcoholism
Anorexia
nervosa
Gastritis
Hiatus hernia
Peptic ulcer
Pregnancy
Pyloric
stenosis
Stomach
disorders

41

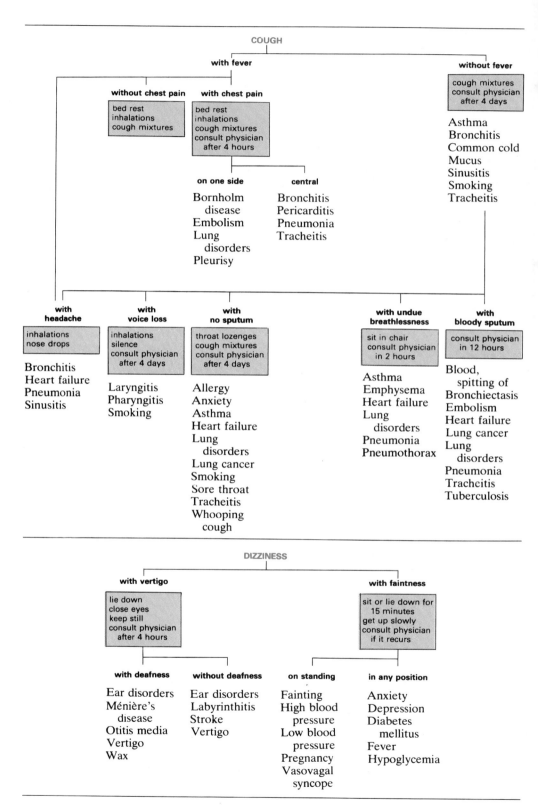

COUGH

with fever

without chest pain

bed rest
inhalations
cough mixtures

with chest pain

bed rest
inhalations
cough mixtures
consult physician
after 4 hours

on one side

Bornholm
  disease
Embolism
Lung
  disorders
Pleurisy

central

Bronchitis
Pericarditis
Pneumonia
Tracheitis

without fever

cough mixtures
consult physician
after 4 days

Asthma
Bronchitis
Common cold
Mucus
Sinusitis
Smoking
Tracheitis

with headache

inhalations
nose drops

Bronchitis
Heart failure
Pneumonia
Sinusitis

with voice loss

inhalations
silence
consult physician
after 4 days

Laryngitis
Pharyngitis
Smoking

with no sputum

throat lozenges
cough mixtures
consult physician
after 4 days

Allergy
Anxiety
Asthma
Heart failure
Lung
  disorders
Lung cancer
Smoking
Sore throat
Tracheitis
Whooping
  cough

with undue breathlessness

sit in chair
consult physician
in 2 hours

Asthma
Emphysema
Heart failure
Lung
  disorders
Pneumonia
Pneumothorax

with bloody sputum

consult physician
in 12 hours

Blood,
  spitting of
Bronchiectasis
Embolism
Heart failure
Lung cancer
Lung
  disorders
Pneumonia
Tracheitis
Tuberculosis

DIZZINESS

with vertigo

lie down
close eyes
keep still
consult physician
after 4 hours

with faintness

sit or lie down for
15 minutes
get up slowly
consult physician
if it recurs

with deafness

Ear disorders
Ménière's
  disease
Otitis media
Vertigo
Wax

without deafness

Ear disorders
Labyrinthitis
Stroke
Vertigo

on standing

Fainting
High blood
  pressure
Low blood
  pressure
Pregnancy
Vasovagal
  syncope

in any position

Anxiety
Depression
Diabetes
  mellitus
Fever
Hypoglycemia

high temperature (over 104°F, 40°C, in children; over 103°F, 39°C, in adults)

cool drinks
sponge with
 warm water
aspirin
consult physician
 if temperature
 persists over 1
 hour

Fever

continued fever

bed rest
aspirin every 4
 hours
increase fluid
 intake

Fever

with rash

consult physician

Chickenpox
Infectious
 diseases
Measles
Mononucleosis
Rocky
 Mountain
 spotted
 fever
Roseola
Rubella
Typhoid
Typhus

for more than five days

consult physician

Endocarditis
Fever
Hepatitis
Mononucleosis
Pneumonia
Pyelitis
Rheumatic
 fever

confusion and delirium

call for medical
 assistance
 urgently
stay with patient
cool drinks
sponge with
 warm water
aspirin

Delirium
Encephalitis
Fever
Hyperthermia
Malaria
Meningitis
Typhoid

See also
Cough p.42
Diarrhea p.41
Headache p.45
Increased
 urination below
Sore throat p.45
Stomachache p.40
Vomiting p.41

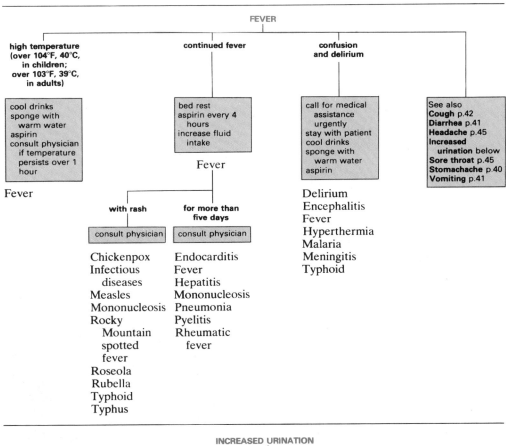

incontinence on coughing

consult physician
in 1 week

Stress
 incontinence

with pain

increase fluid
intake
painkilling drugs
consult physician
in 24 hours

Cystitis
Pyelitis
Salpingitis
Strangury
Tenesmus
Urinary
 disorders

without pain

increase fluid
intake
consult physician
in 24 hours

Diverticulitis
Kidney
 disorders
Pyelitis
Salpingitis

with fever

with blood, with or without fever

with pain

drink much fluid
painkilling drugs
consult physician
in 12 hours
(taking urine
specimen)

Bladder
 disorders
Calculus
Cancer
Cervical
 cancer
Cystitis
Hyper-
 nephroma
Schisto-
 somiasis
Urinary
 disorders

without pain

consult physician
in 24 hours
(taking urine
specimen)

Blackwater
 fever
Bladder
 disorders
Calculus
Cancer
Hematuria
Hemoglobi-
 nuria
Hemophilia
Kidney
 disorders
Nephritis
Prostate
 disorders

with pain

increase fluid
intake
consult physician
in 24 hours

Calculus
Cystitis
Prostatitis
Salpingitis
Strangury
Tenesmus
Urethritis
Urinary
 disorders
Vaginitis

without fever

without pain

(usual fluid intake)
consult physician
in 48 hours

Anxiety
Diabetes
Nephrotic
 syndrome
Prostate
 disorders

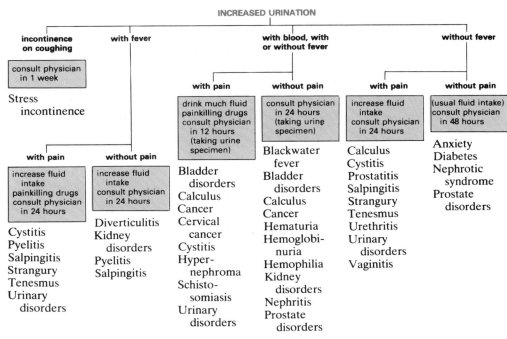

43

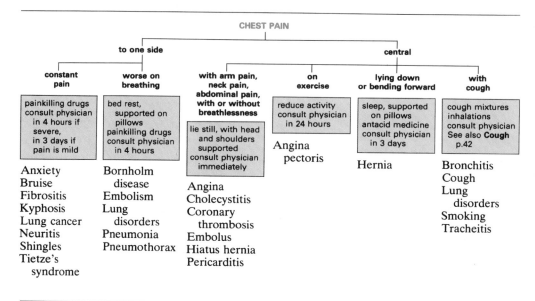

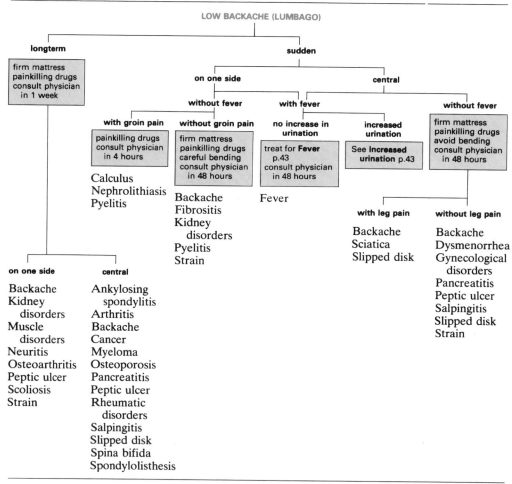

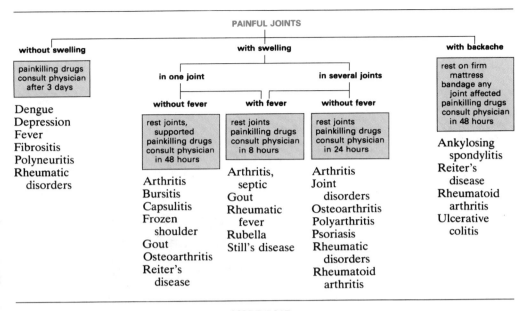

PAINFUL JOINTS

without swelling

painkilling drugs
consult physician
after 3 days

Dengue
Depression
Fever
Fibrositis
Polyneuritis
Rheumatic
  disorders

with swelling

in one joint

without fever

rest joints,
supported
painkilling drugs
consult physician
in 48 hours

Arthritis
Bursitis
Capsulitis
Frozen
  shoulder
Gout
Osteoarthritis
Reiter's
  disease

with fever

rest joints
painkilling drugs
consult physician
in 8 hours

Arthritis,
  septic
Gout
Rheumatic
  fever
Rubella
Still's disease

in several joints

without fever

rest joints
painkilling drugs
consult physician
in 24 hours

Arthritis
Joint
  disorders
Osteoarthritis
Polyarthritis
Psoriasis
Rheumatic
  disorders
Rheumatoid
  arthritis

with backache

rest on firm
  mattress
bandage any
  joint affected
painkilling drugs
consult physician
in 48 hours

Ankylosing
  spondylitis
Reiter's
  disease
Rheumatoid
  arthritis
Ulcerative
  colitis

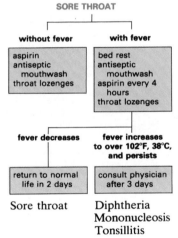

SORE THROAT

without fever

aspirin
antiseptic
  mouthwash
throat lozenges

with fever

bed rest
antiseptic
  mouthwash
aspirin every 4
  hours
throat lozenges

fever decreases

return to normal
life in 2 days

Sore throat

**fever increases
to over 102°F, 38°C,
and persists**

consult physician
after 3 days

Diphtheria
Mononucleosis
Tonsillitis

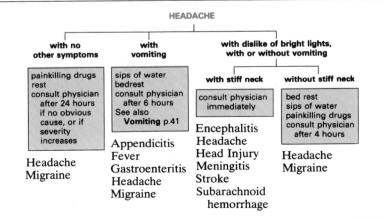

HEADACHE

**with no
other symptoms**

painkilling drugs
rest
consult physician
  after 24 hours
  if no obvious
  cause, or if
  severity
  increases

Headache
Migraine

**with
vomiting**

sips of water
bedrest
consult physician
  after 6 hours
See also
Vomiting p.41

Appendicitis
Fever
Gastroenteritis
Headache
Migraine

**with dislike of bright lights,
with or without vomiting**

with stiff neck

consult physician
immediately

Encephalitis
Headache
Head Injury
Meningitis
Stroke
Subarachnoid
  hemorrhage

without stiff neck

bed rest
sips of water
painkilling drugs
consult physician
after 4 hours

Headache
Migraine

45

Guide to current medical practice

Section contents

For articles in the A-Z of medicine and medical practice that begin with letters I through Z, please consult Volume Two.

Introduction

This section comprises firstly a sort of glossary of word parts (linguistic elements) used in medical terms, and secondly a vast alphabetical compendium of information on all medical topics.

The glossary, entitled **Understanding medical terms**, begins on the next page and has a short introduction of its own. But it is essential to remember, in using the glossary, that it is not a dictionary of words but of word parts: very few of the elements cited and explained can actually stand on their own. With the word parts, however, a truly enormous number of combinations are possible. And the ordinary reader can then use the glossary to "backtrack" for any combination by referring to the elements of that combination.

The **A-Z of medicine and medical practice** is intended as a complete reference work in its own right. Under headings listed in alphabetical order, information is given on medical conditions; the systems, parts, and attributes of the body; and medical equipment, tests, substances, measurements, and studies.

The work has been thoroughly researched and checked by highly qualified experts in the United States and Great Britain, and care has been taken to provide up to date information.

The articles that are concerned with medical conditions generally contain the following information in this order. First, a definition describes the condition and outlines its degree of seriousness; a description of the symptoms then follows, with the causes of the condition. Treatment to remedy the situation is then discussed, and any precautions that could be taken to avoid the condition are given. Finally, further relevant information is given: whether or when to consult a physician, the normal recovery time, and so on.

The articles that describe systems, parts and attributes (such as balance) of the body generally contain the following information in this order. The subject of the article is first located, and its function explained. A list of possible disorders follows, with treatments. Procedures are then outlined, and references made to any other relevant articles.

Other articles describe medical equipment, tests, and studies, or make up tables of useful cross-references to further information.

Understanding medical terms

Few general dictionaries give complete coverage of medical terms. There are thousands of possible combinations of basic word parts (derived mostly from Greek or Latin) that a doctor can use to describe symptoms, disorders, and diseases. But any person who knows the meaning or meanings of the basic word parts can work out the meaning of even the most complicated medical term.

The following pages contain many such word parts, listed one by one in alphabetical order. The meaning of each word part as used in English is also given, and finally in each case there is an example of a medical term that contains the word part. By extension, recognizing and using the word parts, it is possible to "translate" other medical terms that contain them.

For instance: the medical term *cholecystitis* is made up of the parts *chole, cyst* and *itis.* These mean *gall, bladder,* and *inflammation.* So *cholecystitis* means *inflammation of the gall bladder.*

Element/derivation		Meaning	Example
(G = Greek; L = Latin)			
a, an	G	without; with no	amorphous: with no true form
ab	L	away from; off	abnormal: away (deviating) from the normal
ad	L	to; toward	adrenal: toward the kidney
aden, adeno	G	gland	adenitis: glandular inflammation
agogue, agogy	G	producing; promoting	galactagogue: causing the production of milk
alge, algia, algy	G	pain	analgesia: without pain
an *see* a			
andro	G	male; masculine	androgen: a male sex hormone
angi, angio	G	vessel (particularly blood vessel)	angiogram: X-ray record of a blood vessel
ante, ant	G	before; in front of	antecubital: in front of the cubitus (elbow)
anti, ant	G	against; countering	antipyretic: against a fever
apo	G	from; off; down	apoplexy: being struck down
arter, arteri, arterio	G	artery	arteriospasm: spasm of an artery
arthr, arthro	G	joint	arthritis: inflammation of a joint
asthenia, asthenic *see* a *and* sthenia			
ataxia, ataxy *see* a *and* taxia			
auto	G	self	autoplasty: grafting of tissue from another part of the same body
bi	L	two	bicuspid: (tooth) with two cusps
bili	L	bile	biliary: of bile
blast, blasto	G	the germ-plasm	blastogenic: originating in the germ-plasm
blephar, blepharo	G	eyelid	blepharitis: inflammation of the eyelid
bolus, bolism	G	lump	embolus: a lump inside (a vessel)
brachi, brachio	G	arm	brachial: of the arm
brachy	G	short	brachycephalic: short-headed
brady	G	slowness; slowing	bradycardia: slowing of the heart
bronch, bronchi, bronchio	G	bronchial tubes	bronchitis: inflammation of the windpipe
capsul, capsulo	L	envelope of tissue	capsulitis: inflammation of a capsule (such as of the eye lens)
carcin, carcino	G	of cancer; cancerous	carcinogenic: causing cancer
cardi, cardio	G	heart	cardiomyopathy: sickness of the muscle of the heart
cata, cath	G	down	catalepsy: seizure in which the victim falls flat and remains rigid
cele, celo, cel	G	swelling; hernia	cystocele: swelling of the bladder
celi, celio, cel	G	abdomen	celioma: tumor of the abdomen
cephal, cephalo	G	head	acephalous: with no head
cerebr, cerebro	G	brain	cerebrology: study of the brain

Element/derivation		Meaning	Example
cervic, cervico	L	neck	cervicitis: inflammation of the neck of a structure (such as the womb)
chalasia	G	relaxing	achalasia: inability to relax the muscles
cheil, cheilo	G	lip	cheilitis: inflammation of the lips
cheir, cheiro, chiro	G	hand	cheirospasm: spasm of the hand muscles
chiro *see* cheir			
chol, chole, cholia, cholo	G	bile; gall	cholangitis: inflammation of the bile vessels
chondr, chondria, chondro	G	cartilage	chondroma: cartilage swelling
chord, chordo *see* cord			
cirrho	G	wasting	cirrhosis: wasting (of an organ)
col, colo, colono	G	colon	colitis: inflammation of the colon
colp, colpo	G	vagina	colpocele: hernia into the vagina
conidio, conio	G	dust	pneumoconiosis: respiratory disease caused by inhalation of dust
contra	L	against; countering	contraceptive: preventing conception
copr, copro	G	feces; stools	coprolith: a solidified mass of feces
cord, cordo	G/L	cord	cordectomy: removal of a vocal cord
cortico	L	of the cortex, the outer layer of an organ	corticotropin: causing growth of the cortex
cost, costo	L	rib	costal: of the ribs
cox, coxo	L	hip joint	coxitis: inflammation of the hip joint
crani, cranio	G/L	skull	craniotomy: cutting the skull
cry, crymo, cryo	G	cold; freezing	cryosurgery: destruction of tissue by application of extreme cold
crypt, crypto	G	hidden	cryptogenic: of hidden origin
cubit, cubito	L	elbow	cubital: of the elbow
cuta, cuti, cuticul	L	skin	subcutaneous: under the skin
cyst, cysto	G	bladder	cystitis: inflammation of the bladder
cyt, cyte, cyto	G	cell	cytology: study of cells
dent, denti, dento	L	tooth	dentist
derm, dermato, dermis, dermo	G	skin	dermatitis: inflammation of the skin
dextr, dextro	L	right(-hand)	dextrocardia: having the heart on the right(-hand) side
di, dia	G	through	diathermy: heating through
di	G	two	dicephalous: having two heads
dipl, diplo	G	double	diplopia: double vision
dis	L	no longer in a state of	dislocation: no longer properly located
dorsa, dorsi, dorso	L	back	dorsalgia: pain in the back
duct	L	channel; tube	ovarian duct: tube from the ovary
duoden, duodeno	L	of the duodenum	duodenectomy: removal of the duodenum
dys	G	bad; abnormal; painful	dysentery: painful disorder of the intestines
ec, ecto, ectasia	G	out; outward; outer	ectopic pregnancy: a pregnancy in which the embryo grows outside the womb
ectomy (= ec + tomy)	G	cut out; removal	gastrectomy: removal of the stomach
edema	G	swelling	edematogenic: causing edema
em *see* en			
en, endo, em, ento	G	in; inside; within	endoscopy: looking inside
enter, entero	G	intestine	enteritis: inflammation of the intestine
ep, epi	G	upon; on the outside	epidermis: outermost layer of skin
eresis	G	absorption; secretion	choleresis: secretion of bile (by the liver)

48

Element/derivation		Meaning	Example
erythr, erythro	G	red	erythrocyte: red (blood) cell
esthe	G	feeling; sensitivity	anesthesia: with no feeling
estro	G	stimulation; heat	estrogen: a female sex hormone
ex	L	out; (to the) outside	exhale: breathe out
extra	L	beyond; extra	extrasensory: beyond the normal senses
fibr, fibro, fibros	L	fiber; fibrous tissue	fibrositis: inflammation of fibrous tissue
galact, galacto	G	milk	galactophorous: milk-carrying
gastr, gastro	G	stomach	gastritis: inflammation of the stomach
gen	G	originating; creating	cytogenic: forming a cell
gero, geronto, geria	G	old age	geriatric: pertaining to old age
gingiv, gingivo	L	gums	gingivitis: inflammation of the gums
gloss, glosso	G	tongue	glossitis: inflammation of the tongue
glyco	G	sugar	glycopenia: lack of sugar in the tissues
gnosia, gnosis, gnostic	G	knowing; recognizing	prognosis: a forecast
gon, gono	G	seed; semen	gonorrhea: a venereal disease
gon, gony	G	knee	gonyoncus: tumor of the knee
gonad, gonado	G	ovary or testis	gonadectomy: removal of ovary or testis
gram	G	record	cardiogram: record of the heart
graph	G	recorder	encephalograph: device for recording the electrical activity of the brain
gyn, gyne, gyneco	G	female; feminine	gynecomastia: having female breasts
hem, hema, hemat, hemato, hemia, hemo	G	blood	hematuria: blood in the urine
hemi	G	half	hemiplegia: paralysis of one side of the body
hepat, hepato	G	liver	hepatitis: inflammation of the liver
heter, hetero	G	other; different	heteroplasty: grafting of tissue from another person
hist, histio, histo	G	tissue	histology: study of tissue
hom, homeo, homo	G	same; unchanging	homogeneous: of the same origin
hydr, hydro	G	water	hydrophobia: abnormal fear of water
hyper	G	over; excessive	hyperthyroidism: overactive thyroid gland
hypn, hypno	G	sleep	hypnosis: state of apparent sleep
hypo, hyp	G	under; too little	hypoglossal: under the tongue
hyster, hystero	G	womb	hysterectomy: removal of the womb
iatr, iatro, iatry	G	physician; treatment	iatrogenic: originating from the physician or from the treatment
ile, ileo	L	of the ileum (part of the small intestine)	ileocolitis: inflammation of the ileum and colon
ili, ilio	L	of the ilium (the hip bone)	iliac: of the ilium
infra	L	beneath	infracostal: beneath a rib or the ribs
inguin, inguino	L	groin	inguinal hernia: rupture in the groin
inter	L	between	intercostal: between the ribs
intra, intro	L	within; into	intravenous: into a vein
irid, irido, ir	G	of the iris	iridemia: bleeding from the iris
isch, ischo	G	suppression; retention	ischuria: retention of the urine
itis	G	inflammation	nephritis: inflammation of the kidney
kerat, kerato	G	the cornea	keratoectasia: protrusion of the cornea
kin, kine, kino	G	movement	hyperkinetic: overactive in movement
koil, koilo	G	hollow; concave	koilonychia: a disease characterized by concave nails

Element/derivation		Meaning	Example
labi, labio, labr	L	lip	labial: of the lips
lact, lacti, lacto	L	milk	lactogenic: creating milk
laryng, larynge, laryngo	G	of the larynx	laryngitis: inflammation of the larynx
lepsy, lept	G	seizure; attack	narcolepsy: sudden onset of extreme drowsiness
leuco see leuk			
leuk, leuc, leuko, leuco	G	white	leukocyte: white (blood) cell
lingu	L	tongue	lingual: of the tongue
lip, liparo, lipid, lipo, lipomata	G	fat; fatty	lipoma: fatty benign tumor
lith, lithia, litho	G	stone	lithotomy: cutting of a duct or organ to remove a stone
lob, lobo	G	lobe	lobotomy: incision into a lobe (of the brain)
lyo, lysis, lyso, lytic	G	dissolving; breaking down	hemolysis: breaking down of (red) blood cells
ma	G	swelling; tumor	carcinoma: cancerous tumor
macro	G	large	macrocyte: large cell
malacia, malaco	G	softness	osteomalacia: softening of the bones
mamm, mamma, mammo	G/L	breast	mammoplasty: plastic reconstruction of the breast
manu	L	hand	manual: using the hand
mast, masto	G	breast	mastectomy: removal of a breast
melan, melano	G	black	melanuria: dark pigment in the urine
meli, melit	G	sweetness	melituria: sugar in the urine
mening, meningo	G	the membranes round the spinal cord and the brain	meningitis: inflammation of the membranes around the brain
meno, mens, menstru	G/L	monthly	menopause: the end of menstruation
menstru see meno			
mes, meso	G	middle; medium	mesenteron: the mid-gut
met, meta	G	with; alongside; just behind	metacarpals: bones of the hand, just behind the wrist (carpus)
metr, metria, metro	G	womb	metritis: inflammation of the womb
micro	G	small	microcephaly: small head
mon, mono	G	one; single	monocular: with one eye
morph	G	form; shape	mesomorph: person of medium build
motor	L	causing movement	oculomotor nerve: the nerve that controls the eye muscles
muc, mucino, muco	L	of mucus	mucitis: inflammation of a mucous membrane
my, myo	G	muscle; muscular	myalgia: muscle pain
myco, myce, mycet, myceto	G	fungus	mycohemia: fungus in the blood
myel, myelo	G	marrow; center	myeloma: tumor of bone marrow cells
myo see my			
rco, narcotico	G	numbness	narcolepsy: sudden onset of extreme drowsiness
naso	G	nose	nasopharynx: nose and pharynx (area)
	G	death; deadness	necrotic: concerned with death
	G.	new	neoplasm: new growth of tissue
nephro	G	kidney	nephritis: inflammation of the kidney
uro	G	nerve	neurology: study of the nervous system
	L	night	noctambulism: sleep-walking
o	G	night	nycturia: urination at night
mpho	G	the labia minora or clitoris	nymphotomy: surgical cutting of the labia minora or the clitoris

50

Element/derivation		Meaning	Example
ocul, oculo	L	eye	oculist: eye specialist
odont, odonto	G	tooth	orthodontist: one who straightens teeth
odyn, odynia, odyno	G	pain	pleurodynia: pain in the chest wall
olig, oligo	G	few; small; little	oligomenorrhea: small amount of menstrual flow
onco, oncus	G	swelling; bulge	meloncus: swelling on the cheek
onych, onychia, onycho	G	nail	onychopathy: nail disease
oo	G	egg; ovum	oogenesis: formation of the ovum
opathy see path			
ophthalm, ophthalmo	G	eye	ophthalmia: severe inflammation of the eye
opia, opic, opsis, opti, opto	L	eye	optic nerve: nerve from the eye to the brain
orchi, orchid, orchido, orchio, orcho	G	testis (testicle)	orchiectomy: removal of a testicle
orrho	G	serum	orrhotherapy: treatment using serum
orth, ortho	G	straight; correct; upright	orthoptics: straightening vision
oss, osseo, ossi, oste, osteo	G/L	bone	osteitis: inflammation of a bone
ostomy see stoma			
ot, oti, oto	L	ear	otorrhea: discharge from the ear
ov, ovi, ovo	L	egg; ovum	oviduct: tube along which an ovum passes from the ovary
ovar, ovario	L	of the ovary	ovariopathy: disease of the ovary
pachy	G	thick	pachyderma: abnormal thickening of the skin
palat, palato	L	of the palate	palatoplegia: paralysis of the palate
pan, pant, panto	G	whole; complete	pancarditis: inflammation of the entire heart
pancreat, pancreato, pancreatico	G	of the pancreas; pancreatic duct	pancreatitis: inflammation of the pancreas
pant, panto see pan			
par, para	G	beside; beyond	paresthesia: beyond (normal) sensation
paresis, paretic	G	relaxation; weakness	myoparesis: weakness of a muscle
parous, parturi	L	bearing; giving birth	multiparous: having many children
path, pathe, patho, pathy	G	disease; ill condition	pathogen: disease-producer
pector, pectori	L	chest; breast	pectoralgia: pain in the chest
ped, pedia, pedo	G	child; boy	pediatrics: the treatment of children
pelvi, pelvio	L	of the pelvis	pelvisection: cutting of the bones of the pelvis
penia	G	lack; shortfall	leukopenia: shortage of leukocytes (white blood cells) in the blood
pepsia; pepti	G	digestive juices	peptic ulcer: ulcer of the stomach
peri	G	round; around	pericardium: (sac) around the heart
periton, peritone, peritoneo	G	of the peritoneum (abdominal membrane)	peritonitis: inflammation of the peritoneum
pexia, pexis, pexy	G	fixing	organopexy: surgical fixing (by suture) of an organ
phaco, phako	G	lens	phacoid: of the (eye) lens
phage, phago, phagus, phagy	G	eating; consuming	phagocyte: cell that consumes other cells or microorganisms
phako see phaco			
phall, phallo	G	penis	phallodynia: pain in the penis
pharyng, pharynge, pharyngo	G	of the pharynx (throat)	pharyngitis: inflammation of the throat

Element/derivation		Meaning	Example
phil, philia, philo	G	love	hemophilia: bleeding easily ("love of blood")
phleb, phlebo	G	vein	phlebitis: inflammation of a vein
phobe, phobia, phobic, phobo	G	abnormal fear; hatred	agoraphobia: fear of open spaces
phone, phonia, phonic, phono	G	sound	phonocardiograph: device to record the sound of the heart
phor, phore, phoresis, phoria	G	carry; conveying	oophoritis: inflammation of the ovary (egg-carrier)
phot, photo	G	light	photophobia: fear of light
phylac, phylactic, phylaxis	G	protection against infection	prophylaxis: preventive treatment
physo	G	air; gas	physometra: air or gas in the womb
pimel, pimelo	G	fat	pimeluria: fat in the urine
plasm, plasmo, plasti, plasty, plasia	G	(basic) substance which can be added to or shaped	cytoplasm: basic contents of a cell
platy	G	broad	platyrrhine: broad-nosed
plegia, plegic, plexy	G	a stroke; paralysis	hemiplegia: paralysis of one side of the body
pleur, pleuro	G	membrane (pleura) around lungs in chest cavity	pleurisy: inflammation of the pleural membrane
pneuma, pneumato, pneumo, pneumon, pneumono	G	lung	pneumonectomy: removal of a lung
pod, podo	G	foot	podalgia: pain in the foot
polio	G	gray	polioencephalitis: inflammation of the gray substance of the brain
poly	G	many	polyarthritis: inflammation of many joints
post	L	after; behind	postnatal: after childbirth
pre	L	in front of; before	premolar: tooth in front of a molar
pro	G/L	before; forward	progeria: premature aging
proct, procto	G	anus; rectum	proctitis: inflammation of the rectum
prostat, prostatico, prostato	G	of the prostate	prostatectomy: removal of part or all of the prostate
pseud, pseudo	G	false; imagined	pseudocyesis: false pregnancy
psych, psyche, psycho	G	mind	psychology: study of the mind
pulmo, pulmon, pulmono	G	lung	pulmonary: of the lungs
py, pyo	G	pus	pyogenic: forming pus
pyel, pyelo	G	kidney	pyelitis: inflammation of the kidney
pyresis, pyret, pyreto, pyrexia, pyro	G	fever; fire	pyretic: of fever
\chi, rachio	G	spine	rachiopathy: spinal disease
di, radicul	L	root (of nerve or tooth)	radiectomy: excision of the root of a tooth
reno	L	of the kidney	suprarenal: above the kidney
retino	L	of the retina	retinitis: inflammation of the retina
	L	backward; behind	retrobulbar: behind the eyeball
see rachi			
'e rrhage			
rrhea			
ɔ	G	nose	rhinitis: inflammation of the mucous membranes of the nose
gia, rrh	G	outflow	hemorrhage: outflow of blood

Element/derivation		Meaning	Example
rrhea rrhine *see* rhin	G	severe outflow; gush	diarrhea: flow of feces
sacr, sacro	L	of the sacrum	sacralgia: pain in the sacral region
salping	G	Eustachian or fallopian tube	salpingitis: inflammation of a fallopian tube
sapr, sapro	G	putrefaction	sapremia: putrefactive bacteria in the blood
sarc, sarco	G	flesh	sarcoma: fleshy tumor
schisis, schisto, schiz, schizo	G	split; cleft; fissured	schizophrenia: "split mind"
scler, sclera, sclero	G	hardening	arteriosclerosis: hardening of the arteries
scope, scopic, scopy	G	view; look at	ophthalmoscope: instrument for looking at the eye
seba, sebi, sebo	L	fatty secretion of hair and skin	seborrhea: excessive secretion of fatty substances from the skin
sect, section	L	cutting	cesarean section
semeio	G	of symptoms	semeiotic: of symptoms
semi	L	half	semiconscious: half conscious
sepsis, septic	G	decay; putrefaction	septicemia: pathogenic bacteria in the blood
sero	L	of serum (the liquid part of the blood)	serotherapy: treatment by injection of serum
sial, sialo	G	salivary gland	sialitis: inflammation of a salivary gland
sider, sidero	G	iron	sideropenia: iron deficiency
sinistr, sinistro	L	left(-hand)	sinistral: on the left
soma, somat, somato, somi, somia, some	G	body	psychosomatic: of both mind and body, or of one caused by the other
spasmo, spasti	G	of spasm	spasmogen: (substance) producing spasms
sperma, spermato, spermi, spermio, spermo	G	sperm; semen	spermatocele: swelling of a testicle
sphygm, sphygmo	G	pulse	sphygmometer: instrument for measuring the frequency and force of the pulse
spin, spina, spini, spino	L	spine	spinal: of the spine
splanchn, splanchno	G	visceral; intestinal	splanchnic: of the intestine
splen, spleno	G	spleen	splenomegaly: enlargement of the spleen
spondyl, spondylo	G	vertebra	spondylalgia: pain in a vertebra
state, stato, stasia, stasis	G/L	standing	statocyst: organ in the ear that helps people to maintain balance when standing up.
stear, stearo, steat, steato steat, steato *see* stear, stearo	G	fat	steatoma: a fatty tumor
steno	G	contracted	stenosis: constriction (of a tube or vessel)
stern, sterno	G/L	of the sternum (breastbone)	sternalgia: pain in the sternum
steth, stetho	G	chest	stethoscope: device for listening to sounds in the chest
sthenia, sthenic	G	strength; ability	myasthenia: lack of strength in a muscle
stoma, stomat, stomato, stomy	G	mouth; opening	colostomy: making an opening in the body through which the contents of the colon may be emptied
strum, strumi	L	goiter; thyroid gland	strumitis: inflammation of the thyroid gland
sub	L	below; less than	sublingual: below the tongue
super, supra	L	above; more than	superovulation: producing more ova than usual
sy (syl, sym, syn)	G	with; together; the same	synergy: working together

Element/derivation		Meaning	Example
tacho, tacheo, tachy	G	speed; fast	tachycardia: fast heartbeat
tars, tarso	G/L	the margin of the eyelid; the instep of the foot	tarsomalacia: softening of the edge of an eyelid
taxia, taxy	G	coordination; voluntary movement	locomotor ataxia: disease in which coordination of the power to move is increasingly impaired
tel, tele, teleo	G	distance	telesthesia: sensation perceived as though from a distance
ten, teno	G	of a tendon	tenotomy: cutting of a tendon
thalam, thalamo	G	of the thalamus (part of the brain)	thalamectomy: surgical removal of part of the thalamus
thalass, thalasso	G	sea	thalassotherapy: treatment of disease by living near the sea, sea voyages, or sea bathing
therapist, therapeutic therapy	G	treatment for disease	hydrotherapy: treatment in (or with) water
therm, thermo	G	heat; warmth	thermalgia: sensation of burning pain
thoracic, thoraco	G	of the chest, thorax	thoracotomy: cutting into the chest
thrix see tricho			
thrombo, thrombus	G	blood-clotting	thrombus: a blood clot
thyro, thyroid	G	of the thyroid gland	thyroiditis: inflammation of the thyroid
tomy	G	cutting; separating	cystotomy: cutting into the bladder wall
tonia, tonic, toneum	G	stretched; strained	myotonic: being unable to relax a muscle
tonsill, tonsillo	G	of the tonsils	tonsillectomy
tox, toxic, toxico	G/L	poison	toxemia: blood-poisoning
trache, trachea, tracheo	G	windpipe	tracheostomy: making an incision in the windpipe
trans	L	across; from one to another	transfusion: passing (blood) from one person to another
tricho, thrix	G	hair	trichoschisis: splitting of hairs
troph, tropho, trophy	G	nutrition; supply of material for growth	atrophy: lack of growth; wasting
tub, tubo	L	tube (usually uterine)	tubectomy: removal of the uterine tube
tympan, tympano	G	(ear)drum	tympanitis: inflammation of the middle ear
ultra	L	beyond	ultraviolet: electromagnetic radiation just beyond the visible spectrum
ur, ure, uret, uria, urico, urino, uro	G	urine	polyuria: frequent passing of urine
urethr, urethro	G	of the urethra	urethralgia: pain in the urethra
uter, utero	L	womb	uteritis: inflammation of the womb
uvul	G	uvula	uvulitis: inflammation of the uvula
vagin	L	vagina	vaginitis: inflammation of the vagina
vas, vasi, vaso	G	(blood-)vessel; sperm duct	vasectomy: removing part of the vas deferens (sperm duct)
vene, veno	L	vein	venesection: cutting open a vein
vesica, vesicula	G	bladder	retrovesicular: behind the bladder
vir	L	virus	virology: study of viruses
xero	G	dry	xerostomia: dryness of the mouth

A

Abdomen is the body cavity below the chest. It is bordered by the diaphragm above, the pelvis below, and the back muscles and spine behind. The abdomen contains various major organs, including the liver, spleen, pancreas, stomach, small and large intestines, kidneys, adrenal glands, and bladder. In a woman, the abdomen also encloses the reproductive organs; in a man, the abdomen contains the prostate gland.

All the abdominal organs are surrounded by a membrane called the peritoneum. The front and sides of the abdomen are covered by three layers of abdominal muscles. The abdominal aorta (a major artery that carries blood from the heart) and the major veins lie on the back wall of the abdomen.

See also ABDOMINAL PAIN.

A talk about Abdominal pain

Abdominal pain is any pain in the body cavity below the chest. The most common cause in both adults and children is INDIGESTION, as a result of eating too much or eating unsuitable food. Other causes range from the menstrual cramps experienced by many women through more serious ailments requiring prompt medical attention.

Q: *What are minor causes of abdominal pain?*

A: Indigestion is common and generally without serious consequence. It is often accompanied by HEARTBURN, belching, and a sensation of fullness or nausea. Abdominal pain may also be accompanied by diarrhea or vomiting. In most cases, abdominal pain resulting from indigestion ceases within a few hours. If the symptoms persist, however, or if the person stricken is an infant or anyone with a history of serious abdominal illness, a physician should be consulted.

Q: *What are the more serious causes of abdominal pain?*

A: Sudden sharp pain that comes in waves (a condition known medically as COLIC) may be accompanied by vomiting, sweating, and the need to double up. Colic can be caused by several potentially serious disorders, such as intestinal obstruction; inflammation of the peritoneum

(PERITONITIS); or stones (*see* CALCULUS) in the gall bladder (biliary colic) or in the kidneys (renal colic).

Continuous pain that comes on suddenly, together with slight fever, tenderness of the abdomen when touched, and sometimes vomiting and constipation, may be caused by inflammation of the appendix (appendicitis), colon (colitis), pancreas (pancreatitis), or in women a Fallopian tube (salpingitis). In women, an ectopic pregnancy may also be a cause. The presence of cancer in one or more of the abdominal organs may also produce pain.

Q: *What other disorders include abdominal pain as a symptom?*

A: Abdominal pain with backache and frequent, painful passing of urine suggests inflammation of the pelvis of the kidney (pyelitis), or of the bladder (cystitis). There may also be a fever. Recurrent abdominal pain may be caused by a peptic ulcer, cholecystitis, diverticulitis and diverticulosis, or painful menstrual periods (dysmenorrhea). Abdominal pain is also a common symptom of inflammation of the stomach lining (gastritis) or an inflammation of the lining of the stomach and intestinal tract (gastroenteritis).

Q: *Are children especially subject to abdominal pain?*

A: No. The primary cause of stomachache in a child is indigestion. But a child with infection of the middle ear (otitis media) or inflammation of the tonsils (tonsillitis) may complain of a stomachache because

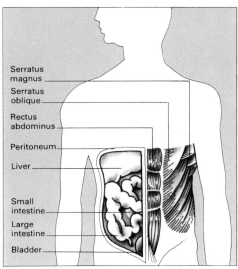

Serratus magnus
Serratus oblique
Rectus abdominus
Peritoneum
Liver
Small intestine
Large intestine
Bladder

Abdomen has three layers of muscle outside the peritoneum and the internal organs.

Abortion

lymph glands near the intestine become tender and swollen. Pneumonia is also a disorder which may cause abdominal pain in children.

Q: *Can pain in the abdomen be a symptom of a disorder elsewhere in the body?*

A: Pain from a heart attack, pleurisy, or pneumonia can be experienced in the upper abdomen. But these disorders have other characteristic symptoms easily recognized by a physician.

See also STOMACH DISORDERS.

Abortion is the termination of a pregnancy before birth. Popularly, the term abortion refers to the deliberate or induced termination of a pregnancy, whereas the spontaneous termination of a pregnancy is commonly called a MISCARRIAGE.

Q: *Why might a physician recommend a deliberate or induced abortion?*

A: A physician might recommend an abortion if tests (for example, amniocentesis) show that the fetus is likely to develop such a severe abnormality as spina bifida or another genetic defect. (*See* GENETIC COUNSELING.) A pregnancy is often deliberately terminated if the mother's health is seriously at risk. But the primary reason for voluntary abortion in the U.S. is birth control. In countries where abortion is permitted, there are strict laws that must be complied with. All states of the U.S. permit voluntary abortion up to the twelfth week of pregnancy (*see* ABORTION LAW).

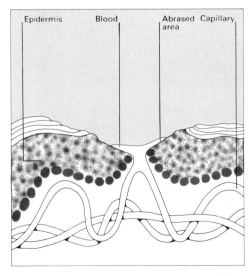

Epidermis   Blood   Abrased Capillary area

Abrasion is an injury to the surface layers of the skin exposing blood capillaries and nerves.

Q: *How is a medically-induced abortion performed?*

A: In early pregnancy, an abortion is generally performed using either minor surgery, such as D AND C (dilation and curettage), or a suction apparatus. When a pregnancy is several months old, a concentrated hormone and salt solution may be injected into the womb. This stimulates the womb to expel the fetus. There are also various drugs, called abortifacients, that are sometimes used to induce abortion, but many of these contain the potentially dangerous drug ERGOT. Alternatively a surgeon performs an operation to open the womb and remove the fetus.

Q: *Is an induced abortion dangerous to the woman?*

A: A medical abortion in early pregnancy, properly conducted, is a safe and minor operation. It can be performed in a clinic or with brief hospitalization.

An abortion performed by an unskilled person and without sterile conditions, exposes the patient to the risk of infection, hemorrhage, or even death.

See also PREGNANCY AND CHILDBIRTH.

Abortion law. In some countries, the deliberate termination of a pregnancy is viewed as a criminal act. Many countries, however, have legalized abortion, although the law differs from country to country and, in the U.S., from state to state. In line with a 1973 decision by the Supreme Court of the U.S., all states permit a woman to have an abortion in the first three months of pregnancy. But the laws regulating abortion after the twelfth week vary from state to state. Some states allow abortion only when the mother's life is in danger, for example, when an embryo develops in the fallopian tube instead of in the womb. Others permit abortion if it is likely that the fetus will be born with serious abnormalities, for example, when a woman contracts RUBELLA during early pregnancy.

See also ABORTION.

Abortus fever is another name for the infectious disease BRUCELLOSIS.

Abrasion is a minor injury in which the skin is scraped or grazed hard enough to make it bleed.

Treatment is to clean the wound immediately with cold water and to apply an antiseptic solution, if available. Apply a dry bandage. The dressing can be removed when a scab has formed, unless there is danger that clothing might rub against it.

See also First Aid, p. 597.

Abscess is a localized collection of pus usually caused by bacterial infection. Bacteria that invade the body are attacked by white blood cells and reduced to pus, which is discharged through the skin. Pimples and boils are surface abscesses. An abscess commonly occurs under the skin and may be caused by an infection of any small gland in the skin (folliculitis), a minor abrasion, or a cut. Abscesses often occur in moist areas of the body, such as the groin or armpit, and are more frequent in persons with DIABETES.

Q: *What are some of the symptoms of an abscess?*

A: Pus forms and the surrounding tissues become red, swollen, and painful as the abscess stretches the area and tries to burst through the skin. Discomfort is relieved when the abscess bursts spontaneously or is lanced.

Q: *What is the treatment for an external type of abscess?*

A: The aim is to encourage the infection to reach the surface of the skin. The customary home treatment is a warm, moist compress. A medical objection to such treatment is that such a compress makes the surrounding tissue more prone to infection. Painkilling drugs, such as aspirin, may be used. The area may be rested, for example, by putting an arm in a sling when there is an abscess in the armpit. A dry dressing should be applied when an abscess comes to a head and discharges.

The abscess may need to be lanced by a physician if there is fever or pain, or if the surrounding skin becomes increasingly red and tender.

Q: *What other kinds of abscesses are there?*

A: There are internal abscesses, usually accompanied by fever, local pain, and a tired, rundown feeling. Such abscesses can occur around a tooth (gumboil), in the breast, in bone (in mastoiditis and osteomyelitis), in the liver (in amebic dysentery), in the vagina (Bartholin's cyst), in the appendix (appendicitis), or in the anal area, between the rectum and the ischium (ischiorectal abscess). In all such cases, a physician must be consulted.

Another kind of abscess is the COLD ABSCESS, which may be caused by tuberculosis. A cold abscess is so called because it is slow-forming and without pain, redness, or heat.

See also BOIL.

Accommodation is the adjustment made by the lens of the eye, by means of its muscles, in order to see clearly objects at various distances. The ability of the lens to focus in this way decreases with age, resulting in the condition called presbyopia.

See also EYE.

Acetabulum is the socket of the hip joint. It is a cup-shaped part of the pelvis into which the head of the thighbone fits. *See* p.4.

Acetaminophen is a mild pain-relieving (analgesic) and fever-reducing (antipyretic) drug; in these respects its effects are similar to those of aspirin and it is often used as an aspirin substitute. Unlike aspirin, acetaminophen is not considered effective in treating inflammation and rheumatic conditions. It does not, however, produce some of the undesirable side effects that aspirin may cause, such as internal bleeding. Acetaminophen is an alternative for persons who are allergic to aspirin. It may also increase the effects of some anticoagulant drugs.

Q: *Can acetaminophen produce any adverse effects?*

A: Yes. In rare cases it may produce skin rashes and other allergic reactions. Blood disorders possibly resulting from its use have also been reported. An overdose of acetaminophen can cause liver damage, and kidney damage may result from prolonged large doses. Acetaminophen should therefore not be used by patients with a disorder of the liver or kidneys.

Acetone is a chemical that is normally formed in the body only in very small amounts. Larger quantities are produced if there is a lack of insulin in the body. This may occur with diabetes, some severe illnesses, or starvation. The chemical can be detected in tests of the urine and blood, and there may be a characteristic odor of acetone (a fruity smell) on the breath.

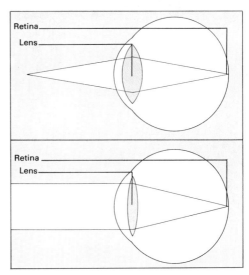

Accommodation is adjustment of the lens in order to focus an image onto the retina.

Acetylcholine

Acetylcholine is a chemical that is produced in nerve endings. It is essential for the transmission of nerve impulses. *See* p.20.

Acetylsalicylic acid is the chemical name for the painkilling drug aspirin. *See* ASPIRIN.

Achalasia is the failure to relax of an area of muscle in the digestive tract. It is caused by nerve damage and occurs most frequently in the esophagus (gullet). Difficulty in swallowing results; food may be held in the esophagus and cause it to expand. Vomiting then brings up the food. Pneumonia may follow if food spills into the lungs.

Q: How is achalasia treated?

A: Treatment is with muscle-relaxant drugs, but a severe attack may need surgery to relax the muscle.

Q: Where else can achalasia occur?

A: A similar condition occurs in the colon (large intestine) of infants. This is known as HIRSCHSPRUNG'S DISEASE, or megacolon.

Achilles tendon is a thick band of connective tissue (tendon) that extends from the calf muscles to the heel bone (calcaneus). Contraction of the muscles attached to this tendon enables a person to stand on tiptoe. The tendon can be torn (ruptured), especially in middle-aged persons, by sudden activity, often with little or no external sign of injury. The tear may have to be repaired by a simple surgical operation.

Achlorhydria is a condition in which there is an absence of free hydrochloric acid in the gastric juice of the stomach. Hydrochloric acid provides a necessary acidity in the stomach and aids the digestion of proteins. There are rarely any symptoms, and specific treatment for the

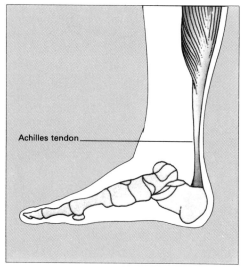

Achilles tendon is the thick connective tissue that attaches the calf muscle to the heel bone.

disorder is not necessary. Often the cause is not known, but it may result from chronic gastritis or PERNICIOUS ANEMIA.

Achondroplasia is an abnormality in the growing areas of long bones such as the thighbone (femur) and upper armbone (humerus). It is caused by a defect in the process that converts cartilage into bone. The condition results in stunted growth, or dwarfism, and can normally be detected at birth. There is no treatment.

Q: Is achondroplasia hereditary?

A: Yes. It is inherited through a dominant gene or from a new gene change (mutation) in a parent.

Q: Are other physical or mental capacities affected?

A: No. The size of the trunk and head are normal. Intelligence is also normal.

Acidosis is a serious condition in which the body's acid-alkali balance is disturbed, and the blood is more acidic than normal. It results from a build-up of carbon dioxide in the blood, often associated with diabetes, a kidney disorder, or starvation. It is treated by treating the underlying cause.

Q: Is acidosis associated with heartburn or indigestion?

A: No, not in the medical definition of the term. In popular usage, however, some people use acidosis to describe any minor stomach disorder, such as indigestion.

Acne is a skin disorder that usually affects the face. The neck, shoulders, chest, and back may also be affected. Acne begins under the skin in glands next to the hair follicles. During puberty, these sebaceous glands enlarge and secrete an oily substance—sebum, a lubricant which keeps skin from drying out. If pores near these glands become clogged with dead skin cells or oily cosmetics, the sebum accumulates underneath, causing inflammation in the surrounding skin. The acne is further aggravated when bacteria multiply in the sebum and add to the inflammation and swelling. Repeated infection can cause a more serious condition, and scarring may result.

Q: Why are young people specifically prone to acne?

A: The exact cause of the correlation between acne and adolescence is unknown. Contributing factors, however, may include the hormonal changes that normally take place at puberty, as well as emotional stress. Diet and cleanliness are now thought by many physicians to be minor factors.

Q: What precautions may minimize acne?

A: Although some physicians recommend the avoidance of foods with a high sugar content and such greasy foods as peanut butter, chocolate, and fried foods, others now feel that dietary restrictions are unwarranted. Most experts agree that greasy or oily cosmetics should be avoided, and the affected areas should be gently cleansed to avoid causing irritation. Spots should not be picked or squeezed, because this may lead to more severe infection.

Q: What specific therapies are effective?

A: Moderate cases of acne may respond to small doses of antibiotics administered over long periods of time. Other therapies that have been found effective include the topical use of vitamin A acid and the oral use of large doses of vitamin A.

In 1983 the Food and Drug Administration approved the general use of Accutane (Trademark), a synthetic chemical related to vitamin A, which has been found to be effective in clearing up even the most serious cases of acne.

Q: Do people other than teenagers suffer from acne?

A: Adults do not get acne as often as do teenagers. But the condition may affect many women before a menstrual period.

Acquired immune deficiency syndrome (AIDS) is a physical condition in which the immune system (*see* IMMUNITY, IMMUNIZATION, and AUTO-IMMUNE DISEASE) becomes defective. The major manifestation of the disorder is a malfunction of the immune system's T-lymphocytes, a type of white blood cell that fights parasites, certain viruses, fungi, and other foreign organisms. AIDS usually begins with a general feeling of being unwell, swollen glands, fever, weight loss, and diarrhea. As the illness progresses, the patient becomes vulnerable to a series of recurring virus infections, such as cold, flu, shingles, and herpes simplex. The most serious of these is the protozoan *Pneumocystis carinii* (PCP), which causes a severe, often fatal, pneumonia. Approximately one-third of AIDS victims also contract a rare form of cancer, Kaposi's sarcoma; other types of cancer have also appeared.

Q: Who get AIDS?

A: The first cases of AIDS were diagnosed in 1981 among homosexual men. Other cases have been found in males or females who take drugs by injection, Haitian immigrants, sexual partners and children of both of these groups, and among hemophiliacs.

Q: What causes AIDS?

A: The source of the syndrome is unknown. Intensive investigation into the source and nature of the disease began in the early 1980's.

Q: How is AIDS passed from person to person?

A: The method of transference is also not understood. Researchers believe that transmission can be made either through intimate physical contact involving the interchange of body fluids, such as saliva or semen, or through the blood stream, that is, via blood transfusions or the re-use of unclean hypodermic needles.

Q: How long does it take before symptoms appear after being exposed?

A: The incubation period for AIDS varies from a few months to more than two years.

Q: Can AIDS be treated?

A: While some of the diseases associated with AIDS can be successfully treated, the underlying immune problem is, apparently, irreversible.

Q: Is AIDS fatal?

A: Approximately 40 percent of AIDS victims die within two years of diagnosis. There is no cure.

Acrocyanosis is a condition in which the fingers and toes turn blue. More common in women than men, it is caused either by insufficient oxygen in the blood, or by low temperature. The result, in either case, is an extreme sensation of cold for the patient. The only treatment is to wear sufficient clothing to keep warm. Persons who suffer also from CHILBLAINS may be helped by drugs that dilate the blood vessels to improve circulation. Smoking may worsen the condition.

Acromegaly is a disorder in which the bones in the arms and legs get thicker and longer, as do those of the hands, feet, jaw, and skull. Facial

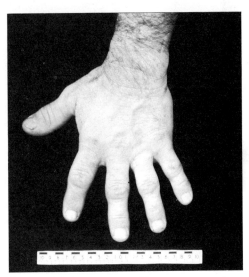

Acromegaly causes normal bone structure to become longer and thicker.

Acrophobia

features become coarser, and the voice may become deeper. The disorder is caused by an excessive production of growth hormone by the pituitary gland, possibly because of a tumor, after puberty. (A related disorder, GIGANTISM, results from overproduction of the growth hormone before puberty.)

In its early stages, acromegaly is almost undetectable. Advanced cases are accompanied by muscular weakness, impairment of vision, and reduced sexual desire.

Q: Can any treatment halt the condition?

A: Skilled medical and surgical care is necessary before too many of the changes become irreversible. X-ray therapy or surgery on the pituitary gland may be recommended.

    See also GIGANTISM.

Acrophobia is an abnormal fear of heights. Occasionally it can be extremely severe and may be a symptom of depression.

ACTH (or corticotropin) is an abbreviation for adrenocorticotropic hormone. It is secreted by the pituitary gland at the base of the brain and is responsible for the stimulation of the cortex (outer layer) of the ADRENAL GLANDS. It makes the adrenal cortex produce the hormones cortisol, corticosterone, and cortisone. Natural or synthetic preparations of ACTH have been used to treat various disorders, such as asthma, multiple sclerosis, and Bell's palsy. It is also used in a test of adrenal gland function.

Actifed (Trademark) is a preparation of the two drugs triprolidine hydrochloride and pseudoephedrine hydrochloride, an antihistamine and a sympathetic nervous system stimulant. It is used to treat coughs, colds, and allergies such as hay fever, which are accompanied by a runny or stuffy nose. It has the effect of inhibiting the secretions of the nose and respiratory tract, thereby lessening breathing difficulties. Actifed may cause drowsiness, lack of coordination, headache, and blurred vision, so it is not advisable to drive an automobile or operate machinery while taking this drug. It may also increase blood pressure and should be used with caution in patients with high blood pressure.

    See also ANTIHISTAMINES.

Actinomycosis is a long-lasting disease caused by a microorganism (*Actinomyces israelii*), which is normally present in the mouth and throat. Infection occurs most commonly in the jaw or neck, and sometimes in the lungs or intestine. Hard, slow-growing swellings form and eventually turn into abscesses. When the abscesses break down, pus is discharged through several openings in the skin. Physicians diagnose the condition by examining the pus under a microscope. Treatment with penicillin is usually effective.

Acupuncture is a method of pain relief and treatment in which the therapist inserts long needles in certain, precisely determined parts of the patient's body. Twirling the free ends of the needles (or sometimes passing a mild electric current through them) induces local anesthesia, providing relief from pain. In China, surgery is performed using acupuncture as a local anesthetic; the patient remains fully conscious during the operation. Its practitioners claim the anesthetic is effective for complicated operations on the stomach, chest, neck, and head.

Q: How does the therapist know where to insert the needles?

A: The needles are located according to the symptoms, following the diagnosis of the practitioner. Many needle points have been charted on the body, and the insertion of needles in one place causes loss of sensation in another. The correct selection of points and the accurate insertion of the needles are essential to the effectiveness of the method.

Q: Are there any advantages in using acupuncture for therapy?

A: Until more medical evidence is available, the success of such treatment is impossible to judge. In any case, acupuncture is generally harmless with conditions such as hay fever, asthma, rheumatoid arthritis, and osteoarthritis. But the possible danger with serious, treatable disorders, such as early forms of cancer, is that any delay in seeking orthodox treatment may result in a worsening of the condition.

Q: Why is acupuncture generally regarded with suspicion in Western countries?

A: Acupuncture is generally regarded with suspicion in Western countries because any scientific basis that it might have has not been demonstrated; neither is the principle fully understood.

Adam's apple is the cartilaginous structure in the front of the neck. It is part of the voice box (larynx) and is usually larger in men than in women. It grows larger in boys during puberty because of one of the effects of the male sex hormone TESTOSTERONE. As a result, vocal cords become longer, and the voice becomes deeper.

Addiction. *See* DRUG ADDICTION.

Addison's anemia is another name for pernicious anemia. *See* PERNICIOUS ANEMIA.

Addison's disease is a rare condition that results from insufficient production by the ADRENAL GLANDS of several vital hormones. It is caused by a disorder of the adrenal glands themselves or by the failure of the part of the pituitary gland that produces ACTH, the hormone that stimulates the adrenal glands, and is most common during middle age.

Q: What are the symptoms of Addison's disease?

A: Common symptoms may include weakness and dizziness caused by low blood pressure, vomiting, loss of weight, and a brownish color of the skin and the membranes lining the mouth. It is difficult to diagnose the condition because it is slow to develop and there may be occasional, temporary improvements in the patient. Tests can reveal the low amount of adrenal hormones in the blood and a disturbance in the balance of salts in the body fluids.

Q: What is the usual treatment?

A: Treatment following a correct, early diagnosis can be highly effective. The missing hormones are replaced and recovery is generally speedy.

Adenitis is inflammation of a gland or lymph node. Mumps is one example of adenitis.

Adenocarcinoma is a cancerous tumor that is situated in the tissue of a gland or duct.

Adenoidectomy is an operation for removal of the adenoids. *See* ADENOIDS.

Adenoids are pads of tissue, resembling tonsil tissue, that form a raised surface at the back of the nasal passage. They trap and destroy bacteria that enter the body through the nose, but are not essential for the body's defense against bacteria. They also help the body to build up resistance (immunity) to future infections.

Q: What can go wrong with the adenoids?

A: In young children, between the ages of four and eight, the adenoids are proportionally larger than at any other age. This sometimes causes the nasal passage to become partly blocked, which may result in snoring, breathing through the mouth (because breathing through the nose is difficult), or the build-up of mucus (catarrh or postnasal drip) in the nasal passage. The swelling or mucus may block the tubes that lead from the nasal passage to the middle ears (the Eustachian tubes), causing hearing difficulties. Ear infection may follow.

Q: What treatment may be prescribed for such conditions?

A: Antihistamine tablets and nasal drops can reduce congestion, but nasal drops should not be used for more than four days at a time. They may cause irritation and excessive dryness in the nose and make the condition worse. If deafness or infection in the middle ear persists, a physician may recommend surgical removal of the adenoids (adenoidectomy). The operation is relatively simple.

Q: Do the adenoids grow again after removal?

A: Yes, but seldom to the original size.

Adenoma is a usually noncancerous (benign) tumor in glandular tissue. By itself, an adenoma causes no symptoms, although various disorders may result if the adenoma presses on a nearby part of the body.

Adenovirus is one of a group of viruses. Adenovirus infections are frequent and include common colds and various minor feverish respiratory illnesses.

Adhesion is a band that connects two sets of body tissues that are not normally connected. Adhesions form in some disorders, following injuries, or following surgery. The sticky healing fluid produced by the damaged internal tissue can solidify to form a band. This band then joins the injured tissue to any body structure or organ with which it comes in contact. Often this is a cavity wall, particularly in the abdomen. Usually this type of adhesion produces no problems. But if the structure so attached is normally free-moving, serious problems may result. The problem can often be relieved by surgery.

Adolescence is the period of body growth and mental development between the onset of puberty and the attainment of physical and emotional maturity. There is a general divergence between the timing of adolescence in young women compared with that in young men. Girls tend to reach puberty earlier and take less time from then on to reach maturity, although their physical changes are greater. Adolescence in

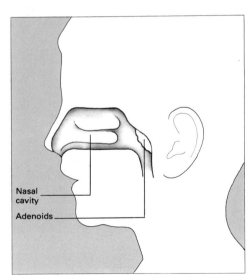

Adenoids at the back of the nose help trap and destroy bacteria, aiding resistance to infection.

Adrenal glands

young women may be considered to last usually from about age twelve through about sixteen. In young men, the corresponding period is from about age thirteen through about age eighteen.

Q: *What physical changes take place during adolescence?*

A: In boys, the genitals increase in size; pubic hair then appears, then armpit hair and facial hair; the voice becomes deeper. In girls, the breasts develop; armpit and pubic hair appears; and menstruation begins.

Q: *What emotional and behavioral changes accompany these physical changes?*

A: Hormonal changes awaken sexual feelings, and most adolescents have some sexual encounters. Early experiences are likely to occur within a group of the adolescent's close friends.

Hormonal changes also account for the moodiness for which adolescents are well known. Inability or extreme reluctance to adjust to changes in outlook leads to depression and sometimes to a consequent apathy. Alternately, there are times when intense physical energy leads to unbounded enthusiasm for particular activities or causes, equally intensely felt.

There may also be a reaction against authority. In modern industrial societies, most adolescents are bound to their parents or guardians for material security. But the individual young person at this time experiences the desire to express his or her own personality, to form a definite character, and to feel as many new sensations as possible.

Some of the experimentation in various activities such as smoking and drinking alcohol that is common among many adolescents also represents a form of determined independence. But the desire for new experiences may, in some cases (as, for example, drug-taking), lead to addiction and eventual premature death.

Q: *How can parents prepare their child for adolescence?*

A: Children should be told frankly and sensibly about the upcoming changes in their body. Information about sex should be provided in a way that is easily understood and that leaves no questions unanswered. This information is best supplied by a parent, or someone with whom the child has an emotionally stable relationship. In many schools, programs are available that highlight the dangers of casual sex, and of smoking, and alcohol and drug addiction.

Q: *How can parents help an adolescent child?*

A: Adolescents come under considerable pressure from the dictates of their own group which encourages them to conform. The bodily processes leading to physical maturity may also give rise to discomfort or embarrassment. One of the best ways that parents and other people can help is to provide understanding, sympathy, advice, and helpful discussion, on all the physiological and psychological problems that accompany this time.

Adrenal glands are two small glands that lie one above each kidney. They are also called suprarenal glands. Each is about two inches (5cm) in diameter. There are two main sections of the gland: the outer layer, known as the cortex, and the central part, or medulla. The gland acts as a hormone-producing center. The medulla produces adrenaline and noradrenaline; the cortex, stimulated by another hormone (ACTH) from the pituitary gland, supplies the body with cortisol and aldosterone. For illnesses associated with disorders in the hormone production of the adrenal gland, *see* ADDISON'S DISEASE; CUSHING'S SYNDROME; PHEOCHROMOCYTOMA.

See also p.21.

Adrenaline, or epinephrine, is a hormone secreted by the central part (medulla) of the ADRENAL GLANDS. It is the hormone that increases the heartbeat and blood pressure in response to stress or anxiety. The flow of blood to the muscles increases, the skin becomes paler, the pupils of the eyes dilate, and energy-producing glucose is released from the liver. These changes prepare the body for immediate action.

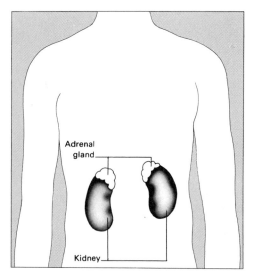

Adrenal glands produce many essential hormones including epinephrine.

Q: Is adrenaline used as a drug?

A: Yes. Natural or chemically-produced adrenaline is injected to treat shock, acute allergy attacks, and asthma. It is also used to slow the absorption, and thus prolong the effect, of local anesthetics.

Aerophagia is the nervous habit of swallowing excessive amounts of air. This may result in belching and swelling of the stomach. The habit is unconscious, and it must be made known to a person before the nervous tension causing it can be reduced. The tendency toward aerophagia is reduced when something hard, such as a pipe, is clenched between the teeth.

Afterbirth is the common name for the PLACENTA and associated membranes that are expelled from the womb, through the vagina, shortly after childbirth. Expulsion of the afterbirth, the third stage of labor, normally occurs within eight to ten minutes of the delivery of the baby. This is followed by a certain amount of bleeding from the womb.

See also PREGNANCY AND CHILDBIRTH.

Afterpains occur in childbirth once labor has ended. They are cramps in the womb as it contracts to return to its normal size. Pains are normally confined to the first forty-eight hours after childbirth and often increase during breast-feeding. If the womb fails to contract and remains soft, prompt medical attention is needed.

Agammaglobulinemia (also called hypogammaglobulinemia) is a rare deficiency or virtual absence in the blood of the antibody proteins called GAMMA GLOBULINS. When the amount of these proteins is low, the body's natural ability to resist infection is weakened. Treatment is by injecting gamma globulin into the bloodstream.

Agglutination is the clumping together of cells, bacteria, or particles within a fluid. Blood corpuscles clump together if they are mixed with other blood of an incompatible type. This example of agglutination is used in identifying blood groups.

Agnosia is a loss of the ability to interpret nerve messages from the senses. It accompanies some brain disorders, such as brain damage from a stroke or a tumor. The sensory organs themselves, such as those in the nose or ears, continue to function normally, but the brain cannot process the messages properly. In most instances only one of the senses is affected.

Agoraphobia is a fear of being in open spaces, sometimes even of going out into the street. It is the opposite of CLAUSTROPHOBIA (a fear of closed spaces). Agoraphobia is sometimes strong and is usually uncontrollable. It may be a symptom of depression or acute anxiety. The sufferer should consult a physician because psychiatric help may be needed.

Agranulocytosis (or granulocytopenia) is an absence of, or deficiency in, white blood cells. It is a serious disorder because the body, lacking white blood cells, can no longer resist infection. The cause of agranulocytosis is not always known, but it most often follows the taking of certain drugs used to treat forms of cancer (such as leukemia). The first signs of agranulocytosis may be infected ulcers on the mouth, throat, rectum, or vagina, accompanied by fever. The patient needs isolation in a hospital and may require transfusions of white blood cells.

A.I.D.S. *See* ACQUIRED IMMUNE DEFICIENCY SYNDROME.

Air sickness. *See* MOTION SICKNESS.

Airway is a natural passage in the respiratory tract through which air passes in and out of the lungs during breathing. The principal airways are the windpipe (trachea) and the two bronchi. The term is also used for an artificial tube used to keep the natural breathing passage open, especially when anesthetics are administered. Such a device is used during surgery on the windpipe (tracheotomy) to correct an obstruction to breathing.

Albino is a person whose body tissues lack the dark coloring matter (pigment) called melanin. Someone who has inherited this relatively rare condition (albinism) has white hair, milky-white skin, and pinkish irises. Albinism is usually caused by the absence of a specific enzyme resulting from a change in the genes; there is no treatment. Because of the absence of melanin, the skin and eyes of albinos are extra sensitive to the sun's rays, and such individuals are

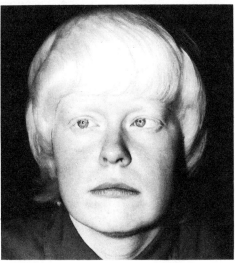

Albino persons lack the pigmentation needed to color skin, hair, and sometimes eyes.

Albumin

advised to avoid direct sunlight and to wear dark glasses.

Albumin is a protein in blood plasma. It is essential for maintaining the correct balance of water in the body. During prolonged disease or when the body is suffering from starvation, the level of albumin decreases. Albumin in the urine (ALBUMINURIA) is usually a symptom of a disorder.

Albuminuria (proteinuria) is the abnormal excretion of the protein ALBUMIN in the urine. It can occur in kidney disease, in heart failure, and with a number of other disorders. Albuminuria should be investigated by a physician; diagnosis is possible only by means of urine tests.

Q: Is albuminuria ever an urgent cause for treatment?

A: In pregnancy, albumin in the urine combined with high blood pressure (hypertension) and swelling, especially of the ankles, signals a serious malfunction.

See also ECLAMPSIA; PREGNANCY AND CHILDBIRTH.

Alcohol is one of a group of liquid organic chemicals of similar structure. Three alcohols only are of medical interest: ethyl alcohol (ethanol), the basic constituent of alcoholic drinks; methyl alcohol (methanol); and isopropyl alcohol (isopropanol). All alcohols are poisonous, but ethyl alcohol is less poisonous than others.

Q: What are the medical uses of alcohol?

A: Ethyl alcohol hardens, cleanses, and cools the skin, and as a rubdown it prevents bedsores.

Methyl alcohol is used as a cooling lotion to the skin, but it is extremely poisonous when drunk and can cause blindness, nerve inflammation (neuritis), and death because of respiratory paralysis.

Isopropyl alcohol is also used as a rubbing alcohol, but it has caused acute intoxication, convulsion, coma, and death in children after sponging for fever.

Q: Are alcoholic beverages dangerous?

A: Alcohol, taken in the form of alcoholic drinks, is the most commonly abused drug in the U.S. Alcohol is addictive, and its repeated use often results in the need to drink more and more to produce intoxication. Other symptoms of alcohol abuse are impaired coordination and, often, aggressive actions. Inflammation of the stomach lining (gastritis), vomiting, and "hangover" are almost inevitable. (See ALCOHOLISM.)

Contrary to popular opinion, alcohol acts as a depressant and reduces self-criticism and anxiety. The prolonged use of alcohol can cause damage to nerves (neuritis) and the liver (cirrhosis), produce mental deterioration (dementia), and increase a tendency toward inflammation of the pancreas (pancreatitis). Chronic gastritis may cause a loss of appetite (anorexia), leading to malnutrition. Alcoholic drinks are rich in calories, although they have little or no nutritive value. For this reason, heavy drinkers often have a weight problem.

Q: Is it safe to drink while taking medicines?

A: No. The effects of alcohol increase the power of drugs contained in, for example, some cough mixtures and sedative drugs such as sleeping pills, antihistamines, tranquilizers, and muscle relaxants. As a result, one drink may have the effect of several and can cause drowsiness and drunkenness. This is dangerous and can be fatal.

Q: When should alcohol be avoided?

A: Alcohol should not be taken by epileptics because it may bring on convulsions. It should be avoided during pregnancy, by diabetics, and by persons with complaints such as gastritis.

Persons killed or injured in motor vehicle accidents involving alcohol				
	Killed % Male	Female	Injured % Male	Female
Age				
0–5	0.6	4.4	1.2	2.7
5–9	1.7	0.0	0.9	2.8
10–14	2.9	0.0	1.3	4.1
15–19	18.3	13.3	20.4	23.5
20–24	23.9	15.6	25.1	19.5
25–34	20.6	22.2	23.4	19.1
35–44	11.4	13.3	12.3	12.6
45–54	10.3	15.6	8.5	8.2
55–64	9.1	9.0	4.4	4.8
65–74	0.6	4.4	2.1	2.3
75—	0.6	2.2	0.3	0.4

Alcoholism can be shown statistically to be related to high motoring fatalities.

A talk about Alcoholism

Alcoholism is a chronic, progressive, and potentially fatal disease. Once it has developed, the individual can not drink ethyl alcohol again without experiencing acute intoxication and inability to stop without assistance. A single cause for alcoholism is not yet known but seems to be the result of the interaction between a possible hereditary predisposition, the effects of ethyl alcohol itself, and the use of alcohol as a means of coping with life.

Approximately ten million people are thought to be alcoholics. The majority can expect to recover with the help of Alcoholics Anonymous and/or an alcoholism treatment program.

Q: *What are the danger signs that point to alcoholism?*

A: The first symptom of alcoholism is an increase in tolerance, that is, increasing amounts of alcohol are needed to produce the same effect that a lesser amount produced in the past. The potential alcoholic may also experience lapses in memory, which are called "blackouts"; he or she may avoid any discussion regarding his or her drinking pattern; a preoccupation with alcohol is exhibited; he or she may hide or sneak drinks to give the impression that less is being consumed; and finally, the potential alcoholic feels "out of control," that is, he or she can no longer stop drinking at will.

Q: *What problems does alcoholism cause?*

A: Alcoholism is physically self-destructive, possibly giving rise to many other forms of illness: delirium tremens, convulsions, heart failure, muscle diseases (myopathy), cirrhosis, and neuritis. Alcoholics become inefficient at work and lose one job after another, often until they become unemployable. Marriages may not endure the strain, and children suffer emotionally and sometimes physically from dealing with a parent who is an alcoholic.

Q: *Is there satisfactory treatment for alcoholism?*

A: Physicians hold out hope for the person who really wants to stop drinking for his or her own self-esteem, if for no other reason. Alcoholics Anonymous (AA), an international self-help group, is often able to give the necessary moral support. A person's local telephone directory or physician's office will give information on how to contact AA. Psychiatrists can help with sedation during the initial "drying out" period, to prevent delirium tremens and to restore the patient's physical health. Some physicians believe that although an alcoholic can stop drinking, he or she cannot return to normal social drinking without the risk of becoming addicted once more.

Antabuse (disulfiram) is a drug that is sometimes given to encourage an aversion to alcohol. When taken in conjunction with alcohol, it causes acute vomiting, severe headache, and flushing. It is successful only if the patient takes it every day, and it should be taken only under close medical supervision.

Aldosterone is a hormone released into the bloodstream by the ADRENAL GLANDS. It helps to control the balance of salts in the body. Excessive production causes high blood pressure (hypertension) due to retention of salt (Conn's syndrome).

See also ADDISON'S DISEASE.

Alimentary canal is the digestive tract, running from the mouth to the anus. It includes the mouth, pharynx (throat), esophagus (gullet), stomach, small intestine, large intestine (colon), and rectum.

Alkali is a type of substance that neutralizes an acid. Most medicines used to relieve "acid stomach," heartburn, and indigestion contain varying amounts of alkalis.

Alkaloid is any one of a group of biologically active substances that contain nitrogen. Alkaloids are found in many plants, and include such drugs as digitalis (from foxglove), atropine (from belladonna), and morphine (from the opium poppy). Most alkaloids have a bitter taste and may be highly poisonous if used incorrectly.

A talk about Allergy

Allergy is a condition in which the body reacts with unusual sensitivity to a certain substance or substances. These substances, which consist of proteins, are called antigens. They stimulate

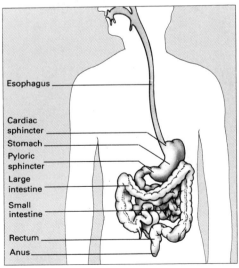

Alimentary canal is the passage down which food travels the entire length of the body.

Esophagus

Cardiac sphincter

Stomach

Pyloric sphincter

Large intestine

Small intestine

Rectum

Anus

65

Alopecia

the body to produce antibodies, which weaken or destroy the invading antigens. In some cases, when an antibody reacts with an antigen, the organic compound HISTAMINE is released from special body cells called mast cells. It is an excess of histamine that results in allergy symptoms.

Q: What are the common allergy symptoms?

A: A runny nose and watering or itching eyes are familiar to many persons who suffer each year from hay fever. In asthma, there is a wheezing; with eczema and hives there is itching, redness, and lumps. Contact dermatitis, an inflammation of the skin, may occur possibly from wearing rubber gloves or touching a certain chemical, such as some kinds of soap. A reaction to antibiotics, particularly penicillin, may be in the form of a RASH.

Q: Why are some people allergic to certain substances and others not?

A: Partly this is due to hereditary factors; some families seem to be more liable to allergies than others, although particular allergies are not necessarily inherited. Emotional disturbances, too, can set off allergic conditions, and many physicians believe that in asthma an emotional factor may be the main reason for starting an attack.

Q: How does a physician determine the cause of an allergy?

A: The physician usually gets a detailed history from the patient to find the most likely source of the problem and may then carry out a skin test. A weak solution of

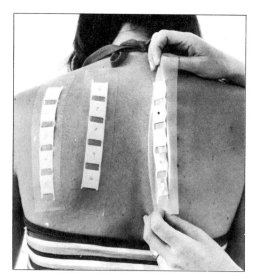

Allergy tests can be done by taping substances to the body and noting reactions.

the substances that are suspected is injected into the skin. A red reaction indicates an allergy to that particular substance. Sometimes a PATCH TEST is done for the same reason.

Q: What treatment can be given for an allergy?

A: When the cause of an allergy is known, the patient can undergo desensitization with injections of the allergen known to cause the symptoms. Beginning with a weak solution, the dose is gradually increased over a period of weeks until a strong solution is reached and the patient is immune to its effects.

If the cause of the allergic reaction is not known, or if the reaction is already taking place, a physician may prescribe ANTIHISTAMINE pills or corticosteroid nasal and lung sprays to control the symptoms.

Q: Are there any dangerous allergic reactions?

A: An allergic reaction to an insect sting or antibiotic drug, such as penicillin, is potentially dangerous and can even be fatal.

A mild reaction usually causes a rash. But in a violent one, called ANAPHYLACTIC SHOCK, the patient finds breathing increasingly difficult. This is an emergency condition, and a physician should be consulted immediately. Fortunately, the condition is not common.

Alopecia is the medical word for baldness. Total loss of hair and patchy loss of hair may occur suddenly at any age. In some people, baldness is due to an abnormal reaction of the body to the hair substance itself. But in many other people the cause is not known. Common male baldness, or male pattern alopecia, results in full scale loss of hair, usually at the temples and the crown of the head; see BALDNESS.

Altitude sickness, also known as mountain sickness, is a condition that some people experience after ascending rapidly to heights of more than about 8,000 feet (2,500m). Others do not suffer until they reach an altitude of more than 13,000 feet (4,000m). The condition occurs because the air at such altitudes contains less oxygen than at lower altitudes.

Q: What are the symptoms?

A: The symptoms include severe headache, shortness of breath, rapid heartbeat, weakness, and nausea with diarrhea. Because not enough oxygen reaches the brain, the patient experiences mental confusion and suffers from poor coordination and insomnia.

No one with heart or lung disease should consider journeys to high altitudes without first consulting a physician.

Alveolus is a small, round body cavity. The term is usually used to describe the microscopic grapelike air cells of the lungs. The plural is alveoli. See p.10.

Alzheimer's diesease, also called presenile dementia, is an abnormal degeneration of the brain that causes loss of memory, similar to that commonly associated with senility in the elderly. In many patients it is accompanied by hallucinations and by difficulty in remembering words (aphasia). It usually occurs in persons of forty to sixty years of age. The disease progresses slowly, but within a few years the patient becomes bedridden and helpless. The cause is not known, and so there is no treatment.

Amalgam is an alloy of mercury and one or more other metals. Dentists use an amalgam to fill a cavity in a tooth.

Amaurosis is the medical term for blindness in which the eye outwardly appears to be normal. It is usually caused by a disorder in the blood supply of the optic nerve or retina. It may accompany the kidney disorder UREMIA.

See also AMBLYOPIA; BLINDNESS.

Amblyopia (lazy eye) is dimness of vision, although the eye outwardly appears to be normal. Amblyopia can occur if one eye is stronger than the other or if the two eyes are not lined up together. The weaker eye then begins to lose vision. The condition is usually corrected by wearing a patch over the strong eye, thus strengthening the weak one. If the condition is not corrected the weak eye can become blind. Amblyopia is often associated with STRABISMUS.

Amebic dysentery is an intestinal disorder caused by the parasite *Entamoeba histolytica*. It is most common in the tropics and subtropics.

See DYSENTERY.

Amenorrhea is the abnormal absence of menstrual periods in a woman. In the years during which a woman normally menstruates, pregnancy is the most common reason for periods to stop. But emotional stress in adolescents can cause amenorrhea, as can depression or the semistarvation of ANOREXIA NERVOSA. There are also physical causes, including endocrine disorders, heart disease, and diseases that affect the ovaries.

With any unexplained stoppage in the menstrual periods, a physician should be consulted and the cause discovered before any treatment is given.

See also MENSTRUATION.

Amenio acid is one of the basic nitrogen-containing substances that go into the making of proteins in living matter. There are more than 20 amino acids required for normal good health, but the human body is not able to make the eight essential ones. These are taken into the body in proteins from foods such as milk, meat, fish, eggs, and cheese.

See also PROTEIN.

Amnesia is the complete or partial loss of memory. General (complete) amnesia may be caused by an injury to the head. Or it can be caused by hysteria after something terrible has occurred and the patient cannot deal with the memory. If the cause is emotional, the forgotten memory can often be recalled when the patient is feeling secure, and especially when in the care of a psychiatrist who tries to bring the suppressed fears out into the open.

Q: What can cause partial amnesia?

A: Forgetting some things, such as names and places, and not others is commonly a sign of aging, depression, or dementia. Certain disorders, such as alcoholism and thyroid deficiency (myxedema), also can be a cause.

Amniocentesis is a method of extracting fluid from the bag of waters (amniotic sac) that surrounds a fetus during pregnancy. The procedure is used to detect possible congenital abnormalities. The sac is punctured with a long needle (after the third month of pregnancy) after the woman has first been given a local anesthetic. There is little danger to the fetus because the location of the placenta is first detected using ultrasound.

The fluid can be analyzed for enzymes and a culture can be made of the cells. If the fetus is found to have a severe disorder, the woman must decide whether to continue the pregnancy. Later in pregnancy the technique is used to test for anemia due to incompatible blood

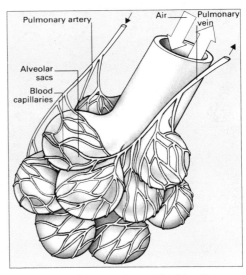

Alveoli in the lungs exchange the blood's carbon dioxide for oxygen from the air.

Amnion

groups in mother and child (*see* BLOOD GROUPS).
Amnion is the membrane lining the womb in which a fetus floats during pregnancy. It is made up of a tough layer of cells and, with the placenta, forms part of the afterbirth.

Amphetamines are a group of drugs that stimulate the central nervous system. They cause a rise in blood pressure, a racing pulse, a feeling of excitement, sleeplessness, and loss of appetite. Amphetamines are used to treat intermittent or cyclic drowsiness (narcolepsy) and excessive muscular and physical activity in children (hyperkinesis).

Q: Are amphetamines addictive?
A: Yes. The stimulative effects of amphetamines have led to abuse and addiction. Physicians now prescribe amphetamines with greater caution and discretion, and supplies are regulated by drug laws.

Ampicillin is a broad-spectrum antibiotic drug which is used to treat infections of the respiratory tract, urinary tract, gastrointestinal tract, and ear, nose, and throat infections, enteric fevers, and gonorrhea.

Q: What are the possible side effects of the use of ampicillin?
A: It may cause diarrhea, nausea, and vomiting. Allergic reactions may also occur; a person allergic to penicillin will probably also be allergic to ampicillin. There is also a specific ampicillin allergy; if a skin rash develops, the patient should consult a physician immediately. Also, because of the strong possibility of a rash, patients suffering from infectious

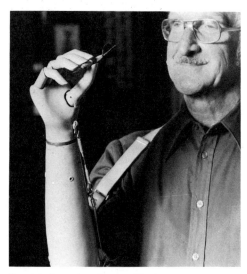

Amputation: the effects of losing a limb can now be minimized by the use of artificial limbs.

mononucleosis (glandular fever) should not use ampicillin. There is a possibility that it may also reduce the effectiveness of oral contraceptives. Rarely, anemia and liver disease may occur.

Ampule, or ampul, is a small, sealed, glass container for keeping a drug sterile.

Amputation is the surgical removal of a limb or other part of the body. The reasons for amputation are either damage or disease. When damage is so serious that repair or healing is impossible, amputation may be a physician's only choice.

Q: What problems face a patient after the amputation of a limb?
A: Emotional stress is a serious problem after an amputation. Also, a patient may experience sensations as if the limb were still there. This can cause confusion and distress and may persist for several months. A good rehabilitation program therefore includes both physical and psychotherapeutic treatment.

Q: What about artificial limbs?
A: When performing an amputation, a surgeon normally tries to leave a stump of bone onto which an artificial limb can be attached. Such a limb can be controlled by brain impulses that remain even after amputation.

Amyloidosis is a disorder marked by deposits of a waxy, clear substance (amyloid) in the tissues of the liver, spleen, kidneys, heart, or tongue. The deposits may be associated with chronic infections or inflammations or some forms of cancer, but sometimes the cause is not known. Amyloid interferes with the normal functioning of the organ in which it is present. There is no known specific cure for the condition, and death results if its presence is not discovered. The only treatment is to deal with the cause, if known.

Amyotrophic lateral sclerosis is a motor neuron disease characterized by progressive degeneration of the cerebral cortex and spinal column. Symptoms of the disease include muscular weakness and spasm. An increase in tendon reflexes and spacticity may precede atrophy in the hands, forearms, and legs. The onset of amyotrophic lateral sclerosis generally begins after age 40, and the incidence is greater among males. Death usually occurs two to five years after the appearance of symptoms.

Analeptics are drugs that stimulate the central nervous system. They are used especially in the treatment of poisoning caused by a drug that has had a serious depressant effect on the nervous system. Analeptics such as caffeine and amphetamines help to restore a person to consciousness.

Analgesics are those drugs or medicines that

relieve pain without loss of feeling or loss of consciousness. They work either by reducing the patient's ability to perceive pain or by altering the appreciation of pain. The oldest of the common analgesic drugs is ASPIRIN. A more recent substitute for aspirin is ACETAMINOPHEN, which is less irritating to the stomach and used by many people for that reason.

Q: *Are aspirin and acetaminophen regarded as safe drugs?*

A: The two drugs are medically safe enough to be readily available without prescription at a drugstore. But physicians advise against excessive or prolonged use or large doses of these, or any other nonprescription analgesics, without prior medical consultation.

Q: *What types of pain need stronger analgesics?*

A: With acute or persistent pain, a physician's advice may well be essential. Physicians prescribe strong analgesics with caution, and dosages are carefully regulated because some analgesics can be addictive.

Anaphylactic shock is a sudden, severe reaction. It is a reaction to the introduction into the body of any substance to which the body is hypersensitive. It may, for example, follow the injection of a drug, or an insect sting. The victim feels faint and becomes pale. The person may vomit and have no control over bowel movements. Wheezy breathing may occur; the patient may collapse into unconsciousness, which may be followed by death. These symptoms can occur in rapid succession.

Q: *What is the treatment for anaphylactic shock?*

A: Emergency treatment is essential and the patient should be hospitalized as soon as possible. Treatment includes injections of epinephrine and the intravenous use of hydrocortisone. The type of aerosol that asthmatics use may be helpful for assisting breathing until skilled help arrives.

Anasarca is the generalized swelling (edema) of the body, especially in the legs and abdomen. It results from the accumulation of fluid in body tissues, often accompanying a kidney disorder. The condition was once known as dropsy.

Anastomosis is the connecting area between two tubes in the body. An artificial anastomosis may be created by surgery, for example, when the open ends of parts of the intestine are joined together after the removal of a diseased section between them.

Androgen is any of a group of substances that produce secondary sex characteristics in the male. TESTOSTERONE, the sex hormone produced by the testicles, is an androgen.

A talk about Anemia

Anemia is any one of the disorders in which the blood has fewer than the normal number of RED BLOOD CELLS, or the red blood cells are deficient in HEMOGLOBIN.

Q: *What are the symptoms of anemia?*

A: Hemoglobin gives blood its red color, and a person with anemia may be noticeably pale, although various other disorders can also cause paleness. Other symptoms of anemia include tiredness, headaches, dizziness, shortness of breath, and palpitations after only slight exertion.

Q: *Is anemia serious?*

A: There are various types of anemia. It may be only minor and give little cause for concern, or it may be a warning sign of a more serious condition. For this reason, a person should not ignore the symptoms, but should seek advice from a physician.

Q: *How is anemia diagnosed?*

A: Physicians diagnose anemia by obtaining a blood count. They take a small sample of blood from the patient and count the number of red blood cells in it. In a healthy person, each cubic milliliter of blood contains between 5 million and 6 million red blood cells, which have a normal life of about three to four months and are replaced continually.

Q: *What are the causes of anemia?*

A: Anemia has three chief causes: (1) loss of blood through bleeding (hemorrhage); (2) failure of the body to make enough new red blood cells; or (3) hemolysis, the

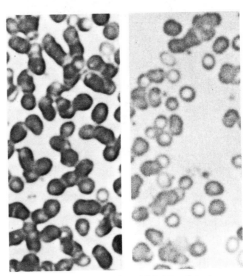

Anemia is a condition in which blood that normally has many red cells (*left*) has few (*right*).

Anesthetics

rapid destruction of the red blood cells in the blood.

Q: *What can prevent the body from making red cells?*

A: Failure of red blood cell production can be caused by faulty diet. Lack of enough iron in the food a person eats leads to insufficient hemoglobin in his or her red blood cells. Lack of vitamin C (ascorbic acid) leads to the anemia that accompanies scurvy. Lack of two essential B vitamins, folic acid and vitamin B_{12}, results in the production of fewer but larger than normal red blood cells (macrocytic anemia). Small amounts of some elements in the diet to aid nutrition, such as copper and manganese, are needed for correct red blood cell formation. Lack of these elements may cause anemia; treatment is to add the missing factor to the diet. In severe cases, a physician may prescribe tablets or injections containing the missing factor.

Manufacture of red blood cells by the red bone marrow can also be slowed by the poisoning effect of an infection, by poisons such as lead, or by cancer. The anemia is made worse if the cancer invades the bone marrow or begins there, as in LEUKEMIA and MYELOMA. Treatment is to try to remove the cause, to prescribe a diet with additional vitamins, and to give blood transfusions if necessary.

Rapid destruction of red blood cells, called hemolytic anemia, occurs in malaria and a few other diseases. It can also arise as a reaction to certain drugs, and in sickle cell anemia, thalassemia, and some other inherited disorders which result in abnormal red cells. Hemolytic anemia can also arise from a blood transfusion with blood of the wrong type or incompatibility of RH FACTOR between a newborn child and its mother. Treatment is aimed at finding the cause, and blood transfusions may be given.

Complete failure to produce red blood cells, the disorder called aplastic anemia, may occur suddenly for no apparent reason. Or it may be caused by sensitivity to a drug that results in destruction of bone marrow cells. Treatment is with corticosteroid drugs, blood transfusions, or sometimes bone marrow transplants.

Q: *Should women routinely take iron tablets?*

A: A well-balanced diet provides sufficient iron for a woman with normal menstrual periods. Such a woman needs about 60 mg of iron per month. If her periods are particularly heavy, or if she is pregnant, her iron intake may not keep pace with her loss and a physician may prescribe additional iron.

A talk about Anesthetics

Anesthetics are drugs that cause a loss of feeling. They are given before medical treatment that would otherwise cause pain. There are many anesthetic drugs and they can be grouped according to the effect they are intended to have on the patient.

Q: *What are the main types of anesthetics?*

A: A general anesthetic, causing loss of consciousness as well as loss of feeling, is given in most surgical operations.
Another group, called local anesthetics, cause a loss of feeling only in the area to be treated. Dentists often use a local anesthetic during the filling or extraction of a tooth. A third group are the topical anesthetics, which remove feeling from a surface area such as an eye or the nose. They make possible medical examinations without pain to the patient.

Q: *On what basis are different general anesthetics given?*

A: It is the task of an anesthesiologist to decide which general anesthetic is best for the patient. The anesthesiologist reviews the patient's medical history and may order tests to help select the anesthetic: the decision is made only after such preparation.

Q: *Are the injections a patient receives when awake part of the anesthetic?*

A: To make the patient relaxed and drowsy,

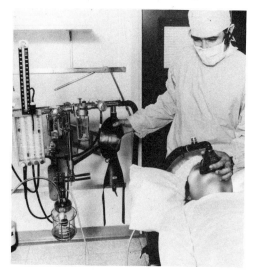

Anesthetics: Boyle's machine is one of the most used and most essential tools in surgery.

Anesthetics

and to dry the mouth and lungs, a sedative injection is given one hour before the operation. Later, immediately before the general anesthetic, an injection of a short period sleeping drug is given in a vein. This takes effect extremely quickly.

Q: *How is a general anesthetic given?*

A: When the patient is asleep after the intravenous injection, a small dose of a drug that relaxes the muscles is generally given. The drugs that continue the general anesthesia are injected or given as gases either through a face mask or a tube inserted through the mouth or nose into the windpipe. The tube is attached to an anesthesia machine, which ensures maximum control over the quantity and composition of the mixture of anesthetic and oxygen.

Q: *What precautions are taken before the anesthetic is administered, and after consciousness has been regained?*

A: The patient is not allowed anything to eat or drink for at least four hours before the operation. This reduces the chances of vomiting and inhaling fluid into the lungs when the anesthetic is being given.

After the operation, the anesthesiologist remains with the patient until consciousness is regained.

Q: *How do local anesthetics differ from general anesthetics?*

A: A local anesthetic is injected either into the tissues surrounding the area to be treated or next to the nerves serving the area. Adrenaline is sometimes added to the injection to increase the time for which the anesthetic is effective.

Q: *What are the various types of local anesthetic?*

A: There are four types of local anesthetic. (1) The most common form of local anesthetic is the type used for a dental injection, in which the loss of sensation affects only a limited area. (2) A local anesthetic that affects a whole section of the body, such as an arm or a leg, produces what is called regional anesthesia. The injection is given close to where the nerves leave the spinal cord. (3) When an injection is given around the spinal cord (epidural anesthesia) or into the cerebrospinal fluid of the spinal cord (spinal anesthesia), the body is anesthetized below the site of injection. Epidural anesthesia is often used during childbirth. (4) Drugs may be injected to produce partial anesthesia combined with amnesia, and the patient becomes peaceful and relaxed. This state, known as TWILIGHT

SLEEP, is a condition favorable for performing examinations, such as that of the inner wall of the stomach (gastroscopy) using a fiberscope.

Anesthetic	Method	Comments
Barbiturates	Injection	Barbiturates produce rapid loss of consciousness, and are effective for short periods. However, they do not cause a loss of pain. For this reason, a barbiturate is used only as a preliminary anesthetic before a general anesthetic is given.
Chloroform	Inhalation	Chloroform was once an extremely common anesthetic, but it is rarely used in surgical procedures today. Chloroform may damage a patient's liver.
Cyclopropane	Inhalation	Cyclopropane is an effective anesthetic, but it is not used as widely today as it once

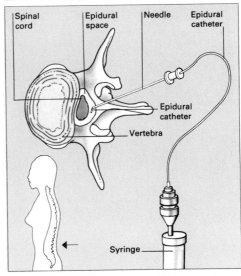

Anesthetics may be introduced into the epidural space between spine and spinal cord.

Anesthetics

Anesthetic	Method	Comments
		was because of its explosive properties. The recovery process from cyclo-propane is speedy, but the patient may become con-siderably excited as he or she regains consciousness.
Ether	Inhalation	Ether was once widely used, but other drugs are considered safer.
Halothane (Fluothane)	Inhalation	Halothane is the most widely used anesthetic today and is considered the most power-ful. It is also safe for use in surgical procedures on persons suffering from asthma.
Nitrous oxide	Inhalation	A drawback of nitrous oxide is that it lacks strength, so large amounts of the drug must be given to produce anesthesia. It is

Anesthetic	Method	Comments
		sometimes known as laughing gas. Although the patient quickly becomes unconscious, anesthesia may not be complete when it is used without oxygen. The patient may remain in an emotionally unin-hibited state, which is often characterized by laughing or crying.

Local anesthetics

Anesthetic	Method	Comments
Procaine hydrochloride (Novocain)	Injection	This is the most widely used local anesthetic. One disadvantage is that its effect wears off quickly. Adrenaline is sometimes mixed with the drug to make the effect last longer.
Carbocaine Nesacaine Xylocaine	Injection	These drugs are more poisonous to the body than procaine, and their use is regulated. One advantage over procaine is that the effect of these drugs lasts longer.
Cocaine Pontocaine Xylocaine	Direct application	Used for surface anesthesia. A solution of the drug is applied directly to the area to be treated.

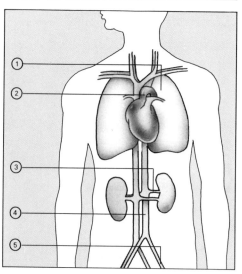

Aneurysms caused by a congenital weakness occur most commonly in these five sites.

Aneurysm is a swelling or ballooning at a weakened point of an artery, a vein, or the heart. More commonly, however, the term aneurysm is used to describe such a swelling in an arterial wall. The weakening of the arterial wall is often a result of hardening of the arteries (arteriosclerosis). A weakness that has been present from birth may also cause aneurysms.

Q: Can an aneurysm be serious?

A: Yes. If an aneurysm bursts (ruptures), it is extremely dangerous. An aneurysm in the aorta, the major blood vessel leading from the heart, may partly rupture (dissecting aneurysm). It usually causes enough pain to act as a warning of impending complete rupture. If an aortic aneurysm ruptures completely, death may result. If the burst occurs in the brain, there is a stroke or brain hemorrhage (subarachnoid hemorrhage).

Q: *Can a ruptured aneurysm be treated successfully?*

A: If treatment can be provided promptly, damage from the rupture may be brought under control. A suspected rupture must be confirmed by an X-ray of the artery (arteriogram). Then a surgical operation is the only treatment.

Angiitis, or angitis, is inflammation of a blood vessel or lymph vessel. It may be caused either by infection (thrombophlebitis or lymphangitis) or by another type of disease, such as thromboangiitis obliterans or polyarteritis nodosa.

A talk about Angina pectoris

Angina pectoris was once the term for any pain in the chest, but it now refers to a specific condition that involves pain from the heart. The pain occurs because not enough oxygen reaches the heart muscle, especially following exercise. There is a tight feeling across the chest, which may later spread into the neck, jaw, shoulders, and to one or both arms as far as the hands. Occasionally, it may also spread to the upper abdomen. In most patients, however, pain is present only in some of these areas. Usually there is shortness of breath and a feeling of faintness.

Q: *What disorders might be associated with angina pectoris?*

A: Coronary heart disease (ARTERIOSCLEROSIS) is the cause of angina pectoris. The condition is not in itself a heart attack, but may be either a warning that one could occur, or the immediate result of one.

Q: *How does a physician distinguish between angina pectoris and other similar pain?*

A: If angina pectoris is suspected, the physician runs a test called an ELECTROCARDIOGRAM (EKG). One of the diagnostic features of angina, however, is that the pain typically occurs during periods of physical activity.

Q: *How is angina pectoris treated?*

A: Overweight patients must lose excess fat, to reduce strain on the heart. Smoking must be discontinued, because nicotine contributes to hardening of the arteries. Regular exercise improves blood circulation to the heart. Before physical effort, drugs such as glyceryl trinitrate (nitroglycerine) help by causing the arteries to expand. Fast-acting capsules of amyl nitrate can be inhaled if pain occurs. Newer drugs called beta-blockers help to prevent pain by reducing the amount of oxygen that the heart muscle needs, and governing the heart rate.

Q: *Should a patient with angina pectoris become less active?*

A: The patient is usually encouraged to lead a normal life. However, the patient should learn to recognize how much exercise he can tolerate without bringing on the pain. He should also avoid emotional upset and cold temperatures.

Angiogram is a series of X-ray films of a blood vessel. A dye that X-rays or other radiation cannot penetrate is injected into a blood vessel, and X-ray pictures are then taken in rapid succession. The series of pictures show up the size and shape of veins or arteries in organs or tissue, and thereby reveal abnormalities such as arteriosclerosis.

Angioma is an abnormal growth of tissue formed by a group of small blood vessels. It may be present on the surface of the skin or internally, and is not usually malignant (cancerous). On the skin, an angioma is a soft, purplish mark called a strawberry nevus. If an angioma occurs in the brain, it can lead to serious conditions such as bleeding (subarachnoid hemorrhage) or a stroke. An angioma that bleeds in the intestine may

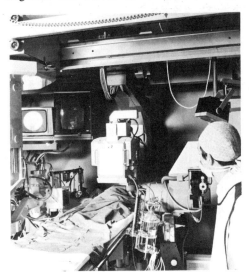

Angiogram is a technique for showing defects in blood vessels by means of X rays.

Angioneurotic edema

cause black stools (melena), the vomiting of blood (hematemesis), or anemia.

Q: What is the treatment for an angioma?

A: A small angioma in the skin may be burned or corroded away (cauterized), but larger ones need plastic surgery. Sometimes it is not advisable to treat an angioma; any disfigurement can be hidden by cosmetics.

Angioneurotic edema (or angioedema) is a form of giant HIVES (urticaria) in which large, irritating swellings occur anywhere on or near the surface of the body. It is thought to be caused by an allergy to a specific food or to a drug. The condition is not usually considered to be serious unless it affects the mouth, throat, or larynx, where it may obstruct breathing. The usual treatment is immediate injection of adrenaline followed by antihistamines. In a more severe attack, a course of steroid drugs may be prescribed.

Ankle is the joint connecting the foot and the leg. The weight of the body is transmitted to the heel bone (calcaneus) of the foot through the strong shinbone (tibia) of the leg. The outer side of the ankle is supported by the slender fibula bone. The ankle joint allows only up-and-down movements of the foot.

Q: What can go wrong with the ankle?

A: One of the most frequent disorders is a sprained ankle, the tearing of the ligaments (bands of fibrous tissue) between the fibula and the side of the calcaneus bone. It is accompanied by pain, swelling, and tenderness. Treatment with painkilling drugs and bandaging, or strapping, for a few days helps it to heal.

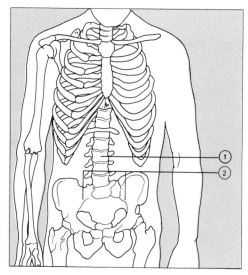

Ankylosing spondylitis, usually begins in the lower spine (1) and sacroiliac joints (2).

A FRACTURE of the ankle may be a break of the fibula alone or of both the fibula and tibia. It is diagnosed by X-ray examination. Treatment consists in restoring the ends of the broken bones to their proper positions, which may require surgery, and then holding them there in a plaster of Paris cast until they heal.

Ankles frequently swell because of excessive fluid in the tissues (edema). Such swelling is common in hot weather, after a person has been standing for a long time, or during pregnancy. Resting with the feet raised generally reduces such swelling.

Ankle sprains, varicose veins, obesity, and local infections may also cause ankle swelling.

Ankylosing spondylitis, also known as bamboo spine, is a condition in which the bones of the spine (vertebrae) fuse together. This causes stiffness and the spine can become bowed. Early symptoms are backache and stiffness in the morning. Ankylosing spondylitis occurs more often in men than in women and usually starts early in adult life. The symptoms gradually worsen but pain need not be continuous. The patient's eyes often become inflamed (iritis), and the joints can become swollen and tender (arthritis).

The cause of ankylosing spondylitis is not known.

Q: Can treatment arrest the progress of ankylosing spondylitis?

A: Yes, but only to the extent that a physician can reduce the pain and stiffness associated with the disorder. Aspirin and some stronger rheumatic drugs are prescribed for the pain or, if it is severe, radiotherapy may be used. Exercises are essential to keep the spine mobile and straight, and physiotherapy (including breathing exercises) is an important aspect of treatment.

Ankylosis is the stiffening of a joint or the fusing together of the bones that form it either through disease or by an operation. If it occurs naturally, the condition may be inherited or it may be discovered at birth. ANKYLOSING SPONDYLITIS is a disease in which the bones of the spine fuse together. Artificial ankylosis (ARTHRODESIS) is a way of stopping some painful joint conditions.

Ankylostomiasis, also known as hookworm disease, is the infestation of the small intestine by small worms (*Ancylostoma duodenale* or *Necator americanus*). These worms, which grow up to 0.5 inches (12mm) long, enter through the skin, travel to the lungs and then to the intestine, and may leave an itching rash. Their eggs are excreted in the feces, and end up living in soil as larvae until they can reenter human skin.

Q: *What are the symptoms of ankylostomiasis?*

A: Symptoms of ankylostomiasis may be pain or diarrhea, and a long infection can lead to anemia with all the symptoms that accompany that disorder. If the disease is undiscovered in children, it may retard growth and mental development.

Ankylostomiasis is diagnosed by testing the feces for eggs and is treated by drug therapy.

Q: *In what parts of the world is ankylostomiasis most likely to occur?*

A: It is more common where a hot climate and damp earth are favorable conditions for larvae to thrive, especially if there is poor sanitation as well. The worms usually enter the skin through bare feet that come into contact with larva-ridden soil. The disorder occurs in tropical areas and in the southern states of the U.S.

Anorectics are drugs that reduce the appetite. Most are AMPHETAMINES or related compounds that, because of their addictive properties, are now used only to treat extreme, life-endangering obesity. As a general rule, drugs should not be used to reduce weight.

Anorexia nervosa is a form of mental illness characterized by a severe loss of appetite not due to any disease. It most commonly is found in young women, but also occurs in older women and men. Researchers believe the disorder is especially likely to develop when parents set excessively high standards or try to exert too much control over their children's lives.

See also BULIMIA.

If forced to eat, the patient may vomit after the meal. Loss of appetite leads to loss of weight, and, in women, menstrual periods cease altogether. The weight loss may be accompanied by extreme wasting. When the anorexic body, which is starved for calories, starts feeding on its own muscle protein, the heart muscles may weaken, leading to irregularities in rhythm or even congestive heart failure.

Q: *Can anorexia be detected in its early stages?*

A: Early diagnosis is difficult. The patient, especially if adolescent, commonly denies that anything is wrong and continues to be cheerful and active. He or she may be deceptive about the quantity of food eaten and deny they are wasting away, continuing to express fear of being fat.

Q: *How is anorexia nervosa treated?*

A: Anorexia needs skilled psychiatric attention. It may be some years before normal health is regained.

Anosmia is the lack of a sense of smell. It occurs in the elderly, in nasal conditions where there is excessive mucus, and sometimes following certain skull fractures.

Anoxia is a lack of sufficient oxygen in the body.

Antacid is a substance that is used medically to neutralize the acid contents of the stomach. Most indigestion mixtures, powders, or pills contain antacids. The antacids may relieve pain, but some may have unpleasant side effects, such as diarrhea or constipation. Prolonged use of antacids should be avoided, except under a physician's advice.

Antenatal is another word for PRENATAL, meaning before birth.

Anthelmintics are drugs that are used to treat disorders caused by infestations with worms.

Anthracosis is a form of PNEUMOCONIOSIS, a lung disorder once common among coal workers.

See also BLACK LUNG.

Anthrax is an infectious disease, now rare, that is transmitted to humans most commonly by farm animals. It can take the form of a characteristic boil on the skin or, if the germs are inhaled, it can cause pneumonia.

Q: *What are the symptoms of anthrax?*

A: Symptoms include a fever and the occurrence of a skin ulcer or boil. Anyone working with animals or animal products who develops an unusual boil should see a physician at once. The boil, caused by *Bacillus anthracis*, is large with a black scab. It forms slowly on the skin and may spread to form more boils.

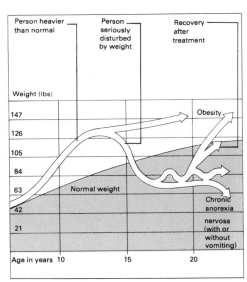

Anorexia nervosa is classically a hyperreaction to being overweight and may be fatal.

Antibiotics

Q: What is the treatment for anthrax?

A: Immediate treatment with penicillin is usually effective. Unfortunately, anthrax bacilli form spores, a resistant form of the germ that is extremely difficult to destroy. Everything in contact with the patient must first be sterilized, and all contaminated animal products must be destroyed.

Antibiotics are drugs that are used to treat various types of bacterial infections. There are many types of antibiotics, and they work either by preventing the infection from growing, or by destroying it. Some antibiotics are produced by a mold or fungus; others are made synthetically.

Q: What are the names of some of the antibiotics and what do they do?

A: PENICILLIN, the first antibiotic (discovered by Sir Alexander Fleming in 1928), destroys multiplying bacteria by making their cell walls burst. There are also a number of newer forms of penicillin, such as ampicillin and amoxyllin.

TETRACYCLINES, another important group, act by interfering with bacterial growth. They are broad-spectrum antibiotics, which means that they are active against many types of bacteria. Other antibiotics of this type include CHLORAMPHENICOL, used to treat typhoid fever, and streptomycin, used in the treatment of tuberculosis.

There are many other groups of antibiotics, each produced to combat specific diseases.

Q: Are antibiotics safe?

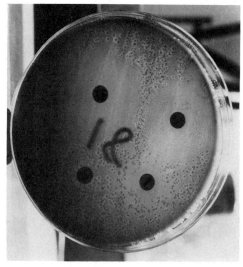

The efficiency of antibiotics is identified by the effect they have on a germ culture.

A: Antibiotics can save lives when prescribed with caution to treat bacterial infection. However, indiscriminate use of these drugs can have serious consequences, and cancel out their usefulness. In the years since 1941 (when antibiotics were first given to patients), a number of bacterial diseases have become resistant to the antibiotics that once were able to control or destroy them.

Some of the drugs, when taken over a long period, may produce unpleasant or damaging side effects. Certain antibiotics may become toxic when stale.

Sometimes, a patient has an allergic reaction to an antibiotic drug. This can be either the serious condition known medically as ANAPHYLAXIS, or a lesser condition that is still important to recognize. Patients who know they are allergic to an antibiotic drug should tell the physician of this fact when being treated for any condition.

Antibody is a substance produced by the body in response to an infection. It combines with an antigen (the foreign substance that activated it) and puts it out of action. Antibodies are part of the development of natural IMMUNITY. They can be produced artificially by IMMUNIZATION.

See also ALLERGY.

Anticoagulants are drugs that interfere with the normal clotting ability of the blood. There are two main groups: direct-acting, such as HEPARIN, which is injected into a vein; and indirect-acting, such as coumarin, which is taken by mouth. Heparin acts quickly but the indirect-acting drugs take up to three days to work.

Q: When are anticoagulants prescribed?

A: They are given to prevent or dissolve a blood clot, such as a blockage in the blood supply to the heart muscle (myocardial infarction) or in a leg vein (thrombosis). They may also be given before certain operations on the female reproductive system, to prevent the clotting in leg veins that tends to occur more frequently than in other operations.

Q: Should a patient who uses anticoagulants observe special precautions?

A: Patients taking anticoagulants require regular blood tests to ensure that the correct dosage is maintained. They should also carry a card naming the anticoagulant drug and stating the dosage, in case they are involved in an accident. Any other tablets or medicines should be avoided, until checked out by a physician or pharmacist, to ensure that they do not alter the anticoagulant effect.

Q: What are the signs of an overdose of anticoagulants?

A: A common indication is the appearance of unexpected bruising in various parts of the body.

Anticonvulsants are drugs used in the treatment of EPILEPSY to prevent the CONVULSIONS that accompany this disorder.

Antidepressants are drugs used in the treatment of mental DEPRESSION. There are two main categories: the monoamine-oxidase (MAO) inhibitor group and the tricyclic antidepressants. If the MAO INHIBITORS are prescribed, the patient is warned to avoid such foods as cheese, broad beans, alcohol, and some yeast extracts, whose chemical properties interact in a dangerous way with this group. The tricyclics are more frequently prescribed because they seem safer and often as effective as the MAO inhibitors, although they act more gradually. A third group, seldom used today is AMPHETAMINES.

Antidepressants should be taken only under a physician's supervision.

Antigen is a foreign substance in the body that stimulates the production of an ANTIBODY. Antigens may be bacteria, viruses, or any other physical agent, such as pollen.

See also ALLERGY; IMMUNIZATION.

Antihistamines are a group of drugs used to counteract histamine, the chemical in the body that is the main cause of allergic reactions. Antihistamines suppress the symptoms without treating the original cause.

Q: In what forms are antihistamines prescribed?

A: They can be obtained in many forms, such as tablets and capsules, injections, nose and eye preparations, and as cream for the skin.

Q: Do antihistamines have unpleasant or dangerous side effects?

A: Antihistamines are powerful drugs and should be used with care. Many of them cause drowsiness, and patients are warned to avoid taking them before driving an automobile. Some patients, however, are stimulated after taking amphetamines and become restless and unable to sleep. Antihistamines often cause a dry mouth and, unless they are taken with food, they irritate the stomach.

See also ALLERGY.

Antinauseants are drugs used to prevent or relieve nausea. There are two main groups: (1) Anticholinergic drugs. These usually contain atropine, which acts on the nervous system to block secretions from the stomach and glands. They may produce blurred vision, a dry mouth, and a rapid heartbeat. Their use should not be prolonged, nor should they be given to patients with GLAUCOMA or to those who may develop urine retention; (2) ANTIHISTAMINES. These usually have a depressing effect on the brain, which produces drowsiness, but may occasionally cause stimulation in children, making them unable to sleep.

Both these types of drugs interfere with the ability to drive an automobile, and should not be taken with alcoholic drinks.

See also MOTION SICKNESS.

Antiperspirants are substances that reduce sweating. They are commonly used to avoid the bad odor associated with perspiration by reducing skin secretions.

Antipruritics are agents that prevent or relieve ITCHING (pruritus). There are many causes of itching, which should be diagnosed before treatment.

Antipyretics are agents (such as aspirin) that help to reduce a fever.

Antiseptic is a substance that prevents the growth of germs and infection. Carbolic acid (phenol) was the first antiseptic to be used, but this has given way to milder modern antiseptics such as cetrimide, alcohol, and iodine-containing compounds.

See also ASEPSIS.

Antiserum is a SERUM containing antibodies made from blood taken from a sensitized human being or animal. It can be injected to give temporary protection against a specific disease, for example, tetanus or diphtheria, in someone who has no immunity to the disease. The antiserum from animals, however, may itself cause an allergic reaction or even severe or fatal shock (anaphylaxis).

See also IMMUNIZATION.

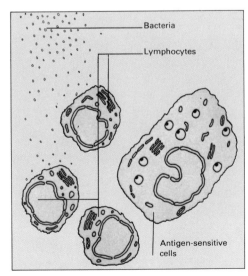

Antibodies are proteins produced by white cells in response to antigens such as bacteria.

Antispasmodics

Antispasmodics are drugs that prevent the contraction of smooth muscle. Antispasmodics are used to treat a variety of conditions, including spastic colon, and bladder and gall bladder disorders.

Antitoxin is an ANTIBODY, formed in the body, that acts against a specific bacterial toxin (poison) by combining with it and neutralizing it.

See also IMMUNIZATION.

Antitussive is a drug used to stop coughing. There are two groups of such drugs, narcotic and nonnarcotic. The narcotic drugs depress the so-called cough centers in the brain, but the patient may become dependent on them if they are used for a long period. CODEINE is the preparation most commonly used in prescription cough suppressants.

There are many nonnarcotic cough suppressants available.

See also COUGH.

Antivenin is a SERUM used to treat poisoning by snake (or other animal) bite. It contains a high concentration of ANTIBODIES, and is injected around the area of the poisonous bite.

See also First Aid, p.519.

Antivert (Trademark) is a preparation of meclizine, an ANTIHISTAMINE. It is used to treat nausea, vomiting, motion sickness, and vertigo. However, the U.S. Food and Drug Administration has rated this product only "possibly effective" against vertigo.

As with all similar drugs, Antivert may cause drowsiness and lack of coordination; persons taking it should not drive an automobile or operate machinery. It has also been reported that high doses of meclizine may produce abnormalities in newborn infants, so the drug should not be used by pregnant women.

Antrum is a cavity within a bone. It is commonly used to describe the air spaces in the bones adjacent to the nose, the SINUSES.

Anuria is a serious malfunction of the kidney in which no urine is produced. Without immediate treatment, anuria is fatal. The kidney failure can be caused by: (1) blockage by a stone (calculus) or tumor; (2) disease, such as acute nephritis; or (3) a decrease in blood pressure during shock.

Treatment is urgent and requires skilled care. Fluids in the diet are restricted and given intravenously. Sometimes, an artificial kidney is used to allow the patient to get rid of the waste products and toxins produced by the body.

See also KIDNEY DIALYSIS; KIDNEY DISEASE.

Anus is the opening at the lower end of the ALIMENTARY CANAL. It is kept closed by a ring of circular muscle called the sphincter. The anus is subject to three common disorders: (1) fissure, a small crack in the skin of the anus; (2) hemorrhoids (external piles), varicose veins outside the anus; (3) pruritus ani (itching), sometimes caused by a neurosis but often caused by a minor disorder of the anal skin (for example, as a result of worms).

The first two complaints may be treated by minor surgery and the last one by a suitable ointment prescribed by a physician.

A talk about Anxiety

Anxiety is a feeling of fearful anticipation and worry, and is a response to possible danger. When fear is exaggerated or has no apparent cause, then, medically speaking, anxiety is an illness needing treatment.

Q: *What are the symptoms of anxiety?*

A: Anxiety is such a common problem that everyone has experienced it at some time and is familiar with the sweating, palpitations, trembling, nausea, and diarrhea that may accompany the condition in various combinations. A medical checkup generally reassures the sufferer that there is not a more serious underlying cause.

Q: *Can anxiety seriously affect a person?*

A: Continued anxiety leads to fatigue and irritability. Sometimes there are sleepless nights (insomnia). Occasionally, anxiety shows itself in the form of a headache, a skin rash, an asthma attack, a peptic ulcer, or a spastic colon.

   Children may regress to wetting the bed, or they may have bouts of vomiting, stomach pains, diarrhea, and nightmares.

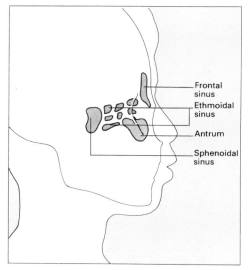

Frontal sinus

Ethmoidal sinus

Antrum

Sphenoidal sinus

Antrum is one of the cavities, called sinuses, in the upper jaw.

Q: Is there any way to get rid of these irrational feelings of fear?

A: Acute symptoms can be helped by TRANQUILIZERS, but these do not cure the underlying condition and often give a false feeling of security. For some people, an in-depth discussion with a friend or a physician may help immediately, but others may need psychiatric help for a longer period of time.

When the patient can be helped to cope with anxious feelings on a regular basis, a cure is in sight.

Aorta is the largest artery in the body, supplying blood to all the organs alongside its course. It starts at the left ventricle of the heart, then arches upwards and backwards, giving off branch arteries to the heart muscles, head, and arms. The aorta then runs down the back of the chest, in front of the spine and esophagus (gullet), to reach the abdomen. There the aorta divides, just above the pelvis, into the common iliac arteries to the legs.

See also p.8.

Aortogram is an X-ray picture of the AORTA, taken after the injection of a special chemical into the blood vessels. It is a type of ARTERIOGRAM.

Apgar score is a rating system that assesses the vital functions in a baby during the first minute after birth. Five functions (heart rate, respiration, muscle tone, color, and reflex response) are each assessed on a zero to two scale and totaled to a possible high of ten. Babies with a total score of eight to ten are given routine postnatal care. The lower the rating under seven, the more special is the attention needed to give the baby a normal start in life.

Aphakia is the condition of an eye in which the lens is absent. In rare cases, aphakia may occur as a congenital abnormality. More commonly, however, aphakia results from an eye injury or following a CATARACT operation.

Aphasia is a condition in which an individual has lost the ability to speak and to understand speech. There is, commonly, also an inability to read and write. The complaint may be only temporary, following a stroke or concussion. Or it may occur briefly after a grand mal attack of epilepsy. Sometimes the condition is partial (dysphasia), and the person retains a usable capacity to write and understand writing.

Aphonia is loss of voice, and is usually a temporary condition. Speech remains possible, although it must be whispered instead of voiced. Aphonia may be the result of (1)

inflammation of the larynx (laryngitis); (2) using the voice too much; or (3) radiotherapy for cancer of the vocal cord. Occasionally, hysteria may be the cause.

Aphrodisiac is a substance that increases sexual desire (libido). There are many substances that are said to have this property, but most of them are ineffectual, and their results often depend on how strongly the individual believes in them. Many so-called aphrodisiacs are harmless, but some may be poisonous, especially if taken in large amounts. Cantharides, a powder of the dried beetle Spanish fly, is highly dangerous when used as an aphrodisiac; consumption of cantharides can be fatal.

Aphthous ulcer is a small whitish sore, usually in the mouth, that is commonly called a canker sore. *See* CANKER SORE.

Apoplexy (for EMERGENCY treatment, *see* First Aid, p.579) is a stoppage of the blood supply to the brain, and is more commonly known as a stroke. *See* STROKE.

Appendectomy is the surgical removal of the APPENDIX, a nonfunctional structure attached to the upper part of the large intestine. The operation is generally performed after diagnosis of APPENDICITIS, a painful inflammation of the appendix.

Q: How is the appendectomy performed?

A: The appendix is removed under general anesthesia, usually through a small diagonal cut in the lower right-hand side of the abdomen. Sometimes the surgeon makes a cut parallel to the middle line near the center of the lower abdomen. With acute appendicitis the appendix may

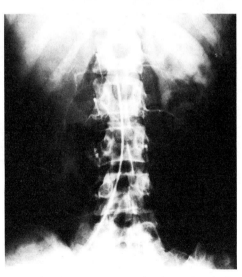

Aortogram is achieved by injecting a chemical into the heart with a catheter.

Appendicitis

burst, and there is the slight risk that the operation itself may cause it to do so. If the appendix bursts and infection spreads to the lining of the abdomen (causing peritonitis), the surgeon leaves a tube in the wound to drain the infection to the surface; after about 48 hours the drain usually can be removed.

Q: *How long does recovery normally take after an appendectomy?*

A: After the operation, recovery is rapid. The stitches are removed about five days later, and the patient is able to leave the hospital within a week. But convalescence may take about a month or more while the various layers of tissue in the abdominal wall heal. In the past an appendectomy was considered a difficult and risky operation, but today the success rate is nearly 100 percent. About one person in ten has the operation.

Appendicitis is inflammation of the appendix, a structure attached to the first part of the large intestine. An early symptom is vague stomach pain around the navel, which becomes more severe and spreads within three or four hours to the lower right-hand corner of the abdomen, sometimes with periods of gripping pain (colic). A feeling of nausea is followed by vomiting, headache, and slight fever. The patient is usually constipated, although occasionally there may be diarrhea. The stomach is tender, and touching it makes the pain worse.

Q: *If appendicitis is suspected, what should be done?*

A: Do not give the patient a laxative. If pain persists after a few hours, a physician should be consulted. Failure to seek prompt medical attention may allow the appendix to burst, thus causing a critical infection of the abdominal lining (peritonitis). With acute appendicitis, the patient is usually admitted immediately to the hospital for an APPENDECTOMY, an operation to remove the appendix.

Q: *Does appendicitis affect certain age groups more than others?*

A: The complaint occurs rarely in children under the age of five, and rarely in adults after the age of fifty.

Appendix is any structure that is attached to a larger or more important part. The term usually refers to the vermiform appendix, which is a worm-shaped structure attached to the first part (cecum) of the large intestine, which lies in the lower right side of the abdomen. It is on average about 3 inches (8cm) long although the size does vary widely. The appendix may also be variably situated; it can be tucked behind the cecum, or hang down into the pelvis. Inflammation of the appendix is called APPENDICITIS.

Appetite is a healthy and natural anticipation of food. It must not be confused with hunger, which is a stronger stimulus.

Many disorders result in or are accompanied by a loss of appetite. Anyone who undergoes a loss of both appetite and weight lasting for more than two weeks should consult a physician. Some diseases, such as overactivity of the thyroid gland (thyrotoxicosis), increase the body's energy requirements and stimulate appetite.

Psychological conditions such as depression may cause either compulsive eating or loss of appetite. ANOREXIA NERVOSA, for example, occurring most often in adolescent girls, makes them unwilling to eat. A child's refusal to eat is commonly not a loss of appetite but a means of upsetting the parents.

It is possible to control appetite with the use of drugs, but this may be extremely dangerous and should be done only on a physician's advice.

Aqueous humor is the watery fluid in the eye, in front of the lens. *See* HUMOR.

Argyll-Robertson pupil is a disorder in which the process for focusing an eye works normally although the reflex response to light is absent. The pupil is commonly contracted and so may appear smaller than normal. The condition is generally a sign of one type of the venereal disease syphilis.

Armpit is the ordinary name for the axilla, the cavity below the shoulder joint. Strong muscles, attached to the chest and shoulder blade, form the front and back walls and help

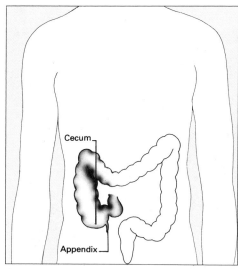

Appendix is a structure, about the size of a little finger, attached to the cecum.

to move the arm. The armpit contains sweat glands, lymph glands, and, in an adult, hairs.

Q: What can go wrong with the armpit?

A: Several common problems can arise there. Heavy perspiration (hyperhidrosis), occurring normally when a person is hot, active, and anxious, can be embarrassing to some people who suffer from the condition all the time. Not much can be done as treatment, apart from using a strong-acting deodorant and antiperspirant preparation.

Other common disorders are abscesses. They may be a consequence of heavy sweating, or not washing the armpit, or too frequent shaving of the hair. They appear more often in persons with diabetes.

Some people have allergic reactions to deodorants, antiperspirants, and perfumes, each of which may produce an area of red, painful skin.

Pain in the armpit may be caused by boils, allergic skin problems, swollen lymph glands or a general lymph gland disorder. Or it may result from a local infection somewhere on the arm, such as that caused by a smallpox vaccination. Swelling in the armpit, with little accompanying pain, is one of the symptoms of Hodgkin's disease, a form of cancer.

Arrhythmia is an irregularity in the heartbeat and therefore also the pulse rate. There are various causes for an irregular pulse. In sinus arrhythmia, a normal occurrence in young people at rest, the pulse rate increases or decreases with breathing. Breathing alters the amount of blood entering the heart and this changes the pulse rate.

See also FIBRILLATION; PAROXYSMAL TACHYCARDIA.

Arsenic is a metalloid chemical element. Its oxide, a grayish white powder, is extremely poisonous. Accumulation of arsenic in the body causes weakness, indigestion, diarrhea, discoloration and peeling of the skin, mental disorders, and loss of sensation in the wrists and ankles. Acute arsenic poisoning may cause death.

Arteriogram is an X-ray picture of an artery. To take the picture, the radiologist first injects the artery with a substance that is opaque to radiation.

See also ANGIOGRAM.

A talk about Arteriosclerosis

Arteriosclerosis is a disorder in which arteries become thick and hard and lose their supple, elastic quality. Usually this happens when fats

are deposited in the vessel walls, a process called atherosclerosis.

Q: What causes the deposits in the arteries?

A: The cause is not fully known, but it is believed to be part of the normal aging process. Arteriosclerosis is more likely to occur or to be severe in any one of the following groups of people: the overweight; smokers; those with high blood pressure (hypertension); the inactive; those with diabetes; and those who have a family history of heart attacks that are connected with increased levels of LIPIDS and CHOLESTEROL in the blood.

Q: Is arteriosclerosis serious?

A: The exact seriousness of the condition depends on which arteries are most affected. A narrowed artery to the heart muscle may cause ANGINA PECTORIS or a HEART ATTACK (myocardial infarction). If the arteries to the legs are affected, the patient feels pain in the calves when walking (intermittent claudication). Affected arteries to the brain may cause a succession of small strokes or a major one (*see* STROKE). Reduced flow of blood to certain areas of the brain may result in PARKINSON'S DISEASE.

Sometimes, when the artery is brittle, a piece of fatty substance (thrombus) breaks away from the inside wall and enters the bloodstream. If the thrombus is sufficiently large, it may block the bloodstream completely and cause a stroke. In one of the limbs, such an obstruction can be extremely serious and requires prompt medical treatment

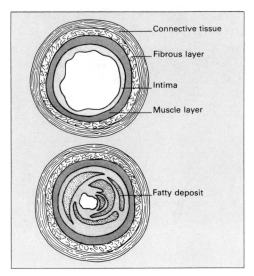
Connective tissue
Fibrous layer
Intima
Muscle layer
Fatty deposit

Arteriosclerosis, hardening of the arteries, develops when fat clings to the artery walls.

Artery

before gangrene (death of tissue) sets in below the blockage.

Q: Can a hardened artery be made to return to its normal size and suppleness?

A: No. If a limb artery has become blocked, after previous treatment has failed to improve circulation, the sclerotic (hardened) section has to be surgically replaced by a section of new artery, either natural or plastic (arterial graft).

Q: What is the treatment for arteriosclerosis?

A: Treatment of arteriosclerosis can only prevent the condition from becoming worse. Special drugs such as clofibrate tend to reduce cholesterol in the blood, and others reduce blood pressure. The patient must lose weight, stop smoking, take regular exercise, reduce the amount of cholesterol-containing foods in the diet, and keep diabetes under control. The same regimen should be followed to help to prevent arteriosclerosis.

Artery is one of the tube-shaped blood vessels that carry oxygenated blood from the heart to the body tissues. Arteries are thick-walled, flexible, and muscular.
See also p. 8.

A talk about Arthritis

Arthritis is a general term for any condition in which joints become inflamed, usually accompanied by pain, swelling, and limited movement. Arthritis has many different forms, but

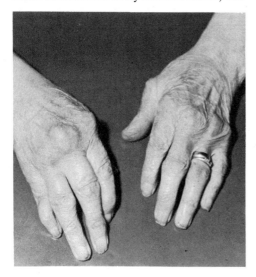

Arthritis is inflammation of the joints that produces the characteristic swelling.

the three most common forms are osteoarthritis, rheumatoid arthritis, and gout. Physicians are not always able to determine the cause of a specific arthritic complaint. In general, arthritis may be caused by infection in a joint, by degeneration of a joint as a person becomes older, or by a disorder of which arthritis is a symptom. The cause of the arthritis determines which course the affliction takes.

Q: What is osteoarthritis?

A: Osteoarthritis is the form of arthritis most common in elderly people. Time takes its toll of joints, which suffer from general wear and tear. The connecting surfaces of the joints become rougher as the cartilage lining the bone deteriorates.
Osteoarthritis most commonly affects those joints that support weight, such as the knees, hips, and spine. For this reason, the condition can be worse in people who are overweight. The effects of the aging process can be hastened if joints have been damaged earlier in life by an accident or injury.

Q: What measures can be taken by the osteoarthritis patient to relieve discomfort?

A: Aspirin is effective for reducing pain, but a physician sometimes prescribes stronger drugs depending on the severity of the condition, for example, piroxican and benoxaprofen. If the pain is in a weight-bearing joint (knee or hip), joint replacement, via surgery, may also be highly effective. Care should be taken when moving. The patient should lose weight, if necessary, and wear soft, rubber-heeled shoes. A living area can be modified to assist an arthritic person: handles near showers, baths, toilets, and beds are all useful aids. A straight-backed chair is easiest to use.

Q: Can a person become crippled with osteoarthritis?

A: Patients with osteoarthritis rarely become bedridden or crippled. The bulbous knobs that may develop on the fingers or toes can be painful and stiff, but serious crippling does not result. Pain flares up with sudden activity after rest, and a bad attack may last for several days. Osteoarthritis of a hip or a knee may prevent a patient from walking normally. If the joints in both legs are affected, the patient may become chairbound.

Q: What is rheumatoid arthritis?

A: Rheumatoid arthritis is painful swelling, usually of the smaller joints, together with the destruction of tissue around them. It most often begins in early adult life, and although an attack may subside, it usually flares up again later. The cause of this affliction remains unknown. There is a risk with rheumatoid arthritis of crippling or other physical deformity. In children, the condition is known as STILL'S DISEASE.

Q: *What is the treatment for rheumatoid arthritis?*

A: Treatment is aimed at providing relief from the symptoms. But the damage to the joints that accompanies the disorder cannot be repaired. Heat, in the form of shortwave diathermy and wax baths, can give short-term relief, and physiotherapy may ease the pain and keep the joints mobile. Salicylate drugs (a category that includes aspirin) and stronger antirheumatic drugs may be prescribed. Some deformities resulting from the disease can be remedied by surgical techniques.

Q: *What is gout?*

A: Gout is a congenital disorder in which the body cannot rid itself of all the uric acid it produces. Excessive quantities of uric acid build up in the bones and joints, as well as in various tissues and cartilage, and this can cause extremely painful attacks of arthritis. A blood test reveals a high concentration of uric acid in the bloodstream. If diagnosis is made early, future attacks may be prevented by the regular use of drugs, such as probenecid.

Q: *What other disorders cause arthritic symptoms?*

A: Joints may become infected as part of a generalized disease, often accompanied by a fever and a feeling of general illness. Bacterial arthritis is the invasion of joint areas by bacteria, causing swelling and inflammation. It occcurs with tuberculosis and gonorrhea. In children, rheumatic fever causes painful joints that become better, then worse over a period of weeks. This is an allergic reaction to streptococcus bacteria. Virus infections, such as rubella (German measles), mumps, and hepatitis, may sometimes produce inflamed joints. Arthritis may also be associated with the spinal disorder ankylosing spondylitis, with ulcers in the colon (colitis), or with inflammation of the urethra (Reiter's disease).

Q: *How effective are hydrocortisone injections for treating arthritis?*

A: Hydrocortisone cannot cure arthritis. Its effect is to reduce the inflammation in a joint, and thereby relieve the pain. Treatment is highly effective for as long as the drug is present, but when the effect wears off, the pain may return. Too many injections are dangerous, because they damage the joint in some instances.

Artificial insemination

Q: *How can surgery help patients with arthritis?*

A: A method of stopping pain in a stiff joint (such as the ankle) is by fusing its bones together in an operation (arthrodesis, or artificial ankylosis). Another possible operation is the replacement of the affected joint by an artificial one made of steel or plastic. This proves highly effective for an arthritic hip or fingers, but is less successful for knee or ankle joints.

Arthrodesis is the deliberate fusing together of the bones of a joint by an operation (artificial ANKYLOSIS). It is used to relieve a painful condition, such as severe osteoarthritis or a joint damaged in an accident.

Artificial heart is a mechanical substitute for the human heart, which can be implanted in a patient to replace a damaged heart. The first successful mechanical heart, the Jarvik-7, was implanted in Barney Clark in 1982. Although Clark, due to medical complications, only survived the implantation for a few weeks, the Jarvik-7 was found to have functioned perfectly.

Artificial insemination is a technique in which sperm is introduced into the neck of the womb (cervix) for the purpose of fertilizing the egg (ovum) by means other than sexual intercourse. This is normally done with a syringe. Artificial insemination is used in some cases of infertility.

Q: *How important is the timing of the insemination?*

A: The timing of the introduction of the

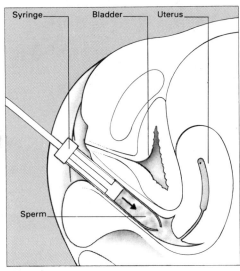

Artificial insemination is the introduction of healthy sperms into the vagina using a syringe.

Artificial kidney

sperm is critical; it should take place during ovulation (when an ovary releases an egg). The timing is estimated by following the woman's morning temperature charts, which show a sudden, slight increase in temperature on the day of ovulation.

Q: *Who supplies the sperm for the insemination?*

A: It is most common for the woman's husband to supply the sperm. This is known as AIH (artificial insemination by husband). The husband, although fertile, may not be able to have sexual intercourse. Or the quantity of sperm produced may be so small that the chances of conception are slight. In this case, sperm is collected and deep frozen until there is a sufficient amount.

Artificial insemination by donor (AID) is the provision of sperm by an unknown male. This is used when the husband is infertile but both partners want a baby of their own. The physician chooses a man with qualities that are compatible with those of the future parents in vital respects, such as race and physical characteristics, absence of congenital abnormalities, and the correct blood group. The practice of artificial insemination is controversial in many countries on legal, religious, and moral grounds.

Artificial kidney is a machine that takes over the function of the natural kidneys when they are damaged by disease and cannot clean the blood of toxic substances. The poisonous substances produce UREMIA, a serious condi-

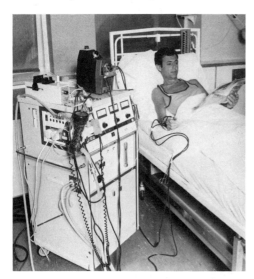

Artificial kidney filters out waste substances in the blood, just like a natural kidney would.

tion that, if left untreated, leads to death.
See also KIDNEY DIALYSIS.

Artificial limb. *See* PROSTHESIS.

Artificial respiration (for EMERGENCY treatment, *see* First Aid, pp.524–529) is any means of inducing breathing in a person whose breathing has stopped. As a part of first aid, it is often the primary treatment. Techniques that are commonly used in artificial respiration include mouth-to-mouth resuscitation, the Holger-Nielsen method, and the Silvester method, all of which are fully illustrated in the First Aid section of these books. An extreme emergency may require a TRACHEOSTOMY, an operation performed by a professional medical person in which a hole is made in the front of the neck into the windpipe (trachea).

Asbestosis is a form of the lung disease pneumoconiosis caused by inhaling asbestos fibers. *See* PNEUMOCONIOSIS.

Ascariasis is an infection of the bowels by roundworms (*Ascaris lumbricoides*). *See* WORMS.

Ascites is an accumulation of fluid in the abdominal cavity. *See* EDEMA.

Ascorbic acid is the chemical name for vitamin C. *See* VITAMINS.

Asepsis is the condition of an environment that is free from infecting organisms. In operating rooms, for example, it is most desirable that there be no airborne infection. To achieve asepsis, the air is filtered and kept at a higher pressure than normal air pressure outside, so that the aseptic air cannot be contaminated by unfiltered air. Operating instruments, surgical clothes, and gloves are all sterilized beforehand, and surgeons scrub their hands and forearms before dressing. Complete asepsis is not possible in a situation where humans are present. In the pharmaceutical industry many drugs are prepared and packaged in closed chambers.

Aspergillosis is infection by any member of the genus of fungi called *Aspergillus*.

Asphyxia (for EMERGENCY treatment, *see* First Aid, pp.524–529) is a condition in which an interference with the breathing process has seriously affected or even stopped the action of the heart and lungs. It is most often caused by SUFFOCATION (choking or obstruction of the air passages). Asphyxia requires urgent treatment because brain damage begins about five minutes after the cessation of the oxygen supply to the brain.

Q: *What are other causes of asphyxia?*

A: Asphyxia can also result from a reduction of the oxygen content in the air, chest injury, paralysis of the lungs, bleeding into the lungs, narcotic drugs, deep anesthesia, or electric shock.

Aspirin, the common name for acetylsalicylic acid, is the most widely used painkilling drug (analgesic). It is also used to reduce fever (as an antipyretic) and is beneficial as an anti-inflammatory in the treatment of the symptoms of such diseases of the joints as rheumatoid arthritis, osteoarthritis, and rheumatic fever.

The usual dose of aspirin is effective for about four to six hours, after which time it is broken down by the liver or excreted in the urine. Despite its almost universal usage, aspirin does not actually cure diseases, but merely relieves symptoms.

Q: *Is aspirin a harmless drug?*

A: When taken according to specified dosages, aspirin is an extremely safe drug. The availability of aspirin without prescription can, however, result in aspirin poisoning if the drug is abused by children, for whom it may be dangerous; adults may also be poisoned by aspirin. Continued use of the drug can cause stomach bleeding and a reduction of blood volume, which may be the beginning of anemia. Also, persons with certain disorders should not take aspirin.

Q: *Which disorders indicate caution with aspirin?*

A: Persons who have peptic ulcers should not use aspirin without medical advice: internal bleeding may occur and blood may be vomited (hematemesis). People who suffer from persistent indigestion and patients taking anticoagulant drugs are also advised against taking aspirin. Mild sensitivity to aspirin may cause an itchy skin irritation (urticaria) or allergic asthma. In such cases, a physician may recommend ACETAMINOPHEN as a safe alternative.

Asthenia is a general condition of weakness, usually arising from muscular or psychological disorders.

A talk about Asthma

Asthma is a disorder in which the patient experiences difficulty in breathing, accompanied by a slight wheezing and a "tight" chest. Additional symptoms can be a dry cough and vomiting (usually in children). An asthma attack may start suddenly, and the fear and worry that this causes can prolong the attack.

Q: *What causes asthma?*

A: Asthma often occurs as an ALLERGY. Many pollens, molds, dusts (especially dust containing the house mite), and animal hair and dander can all cause asthma attacks. Asthmatic symptoms are

sometimes associated with HAY FEVER. Infection in the respiratory system is another cause of asthma.

Exposure to cold, exercise, fatigue, irritating fumes, and certain emotional and psychological states can all trigger an asthma attack. Or these conditions may serve as secondary factors that increase the severity or frequency of attacks. Asthma from these causes may occur in people who have no history of allergic reactions, as well as in those who do.

Q: *How does asthma interfere with breathing?*

A: Air passes through the lungs via tubes (called bronchi) and smaller vessels (bronchioles). With asthma, the smaller bronchi and bronchioles become swollen and clogged with mucus, and the muscles surrounding the bronchioles contract so that the air that should pass through is unable to do so. The body reacts to the lack of oxygen, and the patient forces more and more air into the lungs. But, because of the blockages, there is difficulty in exhaling it. The wheezing noise is caused by air being forcibly exhaled through the narrowed bronchi.

Q: *How long does an asthma attack last?*

A: An attack of asthma may last for a few minutes, but most go on for several hours. A severe, prolonged attack (a form of asthma known as status asthmaticus) may last for a number of hours or even days. A person with status asthmaticus requires hospitalization.

Q: *What immediate help can be given to a person suffering from asthma?*

Age of child	Advised baby aspirin dose. Consult a physician before giving a third dose.	Frequency
6 months		every 3 to 4 hours
1 year		every 3 to 4 hours
2 years		every 3 to 4 hours
3 years		every 3 to 4 hours
4 years		every 4 hours
5 years		every 4 hours

Aspirin dosage must be carefully controlled for children: 4 baby aspirins=1 adult aspirin.

Astigmatism

A: With more severe attacks, it is important that the patient sits upright, either in a chair or in bed and propped up by pillows. A table in front of the patient is useful, because this can be grasped and the arm muscles used to assist breathing. A patient is rarely hungry, but should be encouraged to drink large amounts of liquids. Antispasmodic inhalants from aerosol cans may be helpful in relaxing the muscles of the bronchioles.

Q: *How does a physician treat asthma between attacks?*

A: When the cause is an allergy, ANTIHISTAMINES are often prescribed. Other drugs that may be given, such as terbutaline (Bricanyl), can be taken in tablet form, or in an aerosol spray if an attack seems imminent. Aerosols are generally successful in preventing and treating asthma, but the consequences of overuse may prove fatal because many aerosols contain the drug isoprenaline, which has a stimulant effect on the heart.

A new inhalant drug called cromolyn sodium (Intal) has also achieved some success in preventing asthmatic attacks in some persons.

Q: *What is the treatment for severe asthma (status asthmaticus)?*

A: An attack of status asthmaticus requires urgent hospital treatment. A slow injection of adrenaline may stop the attack quicker than any other treatment.

Patients can be taught how to administer the injection themselves so that time need not be wasted waiting for a physician to administer the dose.

Q: *Apart from taking the appropriate drugs, what other precautions can be taken to prevent an asthma attack?*

A: Several simple measures can reduce the risk of attack. The appropriate medication should be taken prior to events known to trigger an episode—before exercise, for example. A person with allergic asthma should sleep in a room without carpets or rugs. Blankets and pillows of synthetic fiber reduce the risk of house dust and mites. In dry climates, a humidifier can be used to increase the moisture content of the air in the room.

For patients in whom asthma is caused by respiratory infection, breathing exercises may be of value. A physiotherapist can teach the patient the most appropriate ones. These exercises are not only a psychological help in preventing an attack, but when minor respiratory infection does occur, the lungs should function more efficiently.

Q: *Can asthma have any complications?*

A: Because so much air is held in the lungs during an asthma attack, the air cells (alveoli) can become so stretched that the cell walls may tear. This damage causes a gradual loss of elasticity in the lungs and can lead to the condition known as EMPHYSEMA. If the patient coughs too much, the surface of a lung may burst, causing the air to escape into the cavity that encloses the lung (pleural cavity). This condition is known as a pneumothorax.

Other complications can arise from the mucus secretions that do not drain properly during an asthma attack. This can lead to bronchitis and sometimes bronchial pneumonia. Frequent attacks may result in chronic bronchitis.

Q: *What other disorders might be confused with asthma?*

A: A disorder mistakenly known as cardiac asthma has symptoms similar to asthma (gasping for breath, a "tight" chest), but is actually a type of heart disease. Immediate medical attention is required.

Q: *Can asthma be cured completely?*

A: Asthma cannot be cured. The possibility of future attacks can be minimized by drugs and other preventives, but if a person is disposed to asthma, there is always a chance that an attack will occur.

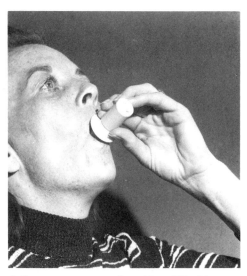

Asthma causes severe breathing difficulties: these may be relieved by means of an inhaler.

Astigmatism is a distortion in vision caused by an irregularity in the curvature of either the outer layer (cornea) of the eye, or the lens. Light rays passing through are not accurately focused on the retina at the back of the eye; the result is a blurring of vision. Astigmatism is found to a small degree in almost everyone. More serious cases can be compensated for by the use of eyeglasses.

Astringent is a substance that helps to stop the outflow of internal body fluids, especially of blood or mucus. Astringents may work in a number of ways: (1) by making the blood vessels smaller; (2) by helping the blood to coagulate; or (3) by removing the water that is essential to the formation of mucus. They are important in treating bleeding from the nose and throat, bleeding from surface wounds, and surface ulcers. The most common astringents are metallic astringents (for example, copper sulfate, silver nitrate, or calcium carbonate); epinephrine, natural and synthetic; vegetable astringents (such as witch hazel); and substances containing alcohol (for example, cologne).

Ataxia is an unsteadiness of movement when muscles fail to work together properly. Ataxia is the result of damage in the brain, especially in the cerebellum, the part of the brain that helps to control balance.

Atelectasis is either complete or partial collapse of a lung. The term refers to two distinct conditions. The first is the failure of the lungs to expand at birth, and the second is the collapsed (airless) condition of a segment of a lung. This collapse is generally caused by an obstruction in the tube (bronchus) leading to the lung, or by excessive secretion of mucus in the lung wall. Such a condition can occur in several respiratory disorders, particularly in pneumonia but also in bronchitis. Pressure from outside the lungs from a tumor or expanded blood vessel (aneurysm), for example, can also press on part of a lung and cause a collapse.

Q: What is the treatment for atelectasis?

A: If the cause of the collapse is a blocked bronchus, such an obstruction may be removed by using a special instrument called a bronchoscope. Atelectasis from other causes can often be corrected by exercises prescribed for the patient by a physiotherapist.

Q: Are there any possible complications of atelectasis?

A: If excessive amounts of mucus are the cause of the collapse, the mucus build-up can become infected.

Atheroma is a condition of the larger arteries in which areas of the arterial walls degenerate into fatty tissue. The condition is part of the blood-vessel disease ARTERIOSCLEROSIS.

Atherosclerosis. *See* ARTERIOSCLEROSIS.

Athlete's foot, or tinea (tinea pedis), is a surface infection of the foot caused by any of a number of fungi. It takes the form of small blisters between the toes. Pain and irritation accompany the infection and, if the surface of the skin breaks, bacterial infections may develop. The fungus grows on moist skin and is usually transmitted in places where many people walk barefoot, such as communal showers and swimming pools.

Q: How is athlete's foot treated?

A: Treatments are available from drugstores without prescription in the form of lotions, ointments, and powders. Finding the most suitable treatment is largely a matter of trial and error. It is important that the infected area be kept dry. Care should be taken to wipe off all moisture after bathing or swimming. If home treatment fails, or if an abscess forms, a physician should be consulted.

Q: Can similar infection occur elsewhere on the body?

A: Yes. Similar infection can appear between the legs (tinea cruris), on the face, under the arms, in the scalp, and especially in the beard area (tinea barbae).

Atopic describes a tendency to acquire allergies. Only the tendency is acquired, not any specific disorder. Hay fever, asthma, and eczema may be atopic allergies.

See also ALLERGY.

Atrium is the medical term for a cavity. It is used most often to describe each of the two blood-collecting chambers in the HEART.

Atrophy is the wasting away of tissue, of an organ, or of the entire body.

Atropine is an alkaloid drug that is extracted from several plants, including belladonna

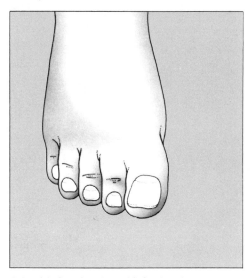

Athlete's foot is a fungal infection that can cause blisters to form between the toes.

Audiogram

(deadly nightshade). It has several applications. It is used as a stimulant for the respiratory system. Its effect of stopping the flow of secretions in the mouth makes it valuable as a preanesthetic drug when the anesthetic is to be inhaled. A weak solution of atropine is often applied to the eye to make the pupil dilate. This makes various eye examinations easier for the physician. Atropine is also used to treat involuntary muscle spasms in the intestine and bladder.

Audiogram is a chart showing the results of a hearing ability test, recorded by a delicate instrument called an audiometer. The test is based on sounds of different frequencies and loudness.

See also DEAFNESS.

Aura is an awareness of an approaching attack of a disorder such as EPILEPSY or MIGRAINE.

Auricle is a term that is used to mean two separate and small parts of the body. It can be either (1) the external projecting part of the ear (also called the pinna); or (2) one of the ear-shaped appendages projecting from each ATRIUM of the heart.

Autism is a severe psychological condition in which experience centers entirely on the self and the person displays an apparent disregard to reality. It appears most often in childhood, usually before the age of three.

Early indications of autism include a vacant stare, a lack of response to affectionate gestures and an apparent insensitivity to pain, perhaps accompanied by acts of self-mutilation. Autistic children may respond with tantrums to changes in their physical surroundings, such as a rearrangement of furniture or toys. Many autistic children are mute, and in others the development of speech is severely restricted, perhaps to a meaningless repetition of a few words.

Q: Can autism be successfully treated?

A: The underlying reason for autism is not fully known, and so treatment is concentrated on the symptoms. In all cases, treatment is long and complex.

Q: Is an autistic person mentally retarded?

A: No. Mental functions are rarely impaired by autism.

Autoimmune disease is a disorder in which the body treats its own tissues or cells as if they were infections and produces antibodies to destroy them. Autoimmunity is known to be the cause of certain types of blood disorders. It is also a suspected factor in such diseases as thyroiditis, multiple sclerosis, ulcerative colitis, and rheumatoid arthritis, although proof of this has not yet been established. In diseases definitely established as autoimmune, treatment includes drugs that suppress the production of antibodies.

Automatism is a state in which a person acts as if automatically, without conscious knowledge (or later memory) of what is happening. Although the person appears normal and functions normally, he or she does not manifest personality, and behavior may be abnormal. The condition commonly represents a hysterical trance or may follow an attack of epilepsy. Sleepwalking is also an example of automatism.

Autonomic nervous system is the part of the nervous system that controls involuntary functions in the body. These functions include gland activity; contraction of involuntary (smooth) muscles; and the action of the heart. Within the autonomic nervous system, there are two divisions: the sympathetic system and the parasympathetic system.

Q: What functions does the sympathetic system control?

A: The sympathetic system controls those activities that prepare the body for sudden activity. These include increasing the blood pressure and heart rate (sending blood to the muscles), increasing glucose production by the liver, reducing the secretion of saliva, causing the erection of hairs on the skin, and causing dilation of the pupils of the eyes.

Q: What functions does the parasympathetic system control?

A: The parasympathetic system produces effects opposite to those of the sympathetic system. It is responsible for a reduction in blood pressure and the

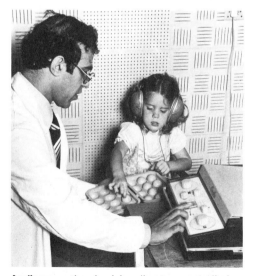

Audiogram: the physician directs a controlled tone through the girl's headphones.

slowing of the heart rate, contraction of the pupils of the eyes, copious secretion of saliva, and increased activity in the stomach and intestines. Thus, after the sympathetic system speeds up the body's responses, the parasympathetic system is the means by which the body returns to its normal calm.

Axilla is the armpit. *See* ARMPIT.

B

Babinski's reflex, or sign, is the turning upward of the big toe and the spreading out of the other toes when the sole of the foot is stroked on the outer edge. Babinski's reflex in an adult indicates damage to the nervous system, such as occurs in a stroke. But it is a perfectly normal reaction in babies under the age of six months.

A talk about Baby care

Baby care. Much of baby care is routine and is best approached in an organized way. The key to this organization is to correctly equip and arrange well the baby's room. Bathing, changing, and feeding a baby should also follow a fixed routine wherever possible. More important than routine are love and affection. Common-sense is also essential, especially concerning safety for the child. Pets should be kept out of the baby's room, as should any member of the family with an infection.

Parents should remember that general advice of the type contained in this article often refers to the average baby. No individual baby is "average" in every respect. Slight variations from the average can be discussed with a physician.

Q: How should a baby's room be organized?

A: The baby's room should be light, warm (70–75°F; 21–24°C), well aired, and close to the parent's bedroom. The crib must be stable so that it cannot easily be knocked over.

A clean sheet should cover a waterproof mattress. Light blankets should be available, but a pillow must never be used because it may smother a young baby.

A table provides an excellent surface for changing and dressing, and for the baby's bath. A nearby shelf should be cleared for diapers, plastic pants, baby powder, soap, towels, cotton balls, cotton swabs, baby oil, cream or ointment for diaper rash, spare sheets, and clean clothing. A bucket is needed for dirty diapers, and an upright chair with supporting back is needed for feeding.

Q: What routine should be followed when changing and bathing a baby?

A: Clothes and diapers should be changed on a firm, flat surface for safety reasons. A newborn baby's neck muscles are too weak to support the head, which must be held while handling the baby. After removing a diaper, gently clean the buttocks with water, soap and water, or baby oil, and rub in some cream to prevent soreness.

Before bathing the baby, test the water (with the elbow) to ensure a comfortable temperature. Always support the baby's head, while he or she enjoys the freedom of kicking in the water. Next take the baby out of the water, soap all over the body, particularly in the armpits and groin, and rinse thoroughly, Dry gently in a soft towel and powder the skin, particularly in the creases. The eyes, nose, and ears can be cleaned with cotton. Any flaking skin on the scalp can be rubbed with oil.

Q: Do the baby's hair, nails, and mouth need any special care?

A: The hair should be brushed twice daily with a soft brush; the nails are soft and can be pared back carefully using small scissors. The mouth should be cleaned with a moist, soft washcloth.

Q: What should a baby be fed?

A: A baby needs food and water. Milk pro-

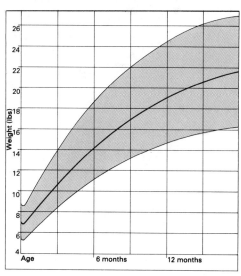

This chart shows the average weight gain of a baby, and normal maximum and minimum.

vides both, and mother's milk supplies, in addition, antibodies that help to protect against disease in the first few weeks of life. Also, mother's milk does not produce the intolerance or allergy that a few babies have to cow's milk.

If the mother is not nursing, she feeds the baby on a formula, as the physician directs.

Solid foods need not be started until the baby weighs at least 10 pounds (4½ kilos) or is 4 to 6 months old. The first solid foods recommended are cereals, e.g., rice cereal. Every 2 months a new type of food may be added. Fruits are generally recommended next. Meats and eggs are last at 9 to 10 months. First portions should be small to avoid diarrhea.

Q: *How much and how often should a baby be fed?*

A: Each day, a newborn baby requires 2½–3 ounces (70–84 grams) of milk for each pound (half-kilo) of body weight. In hot weather or during illness, there is a greater need for water (not food), and so extra water or juice should be given.

The baby should be fed every four hours for the first two weeks of life, but a rigid schedule need not be followed because the baby's hunger may vary.

Q: *How should a baby be fed?*

A: Feeding should take place in a comfortable chair. The temperature of a bottle-feeding should be tested by sprinkling a little on the back of the hand or wrist. Bottle-fed babies must have the nipple removed from the mouth from time to time to allow air to enter the bottle. Too small a hole in a nipple causes excessive swallowing of air, and a hole that is too large feeds too quickly and may produce choking.

Half-way through and after each feeding, the baby should be rested against the parent's shoulder, who should rub the child's back to produce burps, which are the sign of air escaping from the stomach.

Q: *What is the normal weight change in a baby?*

A: It is usual for a baby to lose a few ounces in the first week of life. Then an average gain of 5–7 ounces a week can be expected for the first three months, followed by a more gradual weight gain.

Q: *How much sleep does a baby need?*

A: A newborn baby requires 20–22 hours of sleep a day. He or she should be placed in the crib face down with the head turned to one side. Soft toys must not be left near the face.

Bacillus is a general term for any rod-shaped bacterium of class Schizomycetes, and for bacteria of the genus *Bacillus*. Some bacilli are harmless and found everywhere. Others cause disease, such as *Bacillus anthracis* (see ANTHRAX).

See also BACTERIA.

A talk about Backache

Backache is an extremely common complaint characterized by local or generalized pain anywhere in the spinal region from the neck to the buttocks. It may be caused by various disorders, but the most common are those associated with muscles, ligaments, bones, or nerves.

Q: *How does muscular strain cause backache?*

A: Any sudden strain on the back can cause small tears in the muscles. These tears are felt as local pain. The area is tender when touched and normal movements may be painful for several days while the tears heal.

Q: *Can pain all over the back be due to a muscular cause?*

A: Yes. Pain from generalized muscle ache (myalgia) can sometimes be caused by infection, which triggers off wide areas of muscle spasm. Generalized muscle disorders, particularly in elderly persons, usually start as backache between the shoulder blades. This may be a symptom of the old-age disorder polymyalgia rheumatica. *See* FIBROSTIS.

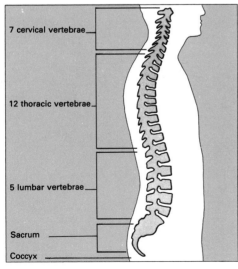

7 cervical vertebrae

12 thoracic vertebrae

5 lumbar vertebrae

Sacrum

Coccyx

Backache can be caused by disorders in any of the divisions of the spine or allied muscles.

Q: *How can backache be caused by ligament problems?*

A: Ligaments are just as susceptible to small tears as are muscles. The tears are again usually caused by unexpected strain, but the pain is more localized than muscular pain and tends to be present continuously. Slight movements can aggravate the tears and make the pain worse.

Q: *Can anything other than sudden strain cause pain in the ligaments?*

A: Yes. Prolonged strain is sometimes put on ligaments from a deformity or weakness that remains from an old fracture. A short leg or muscle weakness may also cause recurrent pain in the ligaments.

Q: *What bone disorders can cause backache?*

A: Several diseases of the vertebrae, including a SLIPPED DISK, cause backache. Old age can cause the bones to become soft (osteoporosis). When this happens the vertebrae collapse slightly, causing compression of the nerves and strain in the ligaments. Both result in backache, and the condition gradually becomes worse. The vertebrae may also collapse, with identical effects, if cancer spreads to the bones.

In OSTEOARTHRITIS, a roughening of the bone edges causes nerve irritation and backache. In young to middle-aged people, a disorder that causes vertebrae to fuse together (ANKYLOSING SPONDYLITIS) produces pain and a gradual stiffening of the back.

Q: *What nerve disorders can cause backache?*

A: A dull deep backache may begin several days before the onset of shingles. A tumor on the spinal cord sometimes causes backache. But the most common form of backache of this type is associated with the inflammation of a nerve (neuritis).

Q: *Apart from causes directly associated with the spine, what other disorders can result in backache?*

A: A low ache in the back often occurs in women before the onset of menstruation, or as part of a painful menstrual period (dysmenorrhea). Other gynecological disorders may also cause backache.

Pain from a kidney infection (such as pyelonephritis) often occurs in the lower or mid back. A dull ache high in the back may be a symptom of a chest disorder.

Q: *What is the treatment for backache?*

A: Painkilling drugs, such as aspirin or acetaminophen, may be taken to relieve the pain due to a minor strain of a muscle or ligament. For more stubborn backache, a physician may prescribe an antirheumatic drug such as phenylbutazone or indomethacin.

Treatment by physiotherapy may include exercises, massage, or local heat. Bone manipulation, sometimes carried out by an osteopath after X-ray examination, may help backache resulting from slipped disk or ligament problems. The spine may be carefully stretched using traction, but the patient has to be hospitalized for this treatment.

Q: *What everyday precautions can relieve back problems?*

A: Correct posture, a firm mattress, and strengthening of the muscles by means of careful exercise can all help to relieve some types of backache. Maintaining correct body weight (by dieting if necessary) also helps to prevent backache, because being overweight puts extra strain on the spine. (*See* DIET.)

Bacteremia (or bacteriemia) is a medical name for a type of blood poisoning. *See* BLOOD POISONING.

Bacteria are a large group of microscopic, single-celled organisms, some of which can cause diseases in humans. There are three different types of bacteria: cocci (*see* COCCUS), which are spherical; spirochetes, which are rigid, flexible, or curved coils (*see* SPIROCHETE); and bacilli (*see* BACILLUS), which are rod-shaped.

Bacterial endocarditis is inflammation of the lining of the heart valves and the heart chambers. It is caused by a bacterial infection and

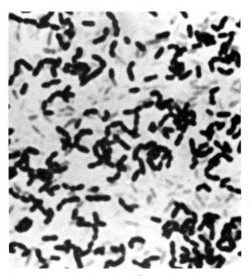

Bacteria can be identified through a microscope after they have multiplied.

Bacterial endocarditis

Bad breath

is particularly likely to occur in persons who have some sort of heart valve deformity, either from birth (congenital deformity) or from damage caused by rheumatic fever. *See* ENDOCARDITIS.

Bad breath is known medically as halitosis. There are many causes but smoking and poor oral hygiene are probably the most common. Adequate dental care and cleaning the teeth after meals should correct most cases of bad breath. If bad breath continues even after such care, a physician should be consulted.

Bagassosis is an asthmalike attack caused by inhaling the spores of a fungus that infects sugarcane. The attack comes several hours after contact, in a person who has worked with the cane for some months. Repeated attacks lead to fine scarring of the lungs and to the development of PNEUMOCONIOSIS. Apart from a change of job or environment there is no treatment.

Bag of waters is a common name for the protective fluid-filled sac that surrounds a fetus in the womb and breaks at the onset of labor. Its medical name is amniotic sac (*see* AMNION).

Balance. Body equilibrium or balance is controlled by the part of the brain called the cerebellum. Changes in body position are detected by the three semicircular canals of the inner ear; by the eyes; and by sensors in the body that send messages to the brain.

Q: What can go wrong with the sense of balance?

A: Various disorders can affect balance. Some are minor or only temporary. For example, some persons traveling by

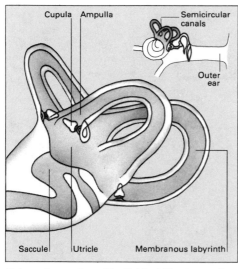

Balance is monitored by fluid within the ears' semicircular canals.

automobile, ship, or airplane experience MOTION SICKNESS. Middle ear infection, known medically as otitis media, can also upset the sense of balance by affecting the semicircular canals. Dizziness or giddiness, caused by an inadequate supply of blood and thus of oxygen to the brain, is the sensation that precedes fainting. It may be due to emotional stress, or it may be a symptom of anemia, heart disease, or a circulatory disorder. Vertigo, in which balance is so severely affected that the room seems to be spinning round, may be a symptom of MÉNIÈRE'S DISEASE or some other ear disorder.

Any person who suffers recurrent or persistent dizziness should consult a physician.

Balanitis is inflammation of the end of the penis (the glans penis), accompanied by itching and a slight discharge. It is caused by a failure to keep the glans clean. For this reason, balanitis is more common in men and boys who have not had a circumcision, particularly if they suffer from PHIMOSIS (the inability to pull back the foreskin). Prevention and treatment depend on keeping the area washed and clean. A physician should be consulted if the disorder does not clear up promptly.

Baldness is the loss of hair that occurs naturally in many men as they grow older. Baldness usually begins at the temples or the crown of the head. A tendency to go bald is inherited and the age at which it begins, and the pattern it takes, are often similar in successive generations.

Q: Do women go bald?

A: Some women experience partial hair loss as they grow older, but complete baldness in women is extremely rare.

Q: Is there any way a man can prevent himself going bald?

A: No. There is no way of preventing the onset of natural baldness. Wigs or hair transplants can disguise the condition. *See also* ALOPECIA.

Bamboo spine is a common name for the condition known medically as ANKYLOSING SPONDYLITIS.

Barber's itch is a form of folliculitis that affects a man's face. *See* FOLLICULITIS.

Barbiturates are a group of sedative and sleep-inducing drugs derived from barbituric acid. Physicians use barbiturates, injected into a vein, as anesthetics. Barbiturates are occasionally prescribed as sleeping pills or used to reduce anxiety or to treat epilepsy.

Q: Can a person become addicted to barbiturates?

BCG vaccine

A: Barbiturates are mildly addictive, and they alter the normal pattern of sleep. Because of the dangers of DRUG ADDICTION and overdosage, physicians prefer to prescribe other kinds of sleep-inducing drugs. Barbiturates should never be taken in combination with alcohol, because of the danger of possibly fatal consequences.

Barium is a metallic chemical element. The metal and its salts, particularly barium sulfate, show up clearly on X-ray photographs. A patient undergoing certain types of X-ray examinations may be asked to swallow a mixture of barium sulfate and water, called a barium meal, which is fairly tasteless unless artificially flavored. A physician can watch by X rays the progress of the barium during and after it is swallowed, as it enters and leaves the stomach, and then as it moves through the small intestine to reach the colon (large intestine). A barium enema, a barium sulfate mixture passed into the rectum and colon, shows the outline of the colon.

Q: Why might a physician ask for a barium test?

A: Barium investigations are used to help diagnose various conditions affecting the digestive tract.

Barotrauma is damage to a part of the body caused by high air pressure. It is particularly common in the middle ear when the Eustachian tube is blocked. (The Eustachian tube connects the middle ear to the back of the throat and acts as a pressure-equalizer.) The barotrauma causes pain in the ear and, in severe cases, may rupture the eardrum. A similar condition may occur in the nasal sinuses.

Bartholin's cyst is caused by a blockage of the duct of BARTHOLIN'S GLAND in the vagina. Its symptoms are a feeling of stretching and sometimes discomfort, particularly during intercourse (the condition called dyspareunia). The usual treatment is surgical removal of the gland in order to prevent repeated infections (Bartholin's abscesses).

Q: How soon after the operation can a woman resume intercourse?

A: A woman should not have intercourse for at least three weeks, and it may be a little painful for a further two months.

Bartholin's gland is one of a pair of lubricating glands at the entrance to the vagina. *See also* BARTHOLIN'S CYST.

Basal metabolic rate (BMR). The metabolic rate is a measure of the speed at which a person "burns" energy while at rest.

Measurement of BMR is seldom used now except in medical research.

Battered child syndrome, also called child abuse, is a recently recognized social problem that involves the physical mistreatment of children by their parents or guardians. It is usually discovered when a physician examines a baby or child and finds evidence of repeated injuries for which the parents make apparently reasonable excuses.

All states require that physicians report suspected cases of child abuse to the appropriate authorities.

Q: Why do some parents abuse their children?

A: The causes of the problem are not known. Most child abusers were themselves abused when they were children. The parents cannot cope emotionally with a crying, demanding child, and sometimes assault the child in an outburst of rage.

Q: What is the solution to the problem?

A: Family counseling by social workers and other experts can often reduce or eliminate the problem. They cooperate with various social and legal agencies to help the parents, who may also benefit from psychiatric therapy. In some cases, the child may have to be removed from the home, although generally this is only a temporary measure.

BCG vaccine (bacillus Calmette-Guérin) is a preparation of harmless TUBERCULOSIS vaccine which is used to give protection against the harmful, natural form of the disease. It was first used by Léon Calmette and Camille Guérin in Paris (1906). In countries where tuberculosis is still common, BCG is given in infancy. A skin test, the mantoux test, is carried out first to show whether natural immunity has been acquired.

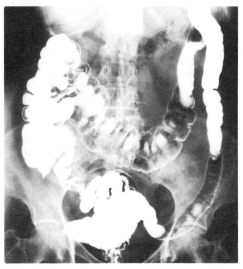

Barium is a radiopaque element the salts of which show up on X-ray photographs.

Bedbug

Bedbug (*Cimex lectularius*) is a small blood-sucking insect that can infest bedding. The insect is red-brown, oval, flat, and wingless. Its bite is painful and causes swelling, itching, and sometimes infection. It may transmit RELAPSING FEVER. A physician can prescribe a cream containing a mild antiseptic such as cetrimide for treating bites. Also, the bedroom furniture should be disinfected.

Bedsore (known medically as decubitus ulcer) occurs in bedridden patients, the elderly or chronically ill, who are unable to move themselves and who have to lie in the same position for long periods of time.

Q: *Where do bedsores form and what do they look like?*

A: The parts of the body most likely to be affected are the pressure areas: the bone at the lower end of the spine (the sacrum), the buttocks, and the heels. The shoulder blades and elbows may also develop these sores. The area first becomes slightly red with cracked skin, which turns dark blue before ulcerating as dead tissues disintegrate.

Q: *Can bedsores be prevented?*

A: Yes. Patients who cannot move themselves must be moved every few hours so that the pressure areas are changed.

Bedclothes must be kept clean, dry, and free from creases. Additional protection can be given to the pressure areas by using rubber rings, foam pads or, even better, real or artificial sheepskin.

Q: *What is the treatment if an ulcer has formed?*

A: The patient must not lie on the ulcer, and this can be awkward. The ulcer should be cleansed with an antiseptic, such as hydrogen peroxide or cetrimide. There is some evidence that zinc salt tablets, in addition to vitamins, may aid recovery. The sores will heal, over a period of time, if they are carefully tended.

A talk about Bed-wetting

Bed-wetting (known medically as nocturnal enuresis) is a common problem of childhood, sometimes causing needless distress to parents and children. A calm, reassuring approach on the part of parents is the key factor in dealing with bed-wetting. Eventually, almost all children become dry.

Q: *At what age does a child usually stop wetting the bed?*

A: As the nervous system matures, the reflexes that control the bladder come under the voluntary control of the brain even while the child is asleep. This occurs at different ages in different children, but by the age of three or four most children are dry.

Q: *What causes bed-wetting in an older child?*

A: Usually the cause of such bed-wetting is emotional. In such a situation, it is wise to consult a physician because the cause needs investigation. Some authorities state that the method by which a child is taught TOILET TRAINING is an important factor in bladder control at night.

In some cases there is a physical cause. There may be a urinary infection, or there may be a structural defect in the urinary tract, present from birth. Rarely, there may be a disorder of the nerves that serve the urinary system.

Q: *What should be done about bed-wetting?*

A: The child should never be scolded or punished. The parents should be calm, rational, and understanding in dealing with the problem.

The child should be given nothing to drink for about an hour or so before bed-time, and should empty the bladder just before going to bed. A physician may be able to help by suggesting methods that other parents have found successful.

Bee sting (for EMERGENCY treatment, *see* First Aid, p.519) can have serious consequences in people who have an allergy to the bee's venom. Desensitizing injections may increase the time between a sting and the development of an allergic reaction, thus

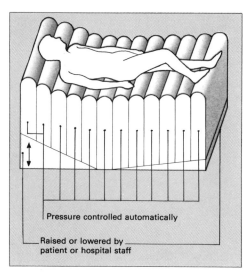

Bedsore problems in an incapacitated patient can be eliminated with a variable-pressure air bed.

Pressure controlled automatically

Raised or lowered by patient or hospital staff

allowing more time for treatment. However, most people are not seriously allergic to bee venom and experience no serious complications from occasional bee stings.

Behavior therapy is a form of psychiatric treatment in which a patient's behavior is modified by a system of rewards and punishments. This is usually used for individuals whose behavior is socially unacceptable.

Belching, sometimes called burping, is the noisy emission of gas from the stomach via the esophagus. It is common for babies to belch after a feeding, but adults also belch, especially if they have eaten too rapidly or taken carbonated drinks. Air swallowing (AEROPHAGIA) is a nervous habit that often results in belching.

Belladonna is an extract of the deadly nightshade plant. It contains ATROPINE, an alkaloid drug used in various forms to treat intestinal disorders and Parkinson's disease. It is also used in eye examinations to dilate the pupils. Side effects include a dry mouth; an overdose may cause an excited, confused mental state and may have fatal consequences.

Bell's palsy is paralysis of the muscles of the face, caused by acute malfunction of, or damage to, the nerve that supplies them.

An attack occurs without apparent cause, although Bell's palsy may be associated with SHINGLES.

Q: What are the symptoms of Bell's palsy?

A: Facial features lose their symmetrical arrangement, and the mouth droops at one corner. Paralysis of the muscles results in loss of control over saliva or tears, so that the patient may dribble or appear to cry.

Q: What is the treatment for Bell's palsy?

A: It is important that a physician is consulted within 24 hours because immediate treatment with corticosteroid drugs may help. Many patients recover spontaneously; about 70 percent recover completely within four to six weeks, and about 20 percent make a partial recovery.

Benadryl (Trademark) is the antihistamine drug diphenhydramine. It causes more drowsiness than many other antihistamines and so is sometimes used to induce sleep.

See also ANTIHISTAMINES.

Bends, also called decompression sickness or caisson disease, is a disorder caused by the formation of nitrogen bubbles in the blood after a person changes too quickly from an environment of high atmospheric pressure to one at normal pressure. Symptoms of the bends include painful joints, tightness in the chest, vomiting, giddiness, abdominal pain, and visual disturbances. Sometimes the victim suffers from convulsions and paralysis may follow. In severe cases, the condition can be fatal.

Q: How are the bends treated?

A: The victim must be returned immediately to a high-pressure atmosphere, either at the original work site or in a recompression chamber. The patient is then brought back very slowly to normal atmospheric pressure. This allows enough time for the dissolved nitrogen to be safely reconverted to its normal gaseous form and breathed out via the lungs.

Q: Can the bends cause permanent damage?

A: Damage to the joints may leave permanent arthritis. The nervous system may also be damaged, causing paralysis or signs of a stroke.

Benign describes a condition that is usually nonrecurrent and seldom causes severe problems. It is the opposite of MALIGNANT.

See also TUMOR.

Benzocaine is a surface, or topical, anesthetic. It is used to make the passage of instruments more comfortable during an examination of internal organs (endoscopy). Benzocaine is also an ingredient in some lozenges used to relieve a sore throat.

(*See* ANESTHETICS.)

Beriberi is a disease caused by a deficiency of vitamin B_1 in the diet. The disease involves nerve degeneration (peripheral neuritis) and muscle disease (myopathy), particularly affecting heart muscle. Beriberi is commonly associated with alcoholism, because many alcoholics fail to eat a properly balanced diet.

Q: What are the symptoms of beriberi?

A: There are two kinds of beriberi, called dry and wet. Dry beriberi results in the

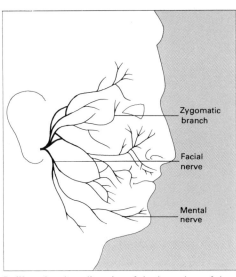

Bell's palsy is a disorder of the branches of the nerves that control the facial muscles.

Zygomatic branch

Facial nerve

Mental nerve

Biceps

loss of strength and of some feeling in the limbs due to nerve degeneration (neuritis). Wet beriberi is caused by accumulated fluid in the limbs (edema) and in the abdomen (ascites) because of heart malfunction; neuritis is commonly present as well.

Q: *How is beriberi treated?*

A: Treatment with vitamin B_1 leads to rapid improvement of heart function, and reduction of the neuritis. Care should be taken to provide the patient with a more balanced diet.

Biceps is a muscle with two heads. The biceps muscle of the upper arm (biceps brachii) is Y-shaped, the single muscle branching into two strands higher up. This muscle bends the arm at the elbow. The biceps muscle of the thigh (biceps femoris) flexes the knee.

Bile, or gall, is an alkaline liquid produced by the liver. The liquid is a dark yellow-green color, and it contains CHOLESTEROL, bile salts, a reddish pigment called bilirubin and a green pigment called biliverdin, some proteins, and urea. It passes down the common bile duct to enter the duodenum (the first part of the intestine). A branch joins the bile duct to the GALL BLADDER, in which bile can be stored until it is needed.

Q: *Why is bile needed?*

A: Bile helps to break down fats in food so that they can be absorbed, and it neutralizes the acidity of the stomach contents when they reach the duodenum. The presence of fats in the duodenum causes the release of a hormone that stimulates the contraction of the gall bladder and the production of bile.

Q: *Are there any bile disorders?*

A: The most familiar is JAUNDICE, in which a blockage of the bile ducts causes bilirubin to circulate in the blood, giving the skin a characteristic yellow color.

See also BILIARY COLIC; CHOLECYSTITIS; GALLSTONE.

Bilharziasis is another name for the parasitic disease schistosomiasis. *See* SCHISTOSOMIASIS.

Biliary colic is an extremely severe pain in the upper right-hand part of the abdomen. The pain, which comes and goes, is often accompanied by sweating and vomiting. It is the result of a spasm of the gall bladder or of obstruction of the bile ducts, either of which is caused by one or more gallstones.

Q: *What is the treatment for biliary colic?*

A: Injections of antispasmodic drugs reduce the pain, which usually ceases altogether when the gallstone passes into the duodenum or lodges at the side of the bile duct. An X ray of the biliary system is taken and the gallstone (and bladder if it is diseased) are removed by an operation.

Biopsy is the removal of a small piece of tissue for the purpose of examining it under a microscope to see whether disease is present.

There are several ways in which a biopsy can be performed: (1) through a small cut in the skin; (2) by a tube passed through the mouth into the intestine to remove a small piece of intestinal lining; (3) through an instrument such as a sigmoidoscope or cystoscope; or (4) with a special needle to reach the liver or kidney.

Biotin, also known as vitamin H, is one of the VITAMINS of the vitamin B complex. It is found in many foods, but particularly rich sources are liver, kidney, milk, egg yolks, and yeast. Biotin deficiency occurs only in association with deficiency of others of the vitamin B group.

Birth control. *See* CONTRACEPTION.

Birth defects. *See* CONGENITAL ANOMALIES.

Birthmark, or nevus, is a blemish on the skin that is present at birth. Birthmarks do not usually cause problems, although there are some abnormal marks, such as a port-wine stain, which may require treatment.

Q: *What are the main types of birthmarks?*

A: The most common birthmark is a simple skin discoloration (nevus pigmentosus), which may be any color from light yellow to black. A mole is typical of this type of birthmark. It does not need treatment, unless it is irritated by clothing or is disfiguring.

Rarer types of birthmarks are generally the result of having a cluster of blood vessels just below the surface of the skin.

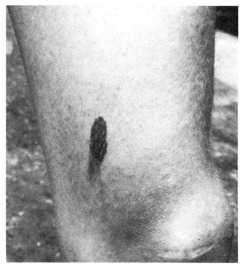

Birthmark of the common, small type needs no treatment unless it causes embarrassment.

Typical of this type is the strawberry nevus. It is a slightly raised reddish or purplish mark that appears most often on the face, head, neck, or arms. It grows rapidly for the first year after birth and then decreases in size. In most children it disappears by the age of five.

A port-wine stain is a complex, flat birthmark. It does not disappear but grows in proportion with the rest of the body. Like a strawberry nevus, it is caused by expanded blood vessels below the surface of the skin.

Q: Why should some birthmarks be removed?

A: If birthmarks of the port-wine stain type are large enough or serious enough to cause danger in case of injury, they may be removed by plastic surgery. In many cases, removal of a birthmark is not medically advised, but cosmetics can be used to reduce any embarrassment that the blemish might cause.

Bites (for EMERGENCY treatment, *see* First Aid, p.519), are punctures or other wounds on the skin caused by animals. The most common bites are those of dogs, snakes, spiders, and various insects. Most bites require only thorough cleansing with an antiseptic and dressing with a small bandage, if necessary. But some bites are serious (such as the bite of the black widow spider) and require specialized medical treatment.

See also RABIES; STING.

Black death is an old name for BUBONIC PLAGUE.

Black eye is a swollen bruise of the eyelids and eye socket. It is usually caused by direct injury, or it may be the result of a fractured skull. The dark color of the skin results from the escape of blood into the eye socket and the thin tissue surrounding it. The blood tends to drain into the eyelids, making the eye difficult to open. It may also spread down the cheek. Cold packs applied with pressure as soon as possible after the injury help the damaged blood vessels to contract, and reduce the swelling.

Blackhead, or comedo, is a plug of hardened secretion in the duct of an oil gland in the skin.

Black lung is the common name for the lung disorder anthracosis. The normal pink color of the lungs is turned black by coal dust or smoke that is inhaled. Once a common disorder only among coal miners, anthracosis is now also found in city dwellers.

Q: What are the symptoms of anthracosis?

A: In the early stages the symptoms resemble those of bronchitis, with coughing and shortness of breath. If the cause is not removed, over a period of years the symptoms gradually get worse. Diagnosis is confirmed by an X-ray examination.

Q: What is the treatment for anthracosis?

A: The lung damage caused by the inhaled dust cannot be repaired, nor can it be treated directly. Breathing clean air halts the progress of the disease and may help to reduce the severity of the symptoms.

Blackout (for EMERGENCY treatment *see* First Aid, p.579) is a temporary loss of consciousness. It is most commonly a condition of FAINTING but may also occur during an epileptic seizure, during a mild stroke, or following heavy drinking.

Bladder is a hollow body structure that collects and stores urine. It is a strong, muscular organ that receives urine from the kidneys, and releases it to be passed out of the body through a tube called the urethra.

Q: How much liquid does the bladder hold?

A: In most adults, the bladder holds a little more than one pint (475ml) of urine. This quantity may be much greater as a result of certain BLADDER DISORDERS. Between 2½ and 3 pints (1.2 and 1.4 liters) of urine are usually excreted each day.

Q: Is the bladder in a child weaker than in an adult?

A: No, but a child's bladder is smaller, and he or she often feels nervous when the bladder is full.

Bladder disorders. The following table lists some common disorders that affect the bladder, grouped according to their chief symptoms. The symptoms may also indicate other clinical disorders; this is not a complete list. A good medical history and physical

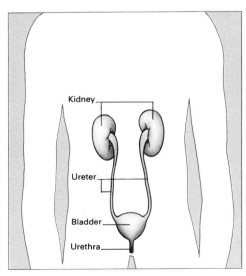

Bladder collects urine from the kidneys, before passing it out through the urethra.

Bland diet

examination by a physician are essential for adequate diagnosis. Each disorder has a separate article in the A-Z section of this book.

Symptom	Disorder
Blood in the urine	CALCULUS (a stone in the kidney, ureter, or bladder)
	CYSTITIS (bladder inflammation)
	TUMOR
Difficult urination	PROSTATE GLAND enlargement
	STROKE (nerve damage affecting bladder control)
Frequent urination	CYSTITIS (bladder inflammation)
	DIABETES (glucose in urine; thirst)
	FIBROIDS (benign tumors in the womb)
	PROSTATE GLAND enlargement
	STRESS INCONTINENCE
	STROKE (nerve damage affecting bladder control)
Painful urination	CALCULUS (a stone in the bladder)
	CYSTITIS (bladder inflammation)
	PROSTATE GLAND enlargement
	URETHRITIS (inflammation of urinary tube)

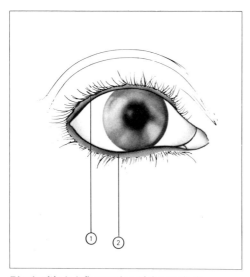

Blepharitis is inflammation of the eyelash oil glands on both rims (1, 2) of the eyelid.

Bland diet is a nonirritating diet of foods such as milk, eggs, chicken, and fish, with little or no salt or spices and minimal roughage. A physician may recommend a bland diet for a patient who is suffering or recovering from a gastrointestinal disorder.

Blastomycosis is a rare infection caused by a fungus. The infection occurs in the lungs causing a slow form of PNEUMONIA with pleurisy.

Bleeding (for EMERGENCY treatment, see First Aid, p.522) occurs from a broken blood vessel as in a cut or other wound, or from internal hemorrhaging (*see* HEMORRHAGE). Blood in mucus that is coughed up, in vomit, or in the stools could be a symptom of an internal disorder, and should be reported to a physician. *See* BLOOD, SPITTING OF; BLOOD, VOMITING OF; HEMORRHOID.

Blepharitis is a disorder affecting the eyelids. Redness and inflammation of the eyelids, soreness, and stickiness are all symptoms. If the lids are infected, a STYE (an infected swelling of a hair follicle) may appear. The cause of blepharitis is usually due to either increased oil secretion from the glands on the lid margins or from an infection of these glands. Sometimes it is a result of allergy.

Q: *What is the treatment for blepharitis?*

A: The eyelids should be cleansed regularly with a warm solution of salt water. A mild antiseptic may be applied to the rims. A physician may prescribe antibiotic or corticosteroid drugs, but continued treatment with these may cause a skin allergy.

Blindness is the loss of vision in one or both eyes. It may be present at birth, or it may occur suddenly in one or both eyes at a later stage in life. Commonly blindness involves a gradual deterioration of vision until the stage when no sight remains. It may be caused by various disorders affecting the eye itself, or may result from a disorder of the visual center of the brain. The medical term for blindness in which the eye appears to be normal is amaurosis. Temporary blindness, commonly called a blackout, can occur with some minor disorders, such as fainting.

Q: *Why are some babies born blind?*

A: Congenital blindness is sometimes caused by infection of the mother by rubella (German measles) at some time during the first three months of pregnancy. The disease causes the lenses in the baby's eyes to be opaque. Other causes of congenital blindness are defects in the formation of the eye and various metabolic disorders.

Q: *What are the causes of gradual blindness?*

A: Any of the following disorders may cause

gradual blindness: pressure within the eyeball (GLAUCOMA); the formation of opaque patches in the eye lens (CATARACT); a retina damaged as a result of high blood pressure (hypertension), diabetes, or degenerative disease of the retina; pressure on the optic nerve from a tumor (for example, pituitary gland ADENOMA); or recurrent ulcers on the cornea, which may be caused by a form of conjunctivitis (TRACHOMA) common in the tropics. Treatment of the cause usually arrests the condition and, in some cases, may restore sight.

Q: What causes sudden blindness?

A: The retina, the part of the eye onto which light rays are focused, may become detached from the layer enclosing it (the choroid), and blindness can result. DETACHED RETINA may be caused by an accidental blow to the eye, or it may occur spontaneously in people with the vision defect MYOPIA. Bleeding behind the retina or inflammation of the optic nerve (RETROBULBAR NEURITIS) may cause blindness in one eye. A blocked vein or artery supplying the eye can also result in sudden blindness.

Sudden blindness in one eye occurs much more frequently than sudden blindness in both. Blindness occurring suddenly in both eyes is usually caused by a stroke that affects the visual center of the brain.

Q: What causes temporary blindness?

A: Temporary blindness may be caused by a spasm of the arteries during a bad migraine headache, by high blood pressure (hypertension), by low blood pressure that precedes fainting, or by a small blood clot (embolus) which is passing through an artery that serves the eye.

Q: How can a blind person lead a normal life?

A: Family and friends should encourage the blind patient to make use of all available resources in making the adjustment to being blind. The patient can learn braille, and discussions with those who are already blind can help the patient to cope with fears and worry. For cases of total blindness, aids such as a white cane, seeing-eye dogs, and even special electronic machines can help to reassure a person that independence can be maintained. For those who are born blind, special schools are available for education and training.

See also AMAUROSIS; COLOR BLINDNESS; NIGHT BLINDNESS.

Blister is a raised area on the skin that contains fluid derived from blood serum. It generally forms as a result of skin irritation, from rubbing, or from pinching. Excessive heat also causes blistering. A blood blister is a purplish area beneath the skin caused by the bursting of blood vessels.

Q: What is the best treatment for blisters?

A: Normal blisters are most effectively treated by applying a mild antiseptic cream and by covering them with a clean, dry pad to prevent further rubbing. If a blister bursts, it should be kept as clean as possible with an antiseptic solution. A blood blister is best wrapped in a firm dressing with a little pressure, to prevent further bursting of blood vessels.

Blood is the body's "transportation system," the medium that carries oxygen and essential nutrients to all parts of the body. It also carries waste products, such as carbon dioxide, to the organs that eliminate them from the body.

Q: What else does blood do?

A: Heat from inner parts of the body is carried in the blood to the skin to keep the temperature of the body stable. The blood also carries defenses against infection (antibodies) to all body tissues, and transports vital chemicals and hormones that are used in the control of body functions. (*See* ANTIBODY.)

Q: How much blood does the body contain?

A: In an adult of average size there is a little less than 10 pints (4.7 liters). The heart pumps about 9 pints (4.2 liters) a minute when the body is at rest.

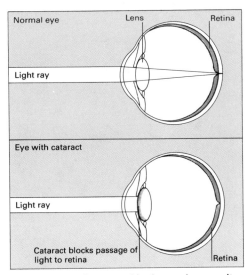

Blindness may be caused by increasing opacity of the eye lens, preventing light penetration.

Blood, spitting of

Q: *What is the composition of blood?*

A: A straw-colored fluid called PLASMA makes up more than half the volume of the blood. Plasma carries red blood cells, white blood cells, blood platelets (essential for clotting), and fat globules. Various chemicals, hormones, proteins, and some gases are also present and are carried either in suspension or dissolved in the fluid. Normal blood is about 78 percent water and 22 percent soilds.

See also BLOOD DISORDERS; BLOOD GROUPS; BLOOD PRESSURE; p.8.

Blood, spitting of (known medically as hemoptysis), is a symptom of bleeding somewhere in the respiratory tract. The blood may come from the nose, mouth, or throat (the upper respiratory passages), the lower respiratory passages, or the lungs. The seriousness of the disorder depends on the cause.

Q: *What can cause the spitting of blood from the upper respiratory passages?*

A: The most common and least serious reason for blood in the sputum (the substance spat out) is that coughing has ruptured a small blood vessel in the mouth or throat. Any infection or damage in the mouth, throat, or back of the nose may also cause bleeding.

Q: *What causes the spitting of blood from the lower respiratory passages?*

A: Bleeding from this region is caused by damage or infection in the trachea (windpipe) or the bronchi (tubes to the lungs). If a bronchus has been subjected to repeated infection, scarring causes deformity that prevents mucous secretions from draining properly, causing bleeding.

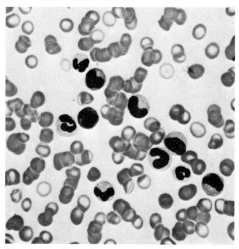

Blood contains microscopic cells of many varieties, as shown by this photomicrograph.

Damage to a bronchus from breathing in a foreign body, such as a peanut or piece of bread, also causes the spitting of blood.

Q: *What causes bleeding from the lungs?*

A: Spitting of blood derived from the lungs may be the first symptom of lung cancer. An inefficiently functioning heart may cause congestion of blood in the lungs, resulting in a bright pink froth at the mouth. Certain other disorders, for example, PNEUMOCONIOSIS, result in a fine, general scarring of the lungs and also cause the spitting of blood.

Q: *When is medical treatment necessary?*

A: A small amount of blood in the saliva should not be cause for alarm. In most cases of hemoptysis, the cause is either obvious or can be easily explained. The unexpected coughing up of blood can be serious, and if the reason is not already known, a physician should be consulted.

Blood, vomiting of (known medically as hematemesis), is a condition that can be serious. Acid in the stomach makes the color of the blood dark, often black. For this reason vomited blood is sometimes described as "coffee grounds."

Q: *What causes vomiting of blood?*

A: The most frequent, and least serious, cause is blood that has been swallowed during a nosebleed. Another common cause of vomiting blood is acute gastritis that occurs after excessive alcohol intake or following a virus infection.

Vomiting blood is more serious if it involves bleeding from a PEPTIC ULCER in the stomach or duodenum, or cancer of the stomach. The vomiting of blood is only rarely associated with hemophilia, leukemia, or other BLOOD DISORDERS.

Q: *What treatment can be given to someone who repeatedly vomits blood?*

A: The person should lie down. Cover him or her with a blanket or coat to treat for shock. Medical assistance should be called immediately.

Blood blister. *See* BLISTER.

Blood clot is a jellylike mass of congealed blood. Clotting is the normal way the body stops bleeding and begins healing following injury. It involves complex chemical reactions between many substances that are present in the blood plasma. Absence of one of these substances results in the disorder HEMOPHILIA. A clot in a blood vessel is called a thrombus.

Q: *When might a blood clot be harmful?*

A: A blood clot can block an artery or vein and stop the flow of blood (THROMBOSIS). Cerebral thrombosis is a blood clot in an artery to the brain, which can cause a stroke. Thrombosis can occur in a leg or pelvic vein (deep vein thrombosis). If this clot dislodges and enters the bloodstream, it may block an artery in the lungs (pulmonary embolus).

Q: *Are some people more susceptible to blood clots than others?*

A: Patients with ARTERIOSCLEROSIS are more likely to get blood clots because the inner walls of the blood vessels are rough. Blood clotting also occurs more easily if the circulation is slow, a condition in those with varicose veins. Other factors which increase the likelihood of blood clots are major injury to the body, the prolonged use of certain drugs such as birth control pills (*see* CONTRACEPTION), smoking, and prolonged bed rest.

Blood disorders. Disorders of the blood are generally categorized by physicians according to the nature of the complaint. There are (1) disorders of blood production; (2) disorders within the blood cells; (3) infections in the blood; and (4) disorders of the blood clotting mechanism.

The following table lists the most common disorders that are caused by blood disease or malfunction. The basic characteristic cited is not intended to denote symptoms, however, but to inform the reader who has heard the name of one of these disorders as to exactly what that condition means with respect to one of the above categories.

(Hodgkin's disease and lymphosarcoma are often considered to be blood disorders but are in fact more accurately regarded as disorders of the lymphatic system.)

Of the conditions listed below, most are serious and require immediate medical treatment. However, many characteristics cited here may also be indicative of some other clinical disorder. A good medical history and physical examination by a physician are essential for adequate diagnosis of a problem. Each disorder listed here has a separate article in the A-Z section of this book.

Disorder	Basic characteristic
ANGRANULOCYTOSIS	Reduced production of white blood cells
ANEMIA	Reduced production or loss of red blood cells
BLOOD POISONING	Infection of blood stream by bacteria
CHRISTMAS DISEASE	Defective blood clotting
HEMOPHILIA	Defective blood clotting
LEUKEMIA	Uncontrolled and disorderly increase of white blood cells
MALARIA	Parasitic infestation of red blood cells

Disorder	Basic characteristic
MONONUCLEOSIS (Glandular fever)	Excess of large white blood cells
MYELOMA	Cancer of the bone marrow
POLYCYTHEMIA	Excessive production of red blood cells
PURPURA	Bleeding under the skin
SICKLE CELL ANEMIA	Deformity of red blood cells in which the cells take on a sickle shape
THALASSEMIA	Deformity of red blood cells
THROMBOCYTOPENIA	Decreased production of blood platelets

Blood groups

Blood groups, or blood types, are classified according to the presence in the blood of particular antigens or proteins. A knowledge of a person's blood group is important when a blood transfusion is necessary, and in preventing problems with newborn children. There are various systems of blood grouping; the two most important are the ABO system and the Rhesus (Rh) system.

Q: *What is the ABO system?*

A: The ABO system distinguishes four blood groups: A, B, AB, and O. All blood can be classified in one of these groups. Group A blood contains proteins that fight against the proteins of the red blood cells from group B or group AB. If a patient of group A is given a transfusion of group B or group AB blood, a serious reaction occurs. The situation is identical for group B blood with respect to A or AB transfusions.

Q: *What is the Rh factor?*

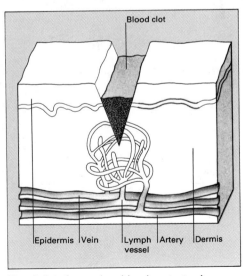

Blood clots form when blood contacts air or fluid from injured tissue.

Blood poisoning

A: The Rhesus system defines two blood types: blood in which the Rh factor is present (Rhesus positive, or Rh+), and that in which it is not (Rhesus negative, or Rh−). In Western countries, about 85 percent of people are Rh+. *See* HEMOLYTIC DISEASE OF THE NEWBORN; RH FACTOR.

The Rhesus system and the ABO bear no correlation whatsoever with each other, but for the sake of clarity the ABO and Rhesus classifications are generally combined when stating a blood group (for example, A+, O−, etc.).

Q: *Is one blood group more common than the others?*

A: Yes. Recent statistics show the following world incidence of blood groups: group O, 46%; A, 42%; B, 8%; AB 4%.

Blood poisoning (also called septicemia or bacteremia) is the presence of bacterial infection in the bloodstream. Once infection has arisen in the blood, it may increase locally or be carried with the blood to other parts of the body (*see also* TOXEMIA). Frequent, intermittent high fever, shivering attacks, and occasionally red streaks leading from a wound and a rash are all symptoms. In extreme cases, abscesses may appear throughout the body, both on the skin and in internal organs such as the liver or brain (*see* PYEMIA). Severe blood poisoning may be fatal if hospital treatment is delayed.

Blood pressure is a measure of the pressure exerted on the wall of any blood vessel, although it is generally recorded for an artery. Two measurements are taken, the highest and lowest values for pressure, which correspond to the two main stages in the pumping action of the heart.

Q: *How is blood pressure measured?*

A: Blood pressure is usually measured by an instrument called a sphygmomanometer. To measure the pressure, an inflatable cuff is placed around the patient's upper arm and a stethoscope is applied to the artery just below the cuff. By listening for changes in the sound of the pulse, a physician knows how much to inflate the cuff to stop blood flowing in the arteries in the arm. Air is slowly let out of the cuff until the blood just starts flowing again. At this stage, the sphygmomanometer records what is called the systolic blood pressure. Further air is let out of the cuff until the sounds become muffled. The instrument then indicates the diastolic pressure. The higher, systolic pressure corresponds to the contraction of the heart muscle, and the diastolic pressure corresponds to relaxation of the heart. The two pressures are expressed in the following way: 120/80.

Q: *What is considered a normal blood pressure reading?*

A: A healthy (normal) blood pressure reading varies with age, activity, and altitude, and from person to person. Bearing in mind these qualifications, values between 100/60 and 145/90 are generally considered normal.

Q: *Are there any disorders that cause blood pressure to rise?*

A: HIGH BLOOD PRESSURE, also called hypertension, is itself a major disorder that requires treatment.

There are several other serious disorders that cause blood pressure to rise well above the normal level.

Q: *What causes low blood pressure?*

A: LOW BLOOD PRESSURE (hypotension) can result from shock and some diseases. It can cause FAINTING.

Blood transfusion is the transference of blood from one person to another. A patient is usually given a transfusion using blood supplied by a blood bank, where the blood has been stored under refrigeration after collection from the donor. Usually in a transfusion, the blood is allowed to flow slowly by gravity into a vein in the patient's arm.

Q: *When is a transfusion necessary?*

A: A transfusion may be carried out because a patient is extremely anemic, either as a result of disease or from a loss of blood through bleeding. A transfusion may also be considered necessary in the treatment of acute shock.

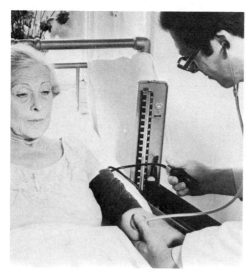

Blood pressure is measured by a piece of apparatus called a sphygmomanometer.

Q: Can a person's blood be completely replaced by a transfusion?

A: Yes. This type of transfusion (exchange transfusion) is sometimes necessary in newborn babies.

See also HEMOLYTIC DISEASE OF THE NEWBORN.

Q: What precautions are taken before transfusing blood?

A: The blood of the donor must be tested to ensure that it is not anemic, nor infected with the germs of diseases. A sample of the donor's blood is mixed (cross-matched) with a sample of the recipient's blood beforehand to make sure that the BLOOD GROUPS are compatible.

Blue baby is a baby born with a congenital heart defect that causes a bluish tinge to the skin. Because of the heart defect, some blood bypasses the lungs and thus misses the normal oxygenation process. Any complication in breathing makes the bluish tinge darker. In many cases, blue babies can be treated by surgery.

See also CONGENITAL HEART DISEASE.

Blurred vision is a common eye disorder. Frequently it is caused by farsightedness, nearsightedness, or astigmatism, all of which can be corrected by eyeglasses or contact lenses. In the elderly, the gradual onset of blurred vision can be caused by a cloudiness in the eye lens (cataract) or degeneration of the retina at the back of the eye.

Q: What can cause sudden blurred vision?

A: There are several possibilities, all of which should be considered by an ophthalmologist. Conjunctivitis is one of the most common. There are other more serious possible causes, including glaucoma, in which there is abnormally high fluid pressure inside the eyeball. Some drugs, including alcohol, may also cause the occurence of blurred vision.

Any case of persistent blurred vision should be discussed with a physician.

Body odor. See BROMHIDROSIS.

Body temperature, even in a healthy person, varies slightly during the course of the day. It is lowest early in the morning and highest later in the afternoon. The highest "normal" temperature, taken using a thermometer placed in the mouth, is generally accepted as being 98.6°F (37°C). The temperature taken in the rectum is more accurate, but tends to be about 1°F (0.5°C) higher than the mouth temperature. The least accurate temperatures are those taken in the armpit or groin.

Q: What can cause variations in normal body temperature?

A: An unexpected variation in body temperature may be a sign of illness (see FEVER; HYPOTHERMIA), or may merely reflect normal changes taking place in the body. Children have a wider range, so a physically active day may raise their temperatures a degree or so above normal without any sign of illness.

Between puberty and the menopause, women experience a rise in body temperature midway through the menstrual cycle when ovulation takes place. This higher temperature continues as the basic normal one until menstruation. Such temperature measurement can be used to time the occurrence of ovulation and improve the chances of conception in a woman who wants to have a baby.

Boils, also called furuncles, are infections of the hair roots or sweat glands caused by the STAPHYLOCOCCUS bacteria. They commonly occur in the armpit, on the back of the neck, in the groin, or on the buttocks, but can appear elsewhere. A red, painful lump forms that gradually grows bigger and then breaks down to form pus in the center. The pus normally discharges spontaneously. Sometimes a series of boils may appear.

Bone is the hard, rigid tissue that forms the body's skeleton. It supports the body and surrounds and protects its internal structures. Bone is made of tough fibers embedded with calcium-containing salts, which make up 95 percent of its substance. Usually hollow, bone acts as a storage place for calcium and the soft, blood-forming tissue called marrow.

See also BONE DISORDERS.

Bone disorders. The following table lists dis-

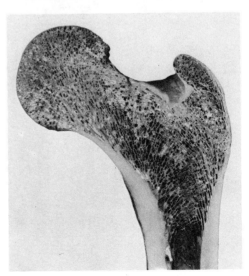

Bone is honeycombed in specific directions for maximum strength, as in the femur.

Booster shot

orders that affect bones, grouped according to cause. Each has a separate article in the A-Z section of this book.

Cause	Possible disorder
Congenital (present at birth)	ACHONDROPLASIA (dwarfism caused by lack of growth hormone)
	OSTEOGENESIS IMPERFECTA (abnormally fragile bones)
Hormone imbalance	ACHONDROPLASIA (dwarfism caused by lack of growth hormone)
Infection	OSTEITIS (inflammation of bone)
Physical damage	FRACTURE (broken bone)
	PAGET'S DISEASE OF BONE (bone deformity of unknown cause)
Tumor	OSTEOMA (nonmalignant tumor of bone)
	OSTEOSARCOMA (malignant tumor of bone)
Vitamin deficiency	OSTEOMALACIA (bone softening in adults due to lack of calcium caused by vitamin D deficiency)
	RICKETS (bone softening in children due to lack of calcium caused by vitamin D deficiency)

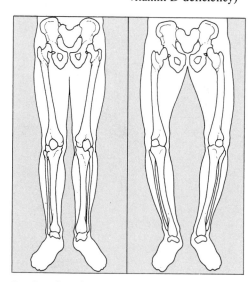

Bowlegs (right), a natural or bone condition, contrasted with normal legs (left).

Booster shot is an additional injection given some time after an initial injection to maintain a person's immunity to a disease. *See* IMMUNIZATION.

Boric acid is a white crystalline powder that was once commonly used medicinally as an antiseptic solution or as an ointment. Large doses taken orally are poisonous and so use of boric acid has been curtailed.

Bornholm disease is another name for epidemic pleurodynia.

Botulism is a rare, severe form of food poisoning. It occurs when food that contains a toxin produced by the organism *Clostridium botulinum* is eaten. Disturbances in vision and general weakness are the most common initial symptoms. Nausea, abdominal pain and diarrhea also occur. The toxin attacks the central nervous system.

Prompt medical treatment is essential, because the disease develops rapidly and has a high mortality rate.

See also FOOD POISONING.

Bowels is the popular name for the intestines. *See* INTESTINE.

Bowlegs (or genu varum) are legs that curve outward, so that when the feet are together there is a gap between the knees. Babies often have bowlegs when they begin to walk. The curvature corrects itself gradually, although sometimes over-compensation in the young child produces knock-knees (genu valgum), the inward curving of the legs at the knees.

By the age of $3\frac{1}{2}$ to 4 years, a child's legs normally become straight.

Q: Can older persons develop bowlegs?

A: Yes. Legs that become bowed later in life may be caused by softening of the bones (OSTEOMALACIA or, in children, RICKETS) or, in elderly people, by PAGET'S DISEASE OF BONE.

Brace is a support, made of metal and other materials, that is used in treating certain growth disorders. Children's teeth are commonly fitted with braces during the growing stage of the jaw to correct any developing irregularities.

Bradycardia is a slow pulse rate. As a medical disorder, bradycardia frequently follows virus illness such as influenza or infectious hepatitis. Bradycardia also occurs with the underactive thyroid disorder myxedema, and with a heart block.

Brain is the large soft mass of nervous tissue enclosed by the skull that regulates and coordinates body activities. It is the primary part of the complicated and refined central nervous system, that controls all the actions of the body, voluntary, involuntary, and reflex. The central nervous system also includes the spinal cord. The largest part of the brain, the CEREBRUM, is the center for voluntary muscular activity, for sensation, and for the highest mental functions as well as for innate instincts. The CEREBELLUM, at the back of the brain, is the center that coordinates movements. Vital functions such as breathing, blood pressure, and hunger are controlled by the HYPOTHALAMUS.

See also p.18.

Brain disorders. The following table lists some disorders that affect the brain, along with basic characteristics of each condition. Each has a separate entry in the A-Z section of this book.

Disorder	Basic characteristic
ABSCESS	Collection of pus in brain tissue
ALZHEIMER'S DISEASE	Premature aging of brain cells, appearing in the middle aged
ANOXIA	Oxygen starvation to the brain during childbirth
BLOOD CLOT	Subdural hematoma pressing on brain
CEREBRAL HEMORRHAGE	Rupture of blood vessel in brain
COMA	Prolonged unconsciousness
CONCUSSION	Temporary unconsciousness following a blow to the head
DOWN'S SYNDROME (Mongolism)	Mental retardation that also produces Mongolian-like features
ENCEPHALITIS	Inflammation of the brain by viral infection
EPILEPSY	Convulsions with or without loss of consciousness
GLIOMA	Malignant tumor of the brain
HYDROCEPHALUS	Abnormal accumulation of cerebrospinal fluid within the skull, causing possible retardation
MENINGIOMA	Malignant tumor of the brain
MENINGITIS	Inflammation of the membranes that surround the brain
MULTIPLE SCLEROSIS	Destruction of material coating the nerves; poor muscle movement and coordination
RUBELLA (in pregnancy)	Possible mental retardation of the newborn

Disorder	Basic characteristic
SPINA BIFIDA	Incomplete development of the spinal cord
STROKE	Rupture of blood vessel in brain or blockage of blood vessel to brain
SYPHILIS (final stage of infection)	Paralysis, loss of sense of position and balance
VITAMIN B DEFICIENCY	Temporary degeneration

Breakbone fever. *See* DENGUE.

Breast is the front of the chest. The same term is used, in the plural, to describe the mammary glands in women. Breast development is one of the secondary sexual characteristics that distinguish women from men. The function of breasts is to produce milk after childbirth to feed the baby. Each breast in an adult female contains 15 to 20 milk glands or lobes (surrounded by fatty tissue), each of which contains a duct (lactiferous sinus) that leads to the nipple. Breasts develop in girls at the onset of puberty in response to hormones produced by the ovaries and the pituitary gland. *See* ADOLESCENCE.

Q: *Is it normal for one breast to be slightly larger than the other?*

A: Yes. The difference is partly caused by a variation in the size of the underlying muscles that supply the shoulder. The muscles tend to be larger on the dominant side (for example, the right side of a right-handed person).

Q: *When do the breasts produce milk?*

A: Milk production is a response to special

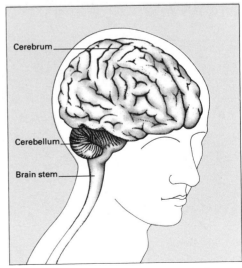

Brain is a specialized section of the spinal cord that receives and interprets sensory stimuli.

Breastbone or sternum

hormones that are produced at the end of pregnancy. The start of milk production in the breasts coincides with the birth of the baby. Early milk is a thin white fluid (colostrum) that differs in composition from normal breast milk that is secreted later. See PREGNANCY AND CHILDBIRTH.

Q: *Do males ever grow female-type breasts?*

A: Such a condition (GYNECOMASTIA) may occur in adolescent boys. A boy should be reassured that the condition will last only for three or four months. In an adult male, hormone imbalance or disease may cause female characteristics.

Q: *Is it natural for the breasts at times to feel different and change in size?*

A: Such changes accompany different stages of the menstrual cycle. Before menstruation, the breasts may feel "tight" and congested; some pain may be experienced, often accompanied by a tingling sensation in the nipples. These changes settle down as soon as the menstrual period begins.

Q: *Why do some women have bigger breasts than others?*

A: Differences in breast size and shape are largely due to inherited factors. Being overweight increases the size of the breasts with extra fatty tissue.

Breastbone or sternum, is the central, vertical bone down the center of the chest, to which most of the ribs are attached.

Breast disorders. The following table lists some disorders that can affect the female breast, and the basic characteristic of each condition. It should be noted that most lumps in the breast are benign (noncancerous) and respond rapidly to treatment. But if a woman does develop such a lump, she should consult a physician as soon as possible. (See also PALPATION.) Hormonal changes caused by the menstrual cycle or taking birth control pills may cause breast pain or tenderness. (See CONTRACEPTION.) Each disorder listed here has a separate article in the A-Z section of this book.

Disorder	Basic characteristic
ABSCESS of breast	Inflammation or rash
ADENOMA	Nonmalignant fibrous growth
CANCER of breast	Malignant tumor
CYST, sebaceous	Nonmalignant growth of fatty tissue
MASTITIS	Inflammation
PAGET'S DISEASE OF NIPPLE	Inflammation of areola and nipple

Breast examination. See PALPATION.

Breast pump is a small suction device that helps to draw milk from a nursing mother's breast. It may be made of plastic or glass and may be operated by hand or by electricity. A mother may need to use a breast pump if a distended breast causes pain, or if a baby has a cleft palate or is premature and therefore unable to suck efficiently.

Breath, bad. See BAD BREATH.

Breathalyzer is an apparatus that is used to analyze exhaled air. The best known breathalyzer is the one used by civil authorities to ascertain whether or not the alcohol content of a motorist's blood is within the legal maximum. One simple type of breathalyzer is a tube containing bichromate crystals that change color when alcohol-rich air is blown through them. A more complicated type used to measure basal metabolic rate analyzes exhaled air electronically.

Breath-holding attack occurs when a child stops breathing during a period of severe crying or in anger (see TEMPER TANTRUM). Such attacks occur most commonly in children between the ages of one and four years. An attack is preceded by a cry or wail, after which the breath may be held for as long as 20 to 30 seconds. The child may turn blue in the face and fall to the ground as if unconscious, making occasional convulsive movements. After recovery, the child may be confused for a further 10 to 15 seconds.

Q: *Is a breath-holding attack serious?*

A: Although these attacks are frightening to witness, they are not serious.

Breathing. See RESPIRATION.

Breathing disorders. See LUNG DISORDERS.

Breathlessness, known medically as dyspnea, is a normal reaction to greater than usual exertion, such as vigorous physical excercise.

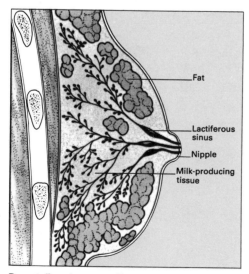

Breast disorders can affect any part of the milk-producing tissue and related breast structures.

Fat

Lactiferous sinus

Nipple

Milk-producing tissue

The normal result of physical exercise is an increase in the amount of carbon dioxide in the blood. Breathing rate automatically increases to get rid of the carbon dioxide through the lungs.

A wide range of lung disorders can be responsible for breathlessness, such as asthma, or pneumonia.

Persons with heart disorders often have difficulty with breathing. A moderate degree of anemia also causes shortness of breath after exercise.

Breech birth is the delivery of a baby buttocks or feet first, rather than head first. *See* PREGNANCY AND CHILDBIRTH.

Brodie's abscess is an area of bone infection filled with pus, usually found in one of the long bones of the arm or the leg. *See* OSTEOMYELITIS.

Bromhidrosis is the medical name for body odor. An offensive smell is caused by the breaking down of stale sweat by bacteria on the skin. Sweat, especially in the armpits and groins, mixes with dead skin cells and decomposes. The odor produced varies from one person to another and depends also on the diet. Treatment is a daily bath or shower and a change of underwear, plus the use of an ANTIPERSPIRANT or DEODORANT.

Bronchial dilators are drugs that widen the airways to the lungs. They enlarge the bronchi and so improve the breathing of patients with bronchial asthma and other chronic chest disorders such as emphysema and bronchitis. Depending on the specific preparation, bronchial dilators may also increase the blood pressure and heart rate and stimulate the respiratory center in the brain. And they may also cause anxiety and muscle tremors.

Bronchial pneumonia, also called bronchopneumonia, is a contagious infection of the lungs. This type of PNEUMONIA is localized mainly in the smaller branches of the bronchial tubes, called the bronchioles.

Bronchial pneumonia can be caused by the pneumoccocus or certain other bacteria or by viruses. The bronchioles become inflamed as they clog with pus and mucus, resulting in one or more of the following symptoms: coughing, chest pains, fever, blood-streaked sputum, chills, and difficulty in breathing.

Treatment is with antibiotic drugs and bed rest. Hospitalization for diagnostic tests may be necessary for some patients.

Bronchiectasis is a chronic disorder of the bronchi and bronchioles, the tubes that carry air in and out of the lungs. The tubes become weakened and stretched, and do not allow normal drainage of fluid secretions from the lungs. This inelasticity of the bronchi may result from an infection, following collapse of the lung (atelectasis), or be an abnormality present at birth.

Q: *What are the symptoms of bronchiectasis?*

A: Bronchiectasis may show few symptoms. Sometimes the patient has a cough with thick phlegm, which occasionally contains blood. There may be a slight fever and a general feeling of being unwell.

Q: *How is bronchiectasis treated?*

A: A physician may prescribe antibiotic drugs at the beginning of any respiratory infection for a patient with a history of bronchiectasis. It is important also to drain the secretions from the lung, and for this reason the patient is taught correct breathing and how to use POSTURAL DRAINAGE. If repeated infections still occur, the physician may recommend a LOBECTOMY, an operation to remove the diseased area.

Bronchiole is any of the many narrow branches of the bronchi, the tubes that carry air to and from the lungs. *See* p.10.

A talk about Bronchitis

Bronchitis is inflammation of the bronchi, the air passages to the lungs. It may be either acute or chronic. Bronchitis often follows a common cold or any infection of the nose and throat.

Q: *What are the symptoms of acute bronchitis?*

A: There is a slight fever, 100 to 102°F (37.8 to 38.9°C), with an irritating, dry, painful

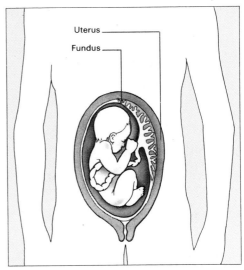

Breech birth occurs when the baby's head stabilizes in the fundus of the uterus.

107

cough that starts to produce thick, yellow sputum after two or three days. At this stage the fever often recedes and the pain from coughing diminishes. Even after the condition improves, a slight cough commonly remains for another week or two.

Q: *What is the treatment for acute bronchitis?*
A: The patient needs bed rest in a warm, humid room with frequent steam inhalations from a vaporizer to soften the infected mucus in the bronchi. Hot drinks should be given; they help the patient cough up and spit out phlegm, and prevent dehydration. Any sedative cough medicine may be taken at night to help the patient sleep. A cough syrup without a sedative may help during the day.

If the condition appears to worsen and the fever increases, a physician should be consulted. An antibiotic may be needed to combat the infection.

Q: *How soon after an attack of acute bronchitis may a person return to work?*
A: All crowded places should be avoided for at least ten days to allow the mucosal lining of the bronchi to heal before taking the increased risk of encountering new infection.

Q: *What causes chronic bronchitis?*
A: Chronic bronchitis is caused by repeated attacks of acute bronchitis. It is aggravated by smoking and by harmful environmental conditions, such as air polluted by chemicals, smoke, and dust.

Q: *What are the symptoms of chronic bronchitis?*
A: The major symptom is a cough which is usually worse in the mornings, when the bronchi have not drained overnight. The patient produces clear, mucus sputum. The sputum becomes thicker and yellow if any additional infection occurs.

The constant, vigorous coughing may break the fine tissues of the lungs and produce a condition called EMPHYSEMA. A patient with emphysema tires quickly and becomes breathless after exercise. HEART FAILURE may occur.

Asthma, obesity, and smoking all complicate and worsen chronic bronchitis. When these conditions are treated as well, the bronchitis usually also improves.

Q: *Can chronic bronchitis be treated?*
A: A close watch is kept on any colds or respiratory infections. The physician usually prescribes antibiotics at the first sign of a bronchitic attack to prevent the possibility of secondary bacterial infection and further damage to the bronchi and lungs. Breathing exercises, and sometimes

POSTURAL DRAINAGE, can help to keep the bronchi clear. The physician will also recommend stopping smoking and, if possible, a change of working conditions.

Bronchogram is an X-ray picture that shows the structure of the lungs. It is taken after a dye (which is opaque to X rays) has been introduced onto the lining of the windpipe (trachea), from where it spreads downward to the lungs.

Bronchopneumonia is also called bronchial pneumonia.
See BRONCHIAL PNEUMONIA.

Bronchoscope is a long thin tube, containing a light, used for examining the windpipe (trachea) and main breathing tubes (bronchi). It can also be used for removing objects that have been accidentally inhaled (such as peanuts) or for clearing mucus from the bronchi.
See also FIBERSCOPE.

Bronchus is either of the two tubes that carry air in and out of the lungs. The bronchi branch from the lower end of the windpipe (trachea), one going to each lung. They are kept permanently open by rings of cartilage and are lined with special hairlike cells that sweep dust and mucus upward toward the throat. The bronchi themselves divide further into narrower branches and finally into the extremely narrow bronchioles.

Brucellosis is an infectious disease, principally of catttle, goats, and pigs, but also occasionally of humans. It is caused by bacteria of the genus *Brucella*, which are found in the milk of infected animals. Human beings contract the disease by consuming infected milk or meat, especially from cattle or by handling diseased animals. In humans, brucellosis is more commonly known as undulant fever or Malta fever.

Bruise is a visible, purplish mark beneath the surface of the skin, caused by the escape of blood from small blood vessels. Most bruises result from a blow or pressure, but sometimes a bruise occurs spontaneously in elderly people. The color of the bruise fades away gradually, becoming purplish blue, brownish, and then yellow, before disappearing.

Bruises may be slightly painful, but they are not usually serious. But a bruise that appears with no apparent cause may be a sign of a disorder such as HEMOPHILIA.

Bubo is a swollen lymph node (a junction of the vessels of the lymphatic system), often containing pus. Buboes most commonly occur in the groin or armpit. They can accompany infectious disease (for example, bubonic plague), and often develop in conjunction with VENERAL DISEASES.

Bubonic plague is a form of PLAGUE in which the lymph nodes become painful, tender, and swollen, forming buboes. Early symptoms are a high fever, restlessness, and mental confusion, which lead to coma and death unless promptly treated.

See BUBO.

Budd-Chiari syndrome is a blockage in the veins that carry blood from the liver, caused by clotting (thrombosis) or the presence of cancer cells. The condition greatly enlarges the liver, which becomes tender, and causes a build-up of fluid in the abdominal cavity (ascites).

Buerger's disease (known medically as thromboangiitis obliterans) is a rare condition of inflammation of the arteries and veins of the arms and legs. It is commoner in men, especially those who smoke. The symptoms vary in intensity. Commonly the disease produces tender, swollen areas over the inflamed veins and then coldness of the feet and hands. Pain occurs in the calves on walking (intermittent CLAUDICATION), due to arterial blockage. The poor circulation may result in GANGRENE.

Q: What is the treatment for Buerger's disease?

A: The patient, if a smoker, stops smoking; this often produces an immediate improvement. A physician may prescribe drugs that dilate the blood vessels.

Bulbar paralysis is paralysis of the muscles of the tongue, lips, palate, and throat. The cause is generally an acute infection that interferes with the coordinating centers in the brain. The patient has difficulty in swallowing and speaking and may inhale saliva and food.

Bulimia is a form of mental illness characterized by an extreme increase in appetite. The victims will typically gorge on food and then purge themselves with laxatives or induce vomiting. Some researchers believe the disorder may develop through excessive parental pressure and standards. But, it also been found that some bulimics display brain chemistry characteristic of certain forms of depression.

Bulimia victims often develop hernias, ulcers, a dependence on laxatives, and loose tooth enamel from the acid in vomit. The violent purging may also upset the body's balance of electrolytes, which can lead to serious cardiac abnormalities.

Q: Can bulimia be detected in its early stages?

A: Usually not. The bulimic typically hides the overeating and purging pattern of the disorder.

Q: How is bulimia treated?

A: Bulimia is usually treated psychiatrically on an outpatient basis. Good results have also been reported from antidepressant drug therapy.

Bulla is a medical term that may describe one of three things: (1) a large fluid-filled VESICLE; (2) a blister; or (3) a space within an organ, such as a lung.

Bunion is the swollen, inflamed condition of the saclike structure (BURSA) adjacent to the joint of the big toe. It causes a thickening of the toe and usually turns it in toward the other toes of the foot (hallux valgus). Loose shoes should be worn and special pads used to protect the bunion from irritation. Bunions may be removed surgically.

See also First Aid, p.585.

Burn (for EMERGENCY treatment *see* First Aid, p.530) is an area of tissue damage caused by heat (including friction and electricity) or cold, by a caustic chemical, or by radiation. Burns are classified according to the depth of the tissue damage.

First-degree burns produce a redness of the skin, and they heal without scarring.

Second-degree burns cause the destruction of deeper structures within the skin, resulting in blistering.

Third-degree burns destroy the full thickness of the skin, leaving an open area; sometimes the deeper tissues (fat or muscle) are also destroyed.

First- and second-degree burns tend to be more painful than third-degree burns, because the nerve endings are damaged but not completely destroyed. Extensive third-degree burns are a life-threatening emer-

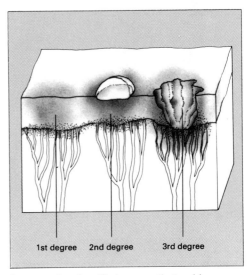

1st degree   2nd degree   3rd degree

Burn can be classified as one that reddens skin (left), blisters skin (center), or destroys it.

Bursa

gency. Large areas of burnt skin cause the loss of body fluid into the surrounding tissues, which can lead to dehydration and the rapid onset of shock, particularly in children. For this reason, intravenous transfusions may be necessary as well as local treatment and painkilling drugs. Second- and third-degree burns often require a skin graft.

Bursa is a small sac-like structure, found mainly in joints, that protects bones and the tissues of muscles and organs where friction may occur (for example, in the elbows and knees). Bursae are filled with a thick compressible fluid.

Bursitis is inflammation of a BURSA. In most cases the cause is unknown, but it can be caused by such factors as injury, infection, and repeated friction. It is treated by rest, use of, heat, anti-inflammatory drugs, and sometimes an injection of a corticosteroid drug.

Byssinosis, also called Cotton workers' disease, or Monday fever, is an allergic reaction to cotton dust. The symptoms are coughing, breathlessness, and constriction in the chest. Symptoms initially occur only on the first working day of each week (hence "Monday fever"). Later, symptoms occur throughout the week, and eventually there is lung scarring and PNEUMOCONIOSIS.

C

Cadmium is a metallic element. Both the metal and its compounds are poisonous. They are widely used in industry, for example, in batteries, electroplating, welding, and also ceramics. If cadmium salts are swallowed, violent diarrhea and vomiting result. More serious poisoning results from prolonged breathing of cadmium oxide fumes. This may cause a cough, pains in the chest, and general weakness. Emphysema may result, causing further difficulty in breathing; it may be fatal if not treated swiftly.

Caesarean section. *See* CESAREAN SECTION.

Caffeine is a stimulant alkaloid drug, present in coffee, tea, and some carbonated drinks. Caffeine increases the pulse rate and stimulates the production of urine from the kidneys. A large cup of strong, freshly ground coffee contains about 100 milligrams of caffeine. Excessive intake of coffee, and therefore of caffeine, may lead to insomnia, a rapid or variable pulse rate, and a feeling of anxiety and apprehension. A sharp reduction in caffeine intake may on the other hand produce acute withdrawal symptoms, such as headache, sweating, tremor, and an inability to concentrate.

Caisson disease. *See* BENDS.

Calamine lotion is a liquid preparation containing zinc oxide. It has a soothing effect when applied to inflamed or irritated skin.

Calcaneus. *See* HEEL.

Calciferol is vitamin D prepared chemically from ergosterol, a substance found in plants and animal tissues. It is used for treating disorders associated with low calcium levels in the body, such as RICKETS.

Calcification is the depositing of calcium salts in body tissues. It occurs normally in bone, especially after a fracture. The temporary build-up of calcium-containing tissue at the site of a bone fracture is called a CALLUS. Calcium compounds may also be deposited in other tissues after injury or infection, causing complications. Torn ligaments surrounding the hips and shoulders are areas most likely to be affected, as also are healed tuberculous areas in the lungs. An excessive intake of vitamin D in certain people, especially children, may cause the deposit of calcium salts in kidney tissue (nephrocalcinosis). This is a serious condition that can lead to kidney failure.

Calcium is a metallic element whose compounds occur in the body and are essential for good health. Ninety-nine percent of body calcium is in the form of calcium phosphate, the chief mineral component of bones and teeth. Calcium is also present in the blood and is needed for the correct functioning of muscles and nerves. Lack of sufficient calcium in the body can lead to bone disorders such as RICKETS.

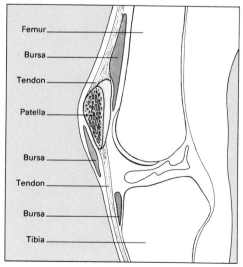

Femur

Bursa

Tendon

Patella

Bursa

Tendon

Bursa

Tibia

Bursa is a fluid filled sac that reduces friction between surfaces that rub against one another.

Children need between 0.36 and 0.54 grams of calcium daily; adults need 0.8 to 1.2 grams. Pregnant women and nursing mothers should increase their calcium intake by about half as much again. The calcium is supplied in the diet and its absorption controlled by vitamin D. Foods rich in calcium include yogurt, milk, cheese, and other dairy products.

Calculus is a stonelike mass that may form in ducts or hollow organs of the body, especially the gall bladder, kidneys, and ureters.

Calculi are composed mainly of crystalline substances: certain salts, cholesterol, and some protein. Because of their hardness, calculi can obstruct a duct or an organ, resulting in inflammation through infection.

Q: Why do calculi form?

A: Calculi formation may be due to a combination of factors, rather than to any one factor. Among such factors are local infection, high levels of calcium or other salts in the blood, and some conditions that cause a reduction in the flow of bodily fluids.

Q: What symptoms might indicate that calculi have formed?

A: Symptoms depend upon the part of the body involved. For example, calculi in the gall bladder (*see* GALLSTONES) may cause no symptoms, or may cause vomiting, jaundice, and severe pain (*see* COLIC) if they lodge in and obstruct the bile duct. The only way to determine if calculi have formed is to conduct tests, including X rays, on parts of the body suspected to be involved (*see* CYSTOSCOPY).

Q: How are calculi treated?

A: Treatment depends upon the site of the calculi and on the severity of the symptoms. For most cases, however, surgical removal of calculi is necessary (*see* LITHOTOMY).

Caldwell-Luc operation is an operation to relieve chronic SINUSITIS by improving the drainage of the maxillary sinus, one of the cavities behind the nose. To improve drainage, a new opening is made through the upper jaw above one of the second molar teeth. This allows drainage of fluid from the sinus into the mouth. Once the sinus has drained, the opening is allowed to heal.

Callus is an area of skin that has become thickened and coarsened as a result of constant rubbing or pressure. The term callus also describes the temporary bonelike tissue that forms between the broken ends of a bone fracture as a normal part of the healing process (*see* CALCIFICATION).

Calorie is a unit of heat energy. In dietetics and medicine, calories are a measure of the energy content of foods. Some foods yield more calories than others when eaten and digested. Individual calorie requirements depend on a person's age, sex, build, and occupation. If a person takes in more calories than he or she needs, a weight gain results.

A talk about Cancer

Cancer is a condition in which certain body cells multiply without any apparent control and destroy healthy tissue and organs.

There are about 100 different types of cancer that affect human beings. The most common forms are breast cancer, skin cancer, lung cancer, and cancer of such digestive organs as the stomach and colon. But cancer can attack virtually any part of the body, including the organs that form blood.

Cancers are grouped into two main scientific classifications: carcinoma, or cancer of the epithelial tissue that forms skin and the linings of internal organs, and sarcoma, or cancer of connective tissue, such as cartilage and bone. Cancer of bone marrow and other blood-forming organs results in the production of cancerous white blood cells, the condition called leukemia. Cancer of lymph glands and other lymphoid tissue is called malignant lymphoma. Both leukemia and lymphoma are often classed as sarcomas, because blood and lymph are forms of connective tissue.

Q: How does cancer develop?

A: In a healthy human, new body cells are produced to enable growth and to replace cells that die through wear and tear. The

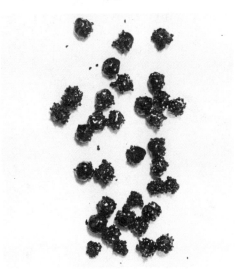

Calculus is a "stone" that forms in hollow organs: these are gallstones.

111

Cancer

new cells are formed when existing cells divide. Normally, the body cells divide at a controlled rate, producing just enough new cells to replace those that die. But cancer cells divide at an uncontrolled rate, forming a cluster of cells called a tumor. Benign tumors do not spread to other parts of the body; malignant (cancerous) ones do.

The spread of cancer (metastasis) occurs when some cancer cells break away from the tumor and travel through the lymphatic system or the bloodstream. These cancer cells may then lodge in other organs or tissues and cause new tumors to form. Once cancer has metastasized, it is very difficult to treat.

Cancer can also spread by invading tissues that surround the tumor. Once formed, cancerous tumors continue to grow.

Q: *What are the symptoms of cancer?*
A: Cancer has no symptoms in its early stages. But symptoms may appear before the cancer begins to spread. The sooner cancer is detected, the better is the chance of a successful treatment. The American Cancer Society lists seven warning signals that may indicate that the disease is developing:
(1) Any changes in bowel or bladder habits. These might indicate cancer of the colon, bladder, or prostate.
(2) A sore that does not heal. This could be a warning that mouth or skin cancer is developing.
(3) Unusual bleeding or discharge. Blood

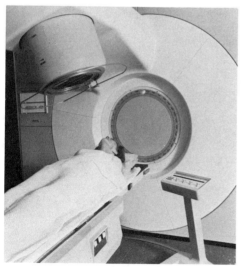

Cancer can be treated with a linear accelerator that disrupts the tumor without damaging skin.

in the urine may be a symptom of bladder or kidney cancer; blood or mucus in the stools may indicate bowel cancer. Any unusual vaginal discharge or bleeding might be a sign of cancer of the reproductive organs.
(4) Thickening or lump in the breast or elsewhere in the body.
(5) Persistent indigestion or difficulty in swallowing. These may warn of stomach cancer or cancer of the esophagus or throat.
(6) Obvious change in a wart or mole. Any sudden change in its size, shape, or color could signal skin cancer.
(7) Nagging cough or chronic hoarseness. A persistent cough, especially if there is spitting of blood and a loss of weight, may be a sign of lung cancer.

Anyone experiencing any of these symptoms should consult a physician promptly. They do not definitely indicate cancer, they are warnings of a possible danger. Only a physician can diagnose cancer.

Q: *How is cancer treated?*
A: Surgery, radiation (radiotherapy), and drugs (chemotherapy) are the most common weapons used to fight cancer. But treatment varies, depending on the nature of the cancer. Surgery is used to remove most tumors, and usually the surrounding tissue, particularly for cancers of the breast, colon, lung, stomach, and womb. Some brain tumors can also be removed surgically. In addition, the patient may receive radiotherapy or chemotherapy before and after the operation.

Some forms of cancer, such as those involving the bladder, cervix, skin, and areas of the head and neck, can be treated with radiotherapy alone. The diseased body part is exposed to radiation from X rays or radioactive substances, such as cobalt 60. Radiation kills normal cells as well as cancerous ones, so care must be taken to administer radiation doses that do not endanger life.

Powerful anticancer drugs are particularly effective against leukemia and lymphoma, but chemotherapy is also used against a variety of cancers. Like radiation, the drugs also kill normal cells and have side effects ranging from nausea to high blood pressure.

Researchers are looking for drugs that will be less harmful to healthy cells. They are also investigating a natural body substance called interferon, which cells produce to protect themselves when a virus invades the body.

Q: What is a cancer patient's chance of survival?

A: The sooner cancer is diagnosed and treated, the better are the chances of survival. Except for malignant pigment-cell tumors (melanomas), skin cancer is the easiest to treat, because it grows slowly and does not spread quickly to other parts of the body; 95 percent of the patients recover. Lung cancer, because it is difficult to detect before it begins to spread, has a high death rate; only 11 percent of the patients recover.

If a patient remains free of cancer for five years after the end of treatment, it is likely that he or she is permanently cured. The five-year survival rate of breast or cervical cancer patients is 71% and 65%; of uterine cancer, 86%; of colon and rectum cancers, 47%; of prostate cancer, 63%.

There are several forms of leukemia and lymphoma, and survival rates vary. But chances of surviving leukemia have increased greatly since the 1970's. Patients with Hodgkin's disease, the most common form of lymphoma, have a survival rate of 68 percent.

Q: Are there any known causes of cancer?

A: Scientists have not found one single cause of cancer in humans, but they know that certain cancer-causing agents (carcinogens) increase the probability of cancer. Carcinogens damage body cells and can eventually cause at least one cell to become cancerous.

Industrial chemicals, such as arsenic, asbestos, and some products of coal and oil, can create hazards for workers. Chemical carcinogens polluting air or drinking water can increase cancer risks for entire communities. Carcinogens have also been found in drugs and food supplies. They include chemicals used in food processing or agriculture. Some natural substances, such as molds that grow on corn and peanut crops, are also suspected carcinogens. Diets that are high in fats may play a role in colon cancer. But the most common chemical carcinogen is the tar found in tobacco smoke.

Overexposure to the ultraviolet rays in sunlight can cause skin cancer, particularly in people with fair, sensitive skin. Large doses of X rays are also a cancer hazard, as are radioactive substances.

Q: Can cancer be inherited?

A: There is an inherited tendency for a few cancers, such as a rare eye cancer that occurs in children under three years of age. Also, cancer of the breast and colon occurs among members of the same family at a higher than average rate.

Q: Does the body have any natural defenses against cancer?

A: Yes. The immune system that protects against invading bacteria and viruses also fights against cancer cells. That is probably why many people never develop the disease. On the other hand, some people may have a weak immune response to cancer cells, and therefore the disease is able to develop.

Q: Can cancer be prevented?

A: Avoiding known cancer-causing agents, such as tobacco smoke, can certainly reduce the risk. But should cancer develop, early detection and treatment is vital. Therefore, regular medical checkups and alertness to the seven warning signs are the best defense against cancer.

See also CERVICAL SMEAR; LEUKEMIA; ONCOLOGY; PALPATION; RODENT ULCER.

Candida is a genus of yeastlike fungi. The species *Candida albicans* is the main infective agent in MONILIASIS (thrush).

Canine describes the four pointed teeth, of which the upper two are known also as the eyeteeth. *See* TEETH.

Canker sore, known medically as aphthous ulcer, is a small and painful whitish ulcer, usually in the mouth or on the lips. It is probably caused by a virus that normally lives in the body cells without causing symptoms.

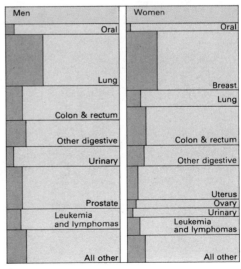

Cancer: colored bands show frequency (height) and death rates (width) of types of cancer.

Cannabis

But in the presence of a disorder, such as a common cold, or even during menstruation, ulcers form.

Various brands of throat drops or ointment stop the pain and help mouth ulcers to heal. Or a physician may prescribe tablets that can be sucked to produce rapid healing.

Cannabis is another name for marijuana. *See* MARIJUANA.

Capillary is the smallest type of blood vessel in the vascular system. Capillaries connect the smallest arteries with the smallest veins, and are so narrow that only one blood cell can pass along them at a time. The function of capillaries is to carry oxygen-containing blood to the tissues, to pass food substances to tissue cells, and to carry away waste products such as carbon dioxide. *See* p.8.

Capsulitis is inflammation of any membrane that encloses an organ. There are various forms of the disorder, but the most common affects the membranes of large joints, especially the hip and shoulder. The inflammation causes stiffness and pain when the joint is moved.

An affected joint should be rested, and a physician may recommend painkilling drugs (analgesics) and antirheumatic drugs for the first few days. If capsulitis takes a long time to improve, the physician may prescribe corticosteroid drugs, physiotherapy, or shortwave diathermy.

Carbohydrate is an organic substance that is an energy-producing constituent of many foods. Carbohydrates are rich in calories—one gram contains 4 calories. The principle carbohydrates are sugars and starch. Common foods containing them include potatoes, bakery products (such as bread), and cane or beet sugar. During the digestion of such foods, the carbohydrates are broken down into the energy-producing sugar glucose (with water and carbon dioxide as waste products).

See also pp. 12–13.

Carbolic acid, also known as phenol, is one of the oldest antiseptics. It was responsible for an important advance in sterile techniques in medicine during the nineteenth century.

Carbon dioxide is a gas that occurs in the atmosphere (0.035 percent by volume) and is produced in body tissues as a waste product of energy-generating processes. Dissolved in the blood, carbon dioxide is carried to the lungs, and from there it is breathed out as a gas. Some carbon dioxide also leaves the body in urine and in perspiration. If the level of carbon dioxide in the blood rises above normal, the brain automatically stimulates the lungs into working faster. The increase in breathing rate is necessary to rid the body of the extra carbon dioxide but it may be harmful in other ways (*see* ACIDOSIS). Solid carbon dioxide (dry ice) is used medically in simple CRYOSURGERY to destroy warts.

Carbon monoxide is a poisonous, inflammable gas that is colorless and, when pure, odorless. It is present in the exhaust fumes from all internal combustion engines, in the gas produced from burning coke, and in sewers. Carbon monoxide is dangerous if inhaled because it is easily absorbed by hemoglobin in the blood, in preference to oxygen, preventing the blood from carrying oxygen. This results in ASPHYXIATION, which can cause death or, if the victim recovers, brain damage.

Q: What are the symptoms of carbon monoxide poisoning?

A: Symptoms vary greatly, but the victim normally has a pink or blotchy face and chest, and complains of dizziness, nausea, faintness, ringing in the ears, and throbbing temples. The pupils of the eyes become dilated, and the victim may lose consciousness.

Q: What action should be taken for carbon monoxide poisoning?

A: Remove the victim as quickly as possible from the source of the fumes. Fresh air and artificial respiration aid the recovery of the victim, but an oxygen mask is the best treatment. For EMERGENCY treatment, *see* First Aid, p.566.

Carbon tetrachloride is a clear, colorless liquid with anesthetic and sleep-inducing (narcotic) properties. In these respects carbon tetrachloride resembles chloroform, but it is too poisonous to be used as an anesthetic. The most com-

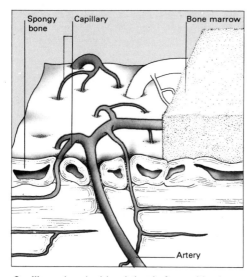

Capillary absorbs blood that is formed in the bone marrow and conveys it to the arteries.

mon uses of carbon tetrachloride today are in the chemical industry.

Q: *What are the poisonous effects of carbon tetrachloride?*

A: Small doses taken orally may cause giddiness, headache, and vomiting, and symptoms of severe kidney and liver damage may occur within weeks. The toxic effects are made worse if carbon tetrachloride is inhaled.

Carbuncle is an inflamed bacterial infection of the skin. It is similar to a BOIL, except that a carbuncle tends to spread locally, sometimes forming clusters with several openings that discharge pus. Carbuncles occur most commonly on the back of the neck, buttocks, and thighs. The infection is usually treated with antibiotics, taken under medical supervision, but sometimes a physician has to make an incision to drain a carbuncle.

Carcinogen is any substance that is known to cause cancer, for example, tobacco tar or asbestos. *See also* CANCER.

Carcinoma is a type of cancer that forms in the epithelial tissue, which covers the inside and outside of various organs, most commonly on the skin and the intestine. *See* CANCER.

Cardiac describes anything pertaining to the HEART.

Cardiac arrest is the sudden stoppage of the heart. *See* HEART STOPPAGE.

Cardiac massage is the manipulation of the heart to restore and maintain the heartbeat. *See* First Aid, p.562; HEART STOPPAGE.

Cardiac murmur. *See* HEART MURMUR.

Cardiac pacemaker is a group of cells in the right ATRIUM of the heart that naturally generates and regulates the impulses that make the heart beat. Artificial devices that can regulate heartbeat disorders are discussed in the article HEART PACEMAKER.

Cardiogram is a graph that records the electrical activity of the heart muscle.

Cardiology is the medical specialty that involves the study of the heart, its functions, and its disorders. *See also* HEART; HEART DISEASE.

Cardiomyopathy is a general term for disorders of the heart muscle that commonly cause palpitations and an irregular pulse. There are various possible causes: (1) genetic factors, (2) infection caused by rheumatic fever or viruses, (3) beriberi and other vitamin B deficiency disorders, and (4) excessive alcohol intake. Usually, however, the cause is unknown.

Cardiopulmonary resuscitation (CPR) is an effective method of treatment for a temporary stoppage of heartbeat. The procedure consists of artificial circulation of the blood and artificial respiration.

To administer CPR to an adult or a large child, the rescuer first applies mouth-to-mouth resuscitation. The rescuer then places the heel of one hand parallel to and over the lower part of the victim's sternum, 1 to 1½ inches (2.5 to 3.8 centimeters) from its tip. The rescuer puts the other hand on top of the first and brings the shoulders directly over the sternum. The rescuer's fingers should not touch the victim's chest.

Keeping the arms straight, the rescuer pushes down forcefully on the sternum. This action, called *external cardiac compression*, forces blood from the heart through the pulmonary artery to other parts of the body. The rescuer alternately applies and releases the pressure at a rate of about 60 compressions per minute. After every 15 compressions, the rescuer briefly gives the victim artificial respiration.

If the victim is a small child, the rescuer uses only one hand for the compressions. Pressure is applied at about the middle of the sternum. To treat an infant, the rescuer exerts pressure with the index and middle fingers at the middle of the sternum. In all cases, the compressions must be accompanied by artificial respiration. Treatment should continue until professional help arrives.

CPR is best performed by two persons. One administers external cardiac compression, and the other provides artificial respiration. The rescuers position themselves on opposite sides of the victim so they can switch jobs easily if either becomes fatigued.

Cardioversion is the restoration of normal rhythm to a disordered heart by means of carefully controlled electric shocks. It may be done when the rhythms normally controlled by the CARDIAC PACEMAKER have been replaced by irregular rhythm, such as atrial FIBRILLATION.

Caries. *See* TOOTH DECAY.

Carotene is a yellow pigment present in many foods (for example, carrots, corn, and eggs). When such a food is digested, the carotene is stored in the liver until it is converted there into vitamin A. *See also* VITAMINS.

Carotid artery is either of the two arteries that lead through the main artery from the heart (aorta) and supply blood to the neck, head, and brain. Each carotid artery divides into an internal and an external artery. *See also* p.8.

Carpal tunnel syndrome is a tingling feeling in the fingers (except the little finger), which may also be weak. The sensation is particularly noticeable at night, and it may be strong enough to wake up a person.

Q: *What causes carpal tunnel syndrome?*

A: A ligament across the front of the wrist becomes swollen and compresses the nerve that supplies the fingers. The condition becomes worse with excessive use of the wrist, before the menstrual period (when fluid normally builds up in ligaments), and with mild arthritis. In

Carpus

rare cases, it may result from hormone disorders.

Q: How is carpal tunnel syndrome treated?

A: Resting the wrist and taking water-removing drugs (diuretics) should improve the condition. If these fail, a physician may inject a corticosteroid drug into the ligament. Sometimes a minor operation is needed to cut free the ligament from the nerve.

Carpus is the medical name for the wrist. A carpal bone is any of the eight small bones in the wrist. *See* WRIST.

Carrier is an apparently healthy person who carries or passes on a disorder without developing its symptoms. This may occur with such diseases as typhoid, diphtheria, and streptococcal infections. A healthy person may also carry a GENE for a disorder, such as hemophilia, which can be passed on to some of the children. A disease-carrying organism, such as a mosquito, is also sometimes known as a carrier.

Car sickness. *See* MOTION SICKNESS.

Cartilage is dense, specialized, semitransparent connective tissue that is capable of withstanding great pressure and tension. Cartilage forms part of the structure of the skeleton in some ribs and between vertebrae of the spine. It is also present in the nose, in the external ear (auricle), and as the gristle covering on joints that makes them move easily. In a developing fetus, cartilage is the major component of the skeleton, and bones are formed later when the cartilage becomes impregnated with deposits of calcium salts.

Q: What is a torn cartilage?

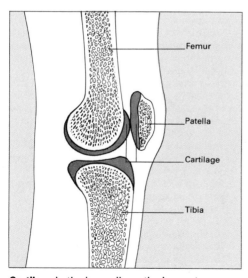

Cartilage in the knee allows the bones to move smoothly against each other.

Femur

Patella

Cartilage

Tibia

A: A torn cartilage commonly refers to a disorder of the knee. The cartilage tears away from the ligament that holds it in position, and a piece of cartilage may become free to move around in the knee joint. This can cause pain, swelling, and sometimes a "locking" of the knee that holds the leg in one position. No weight can be placed on the leg.

Q: How is a torn cartilage treated?

A: A minor tear can be treated effectively with a firm bandage around the knee and by taking as much rest as possible. More serious tears require the removal of the cartilage in an operation (meniscectomy). Osteoarthritis may affect the knee joint later in the patient's life.

Caruncle is a small fleshy lump. A caruncle sometimes appears at the outer opening of the urethra in women. A urethral caruncle may cause bleeding and pain on urination, and may be extremely sensitive to irritation. It is not serious in itself, and can be removed by a minor operation if it causes discomfort.

Castration is the surgical removal of the genital organs. The term is commonly taken to mean the removal of the testicles (ORCHIDECTOMY), although medically it also applies to the removal of the ovaries (OOPHORECTOMY). Castration may be necessary if the growth of a cancerous tumor is stimulated by sex hormones, as happens, for example, with cancer of the prostate or cancer of the breast. The removal of one, or both, testicles or ovaries is sometimes necessary if they have been seriously damaged by infection. In women, the ovaries may be removed at the same time as the womb (HYSTERECTOMY).

Q: Does castration affect sexual desire and fulfillment?

A: The operation in men subdues the sexual drive (libido). Intercourse is still technically possible but unlikely, and the semen does not contain sperm. Growth of body hair is reduced, but the depth of the voice remains unchanged. If a boy is castrated before puberty, secondary sexual characteristics (such as hair growth and deepening of the voice) do not develop.

Castration in women does not reduce a woman's ability to have sexual intercourse or her enjoyment of it, but the possibility of conception is permanently removed.

See also STERILIZATION.

Catalepsy, also called anochlesia, is a prolonged state of immobility in which the patient seems to be in a trance. It is normally associated with psychotic disorders such as SCHIZOPHRENIA, and sometimes accompanies HYSTERIA.

Cataract is an opaque area in the lens of the eye. Cataracts cause a gradual, painless deterioration of sight, beginning with an inability to see detail clearly, and distortion of sight in the presence of bright lights.

Q: What causes cataracts?

A: Cataracts often develop in elderly persons as a result of degeneration of the tissue of the lens. Cataracts may be present at birth (congenital), and the most common reason for this is thought to be rubella infection (German measles) in the mother during early pregnancy. Injury to the eye later in life may also cause cataracts, or they may accompany a disease, particularly diabetes.

Q: How are cataracts treated?

A: If vision is seriously impaired, the lens is removed in an operation. After an initial period of adjustment, clear vision is usually restored with the assistance of strong eyeglasses or contact lenses. In some cases, artificial lenses are placed in the eye at the time the cataract is removed.

Cathartic, or purgative, is a drug that induces one or several watery bowel movements. Castor oil is an example.

See also LAXATIVE.

Catheter is a tube inserted into a body cavity to extract or inject fluids. It is usually made of flexible plastic or rubber.

CAT scanner is an abbreviation of computerized axial tomography scanner, a machine that passes X rays through a patient's body from various angles. This technique enables a computer to build up a three-dimensional image.

The CAT scanner is considered one of the most revolutionary of 20th-century medical advances. It can provide physicians with X rays of parts of the body formerly inaccessible to conventional X-ray techniques. Furthermore, no injection of contrast media into the patient is needed—a procedure that can cause problems in some persons.

Cat-scratch fever is a disorder thought to be caused by a virus transmitted by a scratch or bite of a cat. It develops seven to fourteen days after the scratch or bite. Inflammation of the affected area heals in a few days, but lymph glands in the area remain slightly swollen and tender. A mild fever and general feeling of being unwell may persist from two weeks to a month. There is no specific treatment for cat-scratch fever, which eventually cures itself.

Causalgia is severe burning pain in an area where nerves have been injured, particularly the palm of the hand or the sole of the foot. The surface skin often becomes thinner and reddish, and slight changes such as a cool breeze may aggravate the burning sensation. The patient may become emotionally disturbed. Causalgia is difficult to treat. If pain-killing drugs are not effective, a physician may try local anesthetic injections or surgery to cut the damaged nerves.

Cautery is an artificial way of destroying tissue for medical reasons. It is done using heat, corrosive chemicals, electricity, or (the most recent method) a beam of laser light. Tissue may be cauterized to treat wounds that are likely to become infected or to destroy a lumpy scar. In surgery, an electric cauterizing needle is often used to stop bleeding from small blood vessels. Other examples of cautery are the use of silver nitrate to stop recurrent nosebleeds.

Cecostomy is an artificial opening made by joining the first part of the large intestine (cecum) to the wall of the abdomen. It may be a permanent or temporary measure to treat a blockage of the colon if it is damaged by such conditions as ulcers (ulcerative colitis) or cancer, or after surgery.

See also ILEOSTOMY.

Cecum is the sac-like first section of the large intestine, just beyond the point at which the lower part of the small intestine (ileum) joins the large intestine. Attached to the cecum is the vermiform APPENDIX.

See also p.12.

Celiac disease is a disorder caused by sensitivity to the protein gluten, which is found in wheat, barley, and rye. The cells lining the small intestine are damaged and prevent normal absorption of food, particularly fats. In adults, the disorder is also known as nontropical SPRUE.

Q: What are the symptoms of celiac disease?

A: Babies and young children with the disease fail to gain weight normally, develop a swollen abdomen, and excrete loose, fatty stools. They may also suffer repeated respiratory infections, dry skin, and eventually, signs of anemia, rickets, and other deficiency disorders. Adult patients suffer from tiredness, breathlessness, and muscle cramps. The abdomen is swollen, and the fingers may show clubbing.

Q: What is the treatment for celiac disease?

A: Patients should be put permanently on a gluten-free diet, and treated for the anemia or any deficiency disorder that is present. The diet should also be low in fats, with a high level of protein and vitamins to ensure adequate nourishment.

Cellulitis is a spreading of infection in the tissue under the skin, commonly associated with a small cut, abrasion, or boil. It occurs if

117

Cellulose

the body's defense mechanisms fail to localize the infection. The tissue surrounding the infection becomes red, swollen, and tender, and this area tends to enlarge rapidly. Red lines spreading from the infection toward a local lymph gland are a sign that the lymph vessels have also become infected (lymphangitis). To treat cellulitis, a physician usually prescribes a course of an appropriate antibiotic drug.

Cellulose is a carbohydrate that does not change chemically during the human digestive process. It is present in fiber-containing foods such as green vegetables and whole grain wheat bread. Cellulose aids the elimination of waste products from the intestine. For this reason, it is sometimes used in the treatment of constipation.

Celsius. *See* CENTIGRADE.

Centigrade, or Celsius, is a scale of temperature measurement in which 0° centigrade (written 0°C) is the freezing point of water at sea level, and 100°C is the boiling point of water at sea level. The other common system of temperature measurement is the FAHRENHEIT scale. The normal average human body temperature is 37°C (equal to 98.6°F).

Cerebellum is the part of the brain that lies behind and below the cerebral hemispheres of the brain. It is responsible for the coordination of voluntary movements throughout the body, and it is the center that controls balance.

See also p.18.

Cerebral cortex is the ridged "gray matter" of the brain that forms the outer layer of each hemisphere of the CEREBRUM. The cerebral cortex receives and interprets nerve impulses from the sense organs. It is also concerned with higher mental functions, such as intelligence, memory, and perception.

See also p.18.

Cerebral hemorrhage is a form of apoplexy caused by the bursting of a blood vessel within the brain. This causes bleeding into the brain matter and damage to the surrounding tissue. For symptoms and treatment of a cerebral hemorrhage, *see* STROKE.

Cerebral palsy is a general term for various disorders resulting from damage to the brain that occurs when the brain is deprived of oxygen before, during, or shortly after birth.

However, whatever the origin of this brain damage, all conditions that may be categorized under the term cerebral palsy have one factor in common. There is always some loss of muscle control.

Q: What causes cerebral palsy?

A: There are several possible causes of cerebral palsy. Some of these causes are injury, improper development of the brain, and certain diseases. Furthermore, each of these causes may occur before birth, during the birth process, or shortly after birth. For example, before birth, brain damage to the unborn may result from a disease contracted by the mother during pregnancy, such as rubella. Improper development of the unborn's brain may result if the mother's diet during pregnancy is deficient in certain essential nutrients or if the mother is addicted to such substances as alcohol or other drugs.

During the birth process, brain damage may result if the baby's head is too large to safely pass through the pelvis of the mother. Sometimes the birth process takes so long that the infant's brain cells are deprived of an adequate supply of oxygen. Without that supply, many of the infant's brain cells will die, resulting in permanent loss of function of the parts of the body controlled by those cells.

After birth, an infant can develop cerebral palsy as the result of brain damage caused by a blow to the head. An infant can also develop cerebral palsy as the result of infectious or toxic substances that damage his or her brain cells.

Q: What are some symptoms of cerebral palsy?

A: Some of the more common symptoms of cerebral palsy are lack of balance, clumsy walk, unclear speech, shaking, jerking movements, and convulsions. In some persons with cerebral palsy, there is also mental retardation, learning disability,

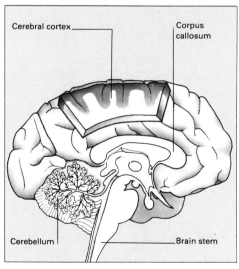

Cerebral cortex and cerebellum coordinate the body and control higher mental functions.

and/or severe hearing and sight problems. Symptoms of cerebral palsy are sometimes apparent at birth. However, in most cases, a definitive diagnosis of cerebral palsy may not be made until the child is between one to two years old.

Q: *How is cerebral palsy treated?*

A: There is no known cure for cerebral palsy. Therefore, treatment for the condition is aimed at helping the victim make best use of his or her physical and mental abilities. Yet the degree of success of treatment of cerebral palsy is largely dependent upon the extent of brain damage involved.

In general, treatment for cerebral palsy usually includes physiotherapy, speech therapy, medications, surgery, biofeedback, and special education. Psychological support is also very important in helping people with cerebral palsy and their families.

For many people with cerebral palsy, a physician may prescribe braces and other devices that provide support and can also aid walking.

Cerebrospinal fluid is a clear, watery fluid that surrounds the brain and spinal cord and helps to protect them from external shock. The fluid, under pressure, assists the supply of nutrients to the brain and the disposal of waste substances.

See also p.18.

Cerebrum is the largest part of the brain, situated beneath the roof of the skull. It consists of two hemispheres that are separated lengthwise by a furrowed division. The outer layer of each hemisphere is the CEREBRAL CORTEX, the section of the brain popularly known as "gray matter."

Within the cerebral hemispheres is white matter consisting of three kinds of fibers that connect the hemispheres, convey impulses to and from the cortex and the spinal cord, and connect different areas of the cortex with each other.

See also p.18.

Cerumen. *See* WAX.

Cervical refers to any cervix, or necklike structure, for example, the upper seven bones of the spinal column (cervical vertebrae) or the neck of the womb (cervix uteri).

A talk about Cervical cancer

Cervical cancer is cancer in the neck of the womb (cervix). There are no symptoms in the early stages of the disease, but bleeding may occur later either between menstrual periods or after sexual intercourse. Local pain may develop, and there may be some difficulty in urinating. Sometimes, blood in the urine is a late symptom.

Q: *Can cervical cancer be detected early?*

A: If a regular CERVICAL SMEAR (Pap test) is made, as gynecologists advise, cervical cancer can be detected at an early stage, although there are no external early symptoms. Diagnosis must be confirmed by further tests, such as biopsy. Immediate treatment following early detection is successful.

If cervical cancer remains undetected until it is in an advanced stage, immediate removal of the womb (hysterectomy) is necessary, and may be followed by radiotherapy. Untreated, cervical cancer is fatal.

Q: *Are some women more likely than others to get cervical cancer?*

A: Yes. Research has shown that cervical cancer is most common in women who have had sexual intercourse from an early age, with several partners, and whose standards of hygiene have been generally low. It is also more likely to occur in women who have had their first baby by the age of twenty. Cervical cancer is rare in women who have not had sexual intercourse.

See also CANCER.

Cervical erosion is an abnormal change in the tissue of an area of the surface wall of the neck of the womb (cervix). Natural healing of the disorder involves the downward growth of tissue cells from the endocervical canal. But it is not uncommon for healing to be incomplete and for the area to become ulcerated. This may cause an abnormal discharge from the vagina, and occasional bleeding, particularly after sexual intercourse.

Q: *What causes cervical erosion?*

A: Infection in the vagina, the stimulus to hormone production resulting from pregnancy, or the use of birth control pills may cause cervical erosion.

Q: *How is cervical erosion treated?*

A: A physician may introduce an antiseptic and antibiotic compound into the vagina to kill the infection and allow the cervical cells to regrow. If this fails, cautery of the damaged area is the usual treatment. This does not usually require hospitalization.

Q: *How soon after cautery can a woman resume sexual intercourse?*

A: A woman should not have sexual intercourse until a further physical examination confirms that the area has healed properly.

Cervical rib

Cervical rib is a small extra rib found in some persons. It is an appendage to the seventh cervical vertebra in the neck. The extra rib need not cause problems. But if it puts pressure on the adjacent nerves and blood vessels, there is pain in the arm and hand, and possibly symptoms similar to RAYNAUD'S PHENOMENON. If a cervical rib causes such symptoms, treatment is to remove it.

Cervical smear (Papanicolaou's test, or Pap test) is a test for the early detection of cancer cells on the neck of the womb (cervix). The test is painless and harmless, and entails the rubbing of a specially shaped piece of wood or plastic across the cervix. This removes some cells, which are examined using a microscope. The test is normally done during a routine gynecological examination. If it reveals abnormal cells, CERVICAL CANCER may be present in an early stage.

Q: How are the results of the test diagnosed?

A: Cells taken in the test are studied (cervical cytology) and then classified into one of four groups: (1) class I cells are normal in structure; (2) class II cells are slightly abnormal, and the possibility of vaginal infection may be investigated; (3) class III cells are definitely abnormal but they are not cancerous; (4) class IV and V cells are cancerous, and the appropriate action should be taken immediately.

Q: How often should a cervical smear be done?

A: Regular gynecological checkups with smear tests are advised for all women over the age of about twenty and for younger women who are sexually active. A smear that is normal should be repeated every three years. After a class II result, a repeat test is advised within three to six months. It is likely that a physician will decide to repeat a class III smear result either at once or within a few weeks. Class II or class III results should not cause alarm, because the cell structures often return to normal.

Cervical spondylosis is an arthritic condition of the upper spine and neck, which tends to become worse with time. A stiff neck may be the only symptom, although pressure on nearby nerves may cause pain and weakness in the arm and hand. Cervical spondylosis is most commonly part of the normal aging process. It can begin earlier in life as the result of back injuries, such as those from playing football or horse riding.

Q: How is cervical spondylosis treated?

A: Heat applied locally to the area, massage, physiotherapy, and antirheumatic drugs all may be of assistance in treating the condition. If these are not successful, it may be necessary to immobilize the neck in a surgical collar.

Cervicitis, also called trachelitis, is the inflammation of the neck of the womb (cervix). The symptoms may be a thick discharge from the vagina, pain during sexual intercourse, bleeding after sexual intercourse, and backache. The cause of cervicitis often remains unknown, but it may be caused by cervical erosion, or by vaginal infections.

Q: What is the treatment for cervicitis?

A: A physician may prescribe antibiotic drugs and recommend abstinence from sexual intercourse and alcoholic drinks. A persistent case of cervicitis may be treated by destroying the infected area using CRYOSURGERY.

Cervix is the neck or any part of an organ that resembles a neck. The cervix of the womb (uterus) is the narrow opening at the base of the womb that protrudes slightly into the vagina.

Cesarean section is the delivery of a baby through a surgical opening in the abdominal and uterine walls into the womb (uterus). This method may be preferable to natural birth through the vagina for various reasons: (1) if the mother's birth canal is too narrow for normal childbirth; (2) if a misplaced placenta blocks the exit from the womb (placenta previa); (3) when the fetus is in an unusual position (for example, head up, feet down); (4) when signs of fetal distress or potential illness occur; or (5) when the mother is ill.

Q: Can a woman who has had a Cesarean

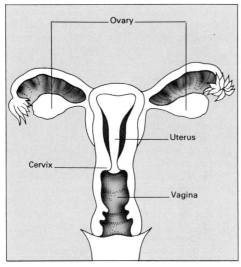

Cervix is the narrow entrance from the vagina leading to the uterus and the fallopian tubes.

section have a normal delivery for her next baby?

A: Yes, unless the reason for surgical delivery was a narrow birth canal or some permanent illness in the mother.

See also PREGNANCY AND CHILDBIRTH.

Cestodiasis is the infestation of the intestine by WORMS of the subclass Cestoda (phylum Platyhelminthes). The most common parasitic worms in this group are tapeworms.

Cetrimide is an antiseptic substance that is used as a cream, solution, or ointment in the treatment of wounds or skin infections. It is also an ingredient of some shampoos and skin cleansers, although cetrimide is poisonous if swallowed.

Chafing is soreness caused by rubbing the skin, usually in fatty areas, on another skin surface, or on wet clothing. The most common areas of chafing are the groin, anal region, neck, wrists, and between the fingers and toes. If the chafed area is kept clean and dry, the irritation heals itself.

Chagas' disease is a disorder transmitted by the bloodsucking bite of a bug that carries the causative agent, *Trypanosoma cruzi*. It is one form of trypanosomiasis. There is a red swelling around the site of the bite which, if on an eyelid, may cause the eye to close. The infection enters through the conjunctiva of the eye, the mucous membranes of the mouth or nose, or a skin abrasion. Symptoms of Chagas' disease are fever, general enlargement of the lymph glands, and a rapid heartbeat. A form of brain inflammation (encephalitis) may develop, with insomnia and irritability. The parasite can also be carried through the bloodstream to the heart and cause an inflammation there, and possibly, heart failure.

Q: What is the treatment for Chagas' disease?

A: There is no effective form of treatment, and the disorder has a high death rate, particularly among children.

Q: Is there a higher incidence of Chagas' disease in some countries?

A: Yes. Chagas' disease is most common in Central and South America, and it occasionally occurs also in the southwest United States.

Chalazion (meibomian or tarsal cyst) is a small hard growth on the eyelid similar to a sebaceous CYST. It forms when an oil-producing gland (a tarsal gland) becomes blocked with secretion. A chalazion is not painful, but if treatment is advised, an ophthalmologist can remove it by cutting it away from the inner side of the eyelid.

See also STYE.

Chancre is a painless ulcer that is an early sign of the venereal disease SYPHILIS. It usually appears on the genitals, but may occur elsewhere depending on the site of the infection, for example, the lips or skin. A chancre appears about three weeks after infection and becomes an ulcerous sore that heals slowly during the next month. It may leave a small scar. It is important to consult a physician about a possible chancre, to receive early treatment of the underlying disease.

Chancroid, also called soft chancre or soft sore, is a highly contagious venereal condition. It is caused by bacteria (*Hemophilus ducreyi*) and is most common in the tropics. About three or four days after contact with the infection, the patient develops a small red ulcerating sore on the genitals. This becomes painful and the local lymph glands swell and may discharge. Other symptoms may be a slight fever and a general feeling of being unwell.

Q: How is a chancroid treated?

A: A course of an appropriate antibiotic drug heals the chancroid effectively. The patient's sexual contacts should be examined for presence of the infection.

See also VENEREAL DISEASES.

Change of life is the time in a woman's life at which menstruation ceases permanently. See MENOPAUSE.

Chapping is a sore, inflamed condition of the skin caused by excessive exposure to cold or wet. Chapped skin should be protected by warm, dry clothing. Preventive measures include the use of water-repellent cream for outdoor activities, and nourishing hand and face creams.

Charleyhorse is a popular term for persistent pain and stiffness in a muscle, usually in the leg. See CRAMP.

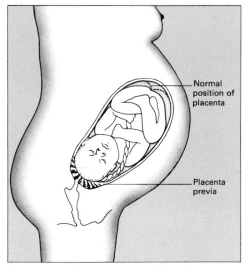

Cesarean section is necessary if the placenta obstructs the birth canal (placenta previa).

Cheilosis

Cheilosis is a reddened condition of the lips, with scaling and cracks at the corners of the mouth, which may become infected. Cheilosis is usually caused by a deficiency of the vitamin B complex, especially riboflavin. Vitamin B tablets and antibiotic skin creams improve the condition.

Chelating agents are substances that combine chemically with heavy metals, such as lead and mercury. They are used, for example, to combat poisoning by such metals. There are various chelating agents, such as penicillamine and EDTA (ethylenediaminetetraaceticacid). A physician decides which agent is best for a particular condition.

Cheloid. *See* KELOID.

Chemosis is excessive swelling of the mucous membranes that line the eyelids (conjunctiva). It is most commonly caused by CONJUNCTIVITIS, or by contact with an irritating substance, for example, chlorine. It may be a temporary reaction, but if the condition does not improve within a few hours, a physician should be consulted.

Chemotherapy is the treatment of disease by chemical agents that have a destructive (toxic) effect on the specific infecting organism. The most common types of chemical-containing agents are antibiotics (for example, penicillin and tetracyclines); antimalarials (for example, quinine); antifungals (for example, nystatin); antivirals (for example, idoxuridine); antiseptics (for example, chlorhexidine and hexachlorophene); and anticancer (cytotoxic) drugs (for example, methotrexate and cyclophosphamide).

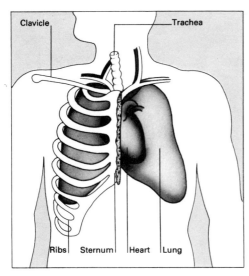

Chest, protected by the ribs, contains most of the respiratory organs, and the heart.

Chest (or thorax) is the upper part of the trunk of the body. It extends from the base of the neck to the diaphragm, which separates the chest from the abdomen. The framework of the chest consists of twelve pairs of ribs, which are connected to the spine at the back, and the intercostal muscles in between them. The upper seven pairs of ribs are connected at the front to the breastbone (sternum). The lower five pairs do not connect directly to the sternum; three pairs are connected indirectly by cartilage, and the other two pairs to the spine only.

The thoracic cavity enclosed by this frame contains the heart; the respiratory apparatus, including the two lungs in their surrounding membrane (pleura), the lower part of the trachea, and the bronchi; various glands; the esophagus (gullet); the two vagus nerves and two phrenic nerves; and the major blood vessels. Movement of the diaphragm and intercostal muscles changes the volume of the thoracic cavity during breathing.

Cheyne-Stokes asthma is breathlessness that occurs in spasms in a patient with a heart disorder. It is also called cardiac asthma. *See* HEART DISEASE.

Cheyne-Stokes breathing is a breathing pattern that is first shallow and infrequent and then increases gradually in depth and speed before fading away again. Before the next cycle begins, breathing may stop for five to fifty seconds. Cheyne-Stokes breathing is often accompanied by alterations in the levels of consciousness, and it most commonly occurs in seriously ill patients with brain or heart disorders.

Q: Is Cheyne-Stokes breathing invariably associated with serious disorders?

A: No. This breathing pattern can occur in elderly people, especially when they have taken sleeping tablets. Poor circulation and acidosis may also be causes.

Q: Is there any treatment for Cheyne-Stokes breathing?

A: If the breathing abnormality is associated with a heart or brain disorder, it improves when the cause is treated. Sometimes, a physician prescribes the drug aminophylline.

A talk about Chickenpox

Chickenpox (or varicella) is a virus infection characterized by a rash of small red spots that appear first on the back and chest and spread to cover the rest of the body. The rash is usually preceded for a few days by a slight fever, sore throat, and discharge of mucus from the nose. The spots develop quickly into clear, oval blisters of various sizes. These become milky in color and within three or four days shrivel up as scabs, which may take another week to fall off. One or two more waves of rashes may occur in the next two to three days. During the acute stage of the disorder, which lasts for three or four days, the patient's temperature may rise as high as 102–104°F (39–40°C), and a physician should be consulted. There is no vaccine against chickenpox.

Q: Is chickenpox contagious?
A: Yes. The first symptoms appear twelve to seventeen days after contact with the disease. The contagious stage extends from about five days before the outbreak of the rash until all of the blisters have crusted. It is advisable to isolate the patient once the spots appear.

Q: How long is chickenpox likely to last?
A: The acute illness lasts for between three and four days, but it is usually another seven to ten days before the spots have disappeared.

Q: Are some people more likely than others to get chickenpox?
A: Yes: children. Adults are less likely to catch chickenpox because, by the age of fifteen, about seventy-five percent of children have had chickenpox, and it is unusual to get the disease a second time. People in poor health and the elderly should avoid contact with a child with chickenpox, because the infection may cause the related disorder SHINGLES (herpes zoster), which is more common in adults.

Q: How is chickenpox treated?
A: Calamine lotion has a soothing effect on the irritating spots, and a physician may prescribe an antihistamine drug (also useful for its sedative effect) to reduce the irritation. It is most important to keep the patient from scratching the spots, because further infection can easily result if the skin is broken. For this reason, babies and small children may sometimes have to wear gloves. A physician may prescribe aspirin, taken every four hours, to reduce the fever and headache. A child must be encouraged to drink plenty of liquids. Nightwear and bedclothes should be light and preferably made of cotton, because wool and synthetic fabrics are likely to be irritating to the skin.

Q: Where else do spots occur apart from the back and chest?
A: Spots may spread to the rest of the trunk and face, as well as to the limbs. Spots may also appear in the mucous membranes, such as those of the mouth and vagina, or in the ears.

Q: Can complications result from chickenpox?
A: Complications are rare, but chest infections, such as bronchitis and pneumonia, sinusitis, and middle ear infection (otitis media) may occur. A more serious possible complication is encephalitis. These can all be treated effectively with prescribed antibiotics.

Q: How long is it before a child is back to normal after chickenpox?
A: A child may be irritable and unusually tired for about a week after the symptoms of chickenpox have disappeared, so it is important that he or she does not return to school too soon after the illness.

Chilblain, known medically as pernio, is a swollen, painful, reddened area occurring on the feet, toes, or fingers, and occasionally on the ears. The complaint occurs in cold, damp weather conditions. The cold damages small blood vessels and nerves in the skin. Some persons are more susceptible than others to such damage, and the condition is more common in men than women. A chilblain may cause aching, burning, and itching, especially when the body becomes warmer. Some chilblains form ulcers that may leave scars after healing.

Q: How is a chilblain treated?
A: Thick, woolen clothing should be worn in cold weather, with adequate covering of the head, legs, and arms, as well as the

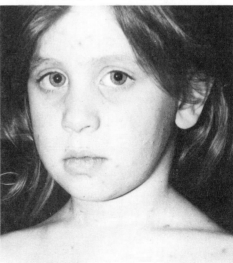

Chickenpox is a highly contagious viral disease that produces a characteristic itchy rash.

Childbirth

rest of the body. Drugs that cause an expansion in the blood vessels are sometimes prescribed. Corticosteroid creams are soothing for itching skin.

Childbirth is the process of having a baby. *See* PREGNANCY AND CHILDBIRTH. For EMERGENCY, *see* First Aid pp.546–549.

Childhood disorders. The following table lists some common illnesses and conditions pertaining specifically to children, or occurring more often in children than in adults, grouped according to symptom. The symptoms may also indicate other clinical disorders; this is not a complete list. A good medical history and physical examination by a physician are essential for adequate diagnosis of a problem. Each disorder has a separate article in the A–Z section of this book.

Symptom	Disorder
Aching joints	EXHAUSTION
	INFLUENZA
	POLIOMYELITIS
	RHEUMATIC FEVER
Breathing difficulty	ASTHMA
	BRONCHITIS
	CROUP
	DIPHTHERIA
	ENLARGED ADENOIDS
	ENLARGED TONSILS
	PERTUSSIS (whooping cough)
Convulsions	EPILEPSY
	FEVER (at the onset of illness)
	MENINGITIS
Cough	ASTHMA
	BRONCHITIS
	COMMON COLD
	CROUP
	CYSTIC FIBROSIS
	DIPHTHERIA
	INFLUENZA
	MEASLES
	PERTUSSIS (whooping cough)
	PNEUMONIA
	TUBERCULOSIS
Diarrhea	CYSTIC FIBROSIS
	FOOD POISONING
	GASTROENTERITIS
	INDIGESTION
	INFLUENZA
	MOTION SICKNESS
Painful ears	EARACHE
	TEETHING
	WAX (in ears)
Rash on the skin	ALLERGY, plant
	CHICKENPOX
	DIAPER RASH
	ECZEMA
	HEAD LICE

Symptom	Disorder
Rash on the skin (continued)	HIVES
	IMPETIGO
	INSECT BITES
	MEASLES
	PRICKLY HEAT
	RINGWORM
	RUBELLA (German measles)
	SCABIES
	SCARLET FEVER
Reading difficulty	HYPEROPIA (farsightedness)
	LEARNING DISABILITIES
	MYOPIA (nearsightedness)
Red, inflamed eyes	ALLERGY
	CONJUNCTIVITIS
	MEASLES
	STYE
	TIREDNESS
	WEEPING
Runny nose	ALLERGY
	COMMON COLD
	INFLUENZA
	MEASLES
	PERTUSSIS (whooping cough)
Sore throat	BRONCHITIS
	COMMON COLD
	DIPHTHERIA
	ENLARGED TONSILS
	INFLUENZA
	MUMPS
	RUBELLA (German measles)
	SCARLET FEVER
Stomachache	APPENDICITIS
	COLIC
	COMMON COLD
	CONSTIPATION
	FOOD POISONING
	INDIGESTION
	INTESTINAL OBSTRUCTION
	INTUSSUSCEPTION
	WORMS
Swollen glands	EARACHE
	MONONUCLEOSIS
	MUMPS
	RUBELLA (German measles)
Vomiting	GASTROENTERITIS
	INDIGESTION
	INFLUENZA
	MIGRAINE
	MOTION SICKNESS
	PERTUSSIS (whooping cough)
	PNEUMONIA
	POLIOMYELITIS
	SCARLET FEVER

124

Chill is a shivering attack and the accompanying sensation of coldness. It is due to an irregular impulse to the part of the brain that regulates body temperature and is a normal reaction to cold. A mild fever sometimes follows a chill, which may be the first indication of an impending infectious illness.

Chiropractic is an alternative, non-orthodox system of medicine in which diseases are thought to be caused by the improper functioning of the nervous system. A major aspect of treatment is spinal manipulation.

Chloasma is a patchy yellowish-brown discoloration of the skin of the face caused by a concentration of the pigment melanin. It often occurs in pregnancy, sometimes in women who take birth control pills, and in ADDISON'S DISEASE.
See also MELASMA.

Chloramphenicol is an antibiotic drug. It is used in the treatment of typhoid fever, some forms of meningitis, and as drops or ointments for skin, eye, or ear infections. It has wide applications, but it is used only with extreme caution because it may cause serious and even fatal damage to the blood-forming cells in the bone marrow.

Chlorhexidine is a disinfectant that is used on its own or with antibiotics to clean wounds or to sterilize the skin.

Chloroform was one of the first general anesthetics and, like ether, was in common use until the 1950s. Since then it has been gradually replaced by safer, less toxic drugs.
See also ANESTHETICS.

Chlorophyll is the pigment in all green plants that absorbs light energy from the sun to convert carbon dioxide and water into carbohydrates. In high concentrations, it can destroy bacteria that produce odors. For this reason it is assumed that chlorophyll acts as a deodorant in toothpastes and aerosol sprays.

Chloroquine is a drug that is taken by persons in malaria-stricken regions to prevent them from getting the disease. The standard preventive dose is 300mg weekly, but larger doses are required if a person actually gets malaria. In some parts of the world, however, the disease is resistant to the drug. Prolonged, high doses may cause permanent eye damage, and regular eye examinations are necessary. Chloroquine has also been used in the treatment of amebiasis, lupus erythematosus, giardiasis, and rheumatoid arthritis.

Chlorpromazine is a tranquilizing drug that is used in the treatment of major psychotic states. It is also used as a sedative drug in anesthesia, and in treating addiction to psychedelic and amphetamine drugs.

Chlor-Trimetron (Trademark) preparations contain the antihistamine drug chlorphenira-mine. It is available as tablets, a syrup, and a liquid for injection. Chor-Trimetron is less likely than other antihistamines to produce drowsiness (often a common side effect with this type of drug), and so it may be prescribed for use during the day. On the other hand, it can stimulate the brain, causing the patient to feel nervous and restless.
See also ANTIHISTAMINES.

Choking (for EMERGENCY treatment, *see* First Aid p.532) is the inability to breathe following the obstruction of the larynx or windpipe (trachea) by food, mucus, or a foreign object that has been swallowed or inhaled.

Cholangiogram is an X ray of the gall bladder and bile ducts, which are made visible by using a dye that blocks X rays. The dye may be swallowed in solution or it may be injected into a vein; the X ray is taken when the dye is excreted in the bile ducts. A gall bladder that is diseased (for example, from infection or stones) may not excrete the dye. A cholangiogram is also taken during an operation to remove the gall bladder (cholecystectomy), in order to ensure that there are no stones in the bile duct.

Cholangitis is inflammation of the bile ducts. It is usually caused by an obstruction of the bile ducts that link the liver with the gall bladder and duodenum. The obstruction may be caused by the presence of gallstones or a cancer, or it may occur following the removal of the gall bladder (cholecystectomy). Pain in the upper abdomen is accompanied by a high fever, often with vomiting, hot and cold sensations, and jaundice. Dark urine and pale feces can be other signs of the disease.

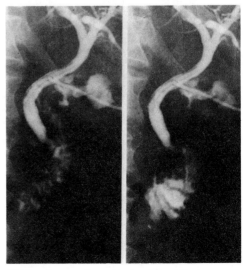

Cholangiogram is an X ray of the bile duct taken after a radiopaque dye is injected.

Cholecystectomy

Q: How is cholangitis treated?

A: Cholangitis may require hospital treatment consisting of antibiotic drugs and intravenous fluids, and an operation to remove the obstruction as soon as the patient is well enough.

Cholecystectomy is the surgical removal of the gall bladder.

Cholecystitis is an inflammation of the gall bladder. Acute cholecystitis is almost always caused by gallstones. Chronic cholecystitis commonly occurs in middle-aged persons, especially women, who are overweight and have gallstones.

Q: What are the symptoms of cholecystitis?

A: In acute cholecystitis, there is usually severe, sudden, or gradual pain in the right upper abdomen, with nausea, chills, vomiting, high fever, and sometimes referred pain in the back or the right shoulder. The symptoms of chronic cholecystitis are less severe and include discomfort in the right upper abdomen, gas, belching, heartburn, or indigestion.

Q: How is cholecystitis treated?

A: Antibiotics and, if vomiting has been severe, hospitalization for intravenous fluids are preliminary treatments for acute cholecystitis. If there is no improvement, the gall bladder is removed (cholecystectomy). Sometimes it is necessary to drain the gall bladder (cholecystotomy) to allow the patient to become well enough for the gall bladder to be completely removed. For patients with chronic cholecystitis, weight loss and a low-fat diet are usually tried first.

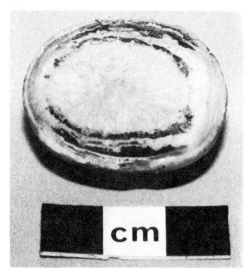

Cholelithiasis is caused by gallstones, which may be about one centimeter in size.

Cholelithiasis is the presence of gallstones in the gallbladder or bile duct. Patients with gallstones usually have too much cholesterol in their bile. When the cholesterol becomes too high and can no longer remain in solution, tiny crystals form that group together to build gallstones. This is somewhat similar to sugar being added to iced tea. The first spoonful will dissolve, but eventually the tea becomes saturated, and the sugar settles to the bottom as crystals. Gallstones occur much more frequently in women than men. A typical gallstone patient is female, middle-aged, and overweight. However, anyone with abnormally high levels of cholesterol has a much greater risk of developing gallstones. One in every four teenagers is affected by gallstones due to diets low in fiber and high in carbohydrate. The most stone-frequent people are those who are overweight, have associated digestive disorders, or are women who take the oral contraceptive pill.

Factors thought to be involved in the formation of gallstones include glandular or genetic predisposition and repeated infections of the bile duct.

Q: What are the symptoms of cholelithiasis?

A: Many gallstones are "silent" (dormant) and produce no symptoms. Symptoms that can occur are pain in the right upper abdomen; gas; belching; a spasm in the bile duct, causing severe pain; sweating, and vomiting, when a stone moves from the gall bladder; and jaundice, if a stone blocks the bile duct. Cholelithiasis increases the chances of damage to the pancreas and cancer of the gall bladder.

Q: How is cholelithiasis treated?

A: The usual treatment for gallstones is the removal of the gall bladder. However, the recently developed Percutaneous Nephroscope machine allows doctors to remove stones through a tiny opening in the patient's back or to shatter them into fragments with bombardments of sound waves.

Cholera is an acute infectious disease caused by bacteria (*Vibrio cholerae,* or *comma*). Symptoms are severe diarrhea and vomiting, with massive loss of body fluids, muscle cramps, and shock caused by dehydration. Cholera is transmitted by water, milk, or other foods, especially shellfish, that have been contaminated by the feces of infected persons. Cholera is mainly an epidemic tropical disease in Asia and Africa.

Q: How is cholera treated?

A: The patient requires replacement of fluids by drinking or by intravenous injection to counteract the dehydration. Antibiotic drugs are also prescribed. During the recovery period, glucose and potassium tablets may be given.

126

Q: *How successful is the treatment of cholera?*

A: When proper treatment is available, it is usually effective and the patient recovers completely within two weeks. The death rate in adults is about five percent, and in children ten percent.

Q: *Can cholera be prevented?*

A: People in epidemic areas are advised to avoid unsterilized water, fresh fruit, and shellfish. Cholera vaccinations provide some protection for at least three months. These consist of two injections given one to four weeks apart. International health regulations make vaccinations a condition of entry to certain countries in which cholera is endemic or of reentry from such countries. Certificates of vaccination are valid for six months.

Cholesterol is a fatty substance found in all animal tissues. The substance makes up an important part of the membranes of each cell in the human body. The liver uses cholesterol to manufacture bile acids, which aid in digestion. Cholesterol is also utilized in the production of certain hormones, including sex hormones.

Q: *How is cholesterol produced?*

A: The human body manufactures most of its own cholesterol. All body cells are capable of production, but most is made by liver cells. Cholesterol also enters the body in food, particularly from butter, eggs, fatty meats, and from organ meats, such as liver and brains.

Q: *How is cholesterol transported in the body?*

A: Three types of special molecules called lipoproteins—high-density lipoproteins (HDL), low-density lipoproteins (LDL), and very low-density lipoproteins (VLDL)—transport cholesterol from the liver through the bloodstream to cells throughout the body.

Q: *Is cholesterol harmful?*

A: Although the body needs cholesterol, high levels of LDL-type and VLDL-type cholesterol have been linked to certain diseases, particularly ARTERIOSCLEROSIS. Because of these problems, many physicians have recommended a diet low in cholesterol. Scientists, however, have also discovered that high levels of HDL-type cholesterol may actually provide protection against heart attack. Cholesterol's role and effect on the body thus remains a source of controversy.

Chondroma is a slow-growing, usually benign tumor of cartilage that may occur wherever cartilage is present in the body. It may or may not cause pain. Depending on its location, it may also increase the chance of breaking a bone. Chondroma occurs most commonly in adolescents and young adults.

Chondromalacia is the softening of cartilage in joints, especially that behind the kneecap (patella). It may cause pain and discomfort, but this usually improves with rest.

Chondrosarcoma is a malignant (cancerous) tumor that forms from cartilage cells. It may develop outside or inside a bone. *See* CANCER; TUMOR.

Chordotomy. *See* CORDOTOMY.

Chorea is a disorder of the nervous system that is characterized by spasm of the facial muscles and involuntary contortions of the limbs. The two common forms of chorea are unrelated: Sydenham's chorea (St. Vitus's dance) and Huntington's chorea.

Q: *What is Sydenham's chorea?*

A: Sydenham's chorea is a disorder in which the small arteries of the brain become inflamed. It is an allergic reaction to streptococcal infection. Sydenham's chorea commonly follows several months after an attack of fever and is most likely to occur in children between the ages of five and fifteen.

   The symptoms of Sydenham's chorea include facial contortions, grunts, and occasionally difficulty in speaking. Sometimes, only one side of the body is affected.

Q: *How is Sydenham's chorea treated?*

A: The disorder is associated with rheumatic fever, and bed rest is essential. Sedative drugs help to control the involuntary contortions, and antibiotic drugs are usually prescribed to fight infection.

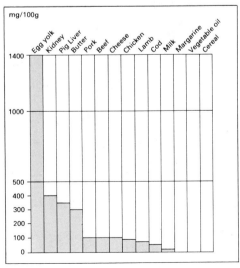

Cholesterol occurs in varying amounts in animal products, but not in vegetable foods.

Choriocarcinoma

The disease is often treated with regular high dosages of aspirin. Recovery may be complete within three or four months, but further attacks occur in about thirty percent of cases.

Q: *What is Huntington's chorea?*

A: Huntington's chorea is a serious inherited disease of the central nervous system, which usually affects persons between the ages of thirty and fifty. The symptoms of Huntington's chorea are the gradual onset of involuntary jerky and contorting movements of the limbs. Mental deterioration and severe change of personality are associated symptoms, and the patient may eventually need institutional care.

Q: *Can Huntington's chorea be treated?*

A: No effective form of treatment has yet been found for the disorder. It affects only males but unaffected females can pass on the gene to their children. The usual medical advice to a person with the disorder is not to have children.

Choriocarcinoma is a malignant growth of the outer layer of the membrane (chorion) that surrounds a fetus in the womb. It is a rare condition that occurs in only one in 50,000 pregnancies. An obstetrician looks for signs of the disease in pregnant women in whom there has been degeneration of an ovum and the formation of a hydatidiform mole. Repeated blood tests are then made to determine the level of certain hormones in the mother's bloodstream. If this level remains above normal, treatment with anticancer drugs (chemotherapy) is given, or the womb may be removed by an operation (hysterectomy).

Choroid is the middle coat of the eyeball that contains the dark coloring matter and blood vessels (*see* p.16). The term choroid plexus is applied to a small group of specialized blood vessels in the cavities (ventricles) of the brain, which produce CEREBROSPINAL FLUID.

Choroiditis is inflammation of the middle coat (choroid) of the eyeball. The symptoms of the disorder are a gradual blurring of vision, with flashes and bright circles of light. There is no pain, unless it is a sudden attack. Untreated, choroiditis may have serious complications.

Christmas disease, or hemophilia B, is an inherited defect in blood clotting which has the same symptoms as classic HEMOPHILIA: prolonged bleeding from slight injuries and internal bleeding without any known cause. Treatment is transfusion of blood plasma containing the correct clotting factor. The condition gets its name from the patient in whom it was first discovered.

Chromosome is a threadlike structure in the nucleus of a cell. It is made up of many hundreds of genes, the messengers that carry the "instructions" that determine a person's hereditary makeup (*see* GENE). There are forty-six chromosomes (arranged as twenty-three pairs) in each human cell except the sex cells, which have only twenty-three chromosomes.

Q: *What happens to the chromosomes when a cell divides?*

A: The chromosomes divide at the same time as the cell, so that the two new cells, each with forty-six chromosomes, are identical to the parent cell. Exceptions are the cells that form sperm and ova, which divide to produce sex cells (gametes) with only twenty-three chromosomes each. This means that when a sperm joins an ovum at fertilization to form a new cell of forty-six chromosomes, it does so with half the genes from the mother and half from the father.

Q: *How do chromosomes decide the sex of an individual?*

A: The male chromosome is called Y. It is smaller, and contains fewer genes than the female chromosome. Each sperm contains either an X or a Y chromosome; each ovum contains a single X chromosome. When a sperm and an ovum combine to form a new individual, the fertilized ovum contains either two X chromosomes (XX) and is female, or it contains an X and a Y (XY) and is male.

Chromosomes of a male consist of 22 pairs (XX), plus one odd set (XY).

Chrysotherapy is the medical term for any treatment that employs gold or its compounds. *See* GOLD.

Chyme is the homogeneous pulp of partly digested food in the stomach. *See* DIGESTIVE SYSTEM.

Cicatrix is the medical name for a scar. *See* SCAR.

Cilia are the fine, hairlike projections of many cells of the body that sweep particles along. Microscopic cilia are found, for example, in the airways to the lungs (bronchi). Eyelashes are an example of large cilia.

Circadian rhythm is the daily biological pattern in which sleep, hunger, and variation in body temperature occur. Moving to a distant time zone may disturb the rhythm, and the body may take ten days to adjust completely to the change.

Circulation, in medicine, usually means the flow of blood from the heart, through the arteries and capillaries, and back to the heart through the veins. The term may also be applied to the circulation of the cerebrospinal fluid around the brain and spinal cord, to the aqueous circulation of the eye, or to the lymphatic system.

Q: *Does all the blood go round one single circulation system?*

A: No. The systemic circulation is the passage of blood around the body. The pulmonary circulation is the passage of the blood through the lungs and back to the heart. In the fetal circulation, the blood by-passes the lungs from the pulmonary circulation into the systemic circulation through a special duct (ductus arteriosus). The placental circulation passes blood through the placenta of the fetus.

There are also the two portal circulation systems in which the blood flow starts and ends in the capillaries. One flows from the intestine to the liver (the hepatic portal system) and the other from the hypothalamus of the brain to the anterior lobe of the pituitary gland.

See also p.8.

A talk about Circumcision

Circumcision is the surgical removal of all or part of the FORESKIN (prepuce) of the penis. In infancy, it is usually carried out for social or cultural reasons. In later life it is less common, and usually performed for medical reasons.

Q: *How is circumcision carried out?*

A: There are two common methods. (1) A specially shaped piece of plastic is applied over the end (glans) of the penis and the foreskin is stitched over it before being cut off. (2) The foreskin is carefully cut and then stitched. An anesthetic is not used for newborn babies, but is used for a child or an adult.

Q: *Are there any risks involved in the circumcision operation?*

A: Mistakes are extremely rare, but can occur. Too much skin, or not enough, may be removed, as may part of the glans itself. Damage may be caused to the urethra, or severe bleeding may occur.

Q: *What are the medical reasons for circumcision?*

A: In some rare instances, the foreskin is unusually long and the exit unusually narrow (phimosis) at birth. Or the glans, inside the foreskin, may become infected by bacteria (*see* BALANITIS) or from diaper rash. This causes the foreskin to become scarred and abnormally tight. Sometimes the foreskin stays retracted (paraphimosis). All of these conditions can be corrected by circumcision.

Q: *What are the social reasons for circumcision?*

A: These differ from culture to culture. Often circumcision forms part of a religious rite or an initiation into adulthood. Frequently, circumcision may seem desirable because it is in the tradition of the family or because the majority of boys in the neighborhood are circumcised.

Q: *What possible advantages are there in not being circumcised?*

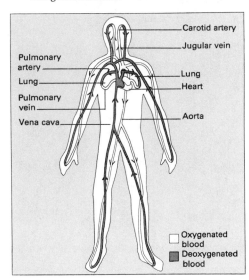

Circulation uses two main circuits, the systemic to the body; the pulmonary to the lungs.

Cirrhosis

A: Ulceration of the glans is commoner in those who are circumcised than in those with a foreskin.

Q: *Does circumcision have any effect on the incidence of cancer of the penis or cancer of the cervix?*

A: There is some evidence, although it is not conclusive, that cancer of the penis is commoner in the uncircumcised and that circumcision reduces the possibility of cancer of the cervix (the internal opening to the womb) in the man's sexual partner.

Cirrhosis is a type of permanent and progressive liver damage. Any chronic liver disease, especially those caused by alcohol abuse or viral hepatitis, can lead to the formation of fibrous scars and nodules that connect to involve large areas of the liver. Once present, cirrhosis is permanent, but its progress can be stopped if the cause is removed. Untreated, it can be fatal.

Q: *What are the causes of cirrhosis?*

A: In the U.S. the commonest cause of cirrhosis is alcohol abuse. Other causes include infections, such as HEPATITIS and CHOLANGITIS; AUTOIMMUNE DISEASE; some rare inherited diseases (such as WILSON'S DISEASE and HEMOCHROMATOSIS); and some drugs and chemicals, such as CARBON TETRACHLORIDE. In some parts of the world, virus infections or parasites such as liver flukes are more common causes.

Q: *What are the symptoms of cirrhosis?*

A: Early symptoms can include weakness and a feeling of tiredness, loss of appetite, nausea and vomiting of blood, and constipation or diarrhea. Symptoms of advanced cirrhosis include jaundice, broken blood vessels, a hard liver, a swollen abdomen, and swollen ankles. Some men suffering from the disorder experience an enlargement of their breasts, loss of pubic hair, and shrinking of the testicles (causing impotence).

Q: *How is cirrhosis treated?*

A: In cirrhosis caused by drinking alcohol, the only useful treatment is to stop drinking completely.

In cirrhosis caused by autoimmune disease, steroids and immunosuppressive drugs may be prescribed. Specialized care over a long period includes a high-protein diet with extra vitamins. Antibiotic drugs may be prescribed if there is infection (cholangitis). Occasionally the accompanying high blood pressure in the liver can be reduced by a surgical by-pass operation.

Q: *Can cirrhosis cause complications?*

A: Cirrhosis results in a kind of scar tissue that interferes with the flow of blood through the liver. This raises the blood pressure in the veins within the abdomen, especially at the lower end of the esophagus, which becomes dilated and congested (esophageal varices), and the rectum (hemorrhoids). If these veins burst, severe internal bleeding and vomiting of blood (hematemesis) can result.

Other complications of cirrhosis include jaundice, coma, bleeding disorders, peptic ulcers, and accumulation of fluid in the abdomen (ascites).

Claudication is the medical term for limping or lameness. Intermittent claudication is pain in the legs that is a symptom of arterial disease; the pain occurs only during exercise.

Claustrophobia is an abnormal fear of being in any confined area or enclosed space, such as a windowless elevator. It is the opposite of AGORAPHOBIA.

Clavicle, or collarbone, is one of two bones that connect the breastbone (sternum) with the shoulder blades (scapulas).

Claw hand is a deformity of the hand characterized by widely spread fingers, so that the hand resembles a claw. It is usually the result of a nerve injury.

Cleft palate is an abnormal fissure in the palate of the mouth that is present at birth. It is caused by faulty development of the facial structure of the fetus. Often, a cleft palate is accompanied by a similar division in the upper lip, called a harelip. In normal development, separate tissues fuse together to form the palate, upper lip, and upper jaw.

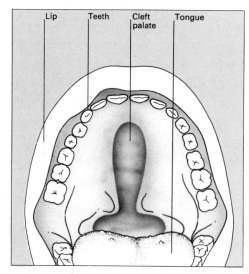

Cleft palate occurs because the roof of the mouth does not develop completely.

Q: Does a cleft palate cause feeding problems for a baby?

A: Yes. A cleft palate and harelip interfere with the natural sucking ability of a newborn baby, and the child must be fed with a bulb syringe or spoon, or with a special long nipple on a baby bottle.

Q: Can a cleft palate be corrected?

A: Most cases of cleft palate can be repaired by a series of operations during childhood. Plastic surgery is necessary to repair a harelip. If proper treatment is not started at a reasonably early age, the child may develop speech difficulties. Speech therapy may be necessary in any case for a person with a cleft palate.

Climacteric is the medical term for the time in a man's life when sexual activity naturally begins to decrease. In women, climacteric describes the changes that take place during the menopause (*see* MENOPAUSE).

Clitoris is a small, soft, sensitive area of tissue that is part of the female genitalia. It is situated below the pubic bone and is partially enclosed by the thin folds of the labia minora (*see* LABIUM). The clitoris plays an important part in the sexual stimulation of the female and, like the male penis, it becomes erect during sexual excitement.

Clonic refers to the alternate rapid contraction and relaxation of muscles.

Clostridium is a genus of spore-bearing, rod-shaped or spindle-shaped bacteria that are able to grow in the absence of oxygen. These bacteria are common in soil and in the intestines of animals. Some species are harmless to humans, but others produce toxins that are highly dangerous and may be fatal (*see* FOOD POISONING).

Clot is the jellylike substance formed when a liquid coagulates. In medicine, the term is normally used to mean a blood or lymph clot (*see* BLOOD CLOT).

Clubbing is a condition of the ends of the fingers or toes, which become rounded and alter the shape of the nails. In most cases, clubbing is a sign of a serious underlying heart or lung disorder. It may also be a symptom of CELIAC DISEASE. If the cause is found and successfully treated, clubbing may disappear.

Clubfoot (known medically as talipes) is a deformity of the foot, present at birth. In the most usual form (talipes equinovarus), the sole of the foot is turned inward and the heel upward. It is more common in boys than in girls, and may affect both feet.

Treatment is most effective when started soon after birth. The foot is held in the correct position by a metal brace or a plaster of Paris cast. An orthopedist may recommend an operation to correct the condition.

Coagulation is the formation of a clot in blood, lymph, or other liquid. It is a normal part of the healing process following an injury or surgery. Blood coagulation is a complicated process involving many factors to produce a BLOOD CLOT. If any of these factors is missing, coagulation occurs slowly or not at all. Hemophilia is an example of a disease caused by a missing coagulation factor.

See also AGGLUTINATION.

Coarctation is a narrowing in a tube. The term usually refers to the narrowing of the aorta, the chief artery leading from the heart. This is usually a congenital defect (present at birth). Coarctation of the aorta prevents normal blood flow, causing high blood pressure in the head and arms, and low blood pressure in the rest of the body. It may be treated by surgery, in which the narrowed section of the aorta is removed.

Cobalt bomb is a bomb-shaped lead casing that contains the radioactive isotope cobalt-60. The bomb is used to treat cancer by directing radiation from the cobalt-60 at a tumor.

Cocaine is a drug obtained from the leaves of the coca tree. The drug acts as a stimulant. Cocaine is used as a local anesthetic in the treatment of minor conditions of the ears, eyes, nose, and throat. Cocaine is sometimes combined with opiate drugs in treating the painful, terminal stages of cancer. Large doses of cocaine cause striking stimulation and trembling. In some patients, a marked sensitivity to cocaine can bring on serious allergic symptoms immediately.

Q: Can a person become addicted to cocaine?

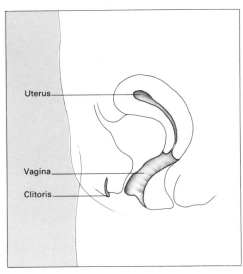

Clitoris, part of the female genitalia, is made of erectile tissue similar to the male penis.

Coccus

A: Many scientists do not believe the drug produces physical dependence. Repeated use of cocaine, however, causes a strong psychological craving and a sense of suspicion and fearfulness. Constant users see and hear things that do not exist. They believe they have special mental powers and enormous physical strength. Prolonged use of cocaine also causes nausea, sleeplessness, and loss of appetite and weight.

Coccus is a spherical type of bacteria, which can be the cause of many infections. Streptococcus, pneumococcus, and gonococcus are examples of this group of bacteria.

Coccygodynia is a severe pain in the region of the coccyx, at the base of the spine. It may occur after an injury or as a form of neuralgia. Treatment is generally with painkilling drugs or local anesthetic. If this fails, the coccyx may be removed by surgery.

Coccyx is the final bone of the spine, usually formed from four small bones fused together and joined to the sacrum. The coccyx is sometimes called the tailbone.

Cochlea is the spiral-shaped portion of the ear which contains the inner ear parts. These include the sensory cells (hair cells) and the nerve endings that transmit sound to the brain. *See* p. 16.

Codeine (known medically as methylmorphine) is a drug derived from opium. It is used as a painkiller, a cough suppressant, and a treatment for diarrhea. Prolonged use of large quantities may produce mild addiction. Many painkilling preparations contain a small amount of codeine in addition to acetaminophen or aspi-

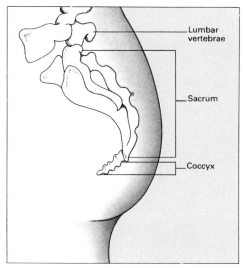

Coccyx is a small bone at the base of the spine formed from four rudimentary vertebrae.

rin. Codeine is available only by prescription.

Cod-liver oil is purified from the fresh livers of codfish. The oil contains a high concentration of vitamins A and D and was once used to supplement children's diets.

Coil is the common name for a type of intra-uterine device (IUD) used in contraception. *See* CONTRACEPTION.

Coitus. *See* SEXUAL INTERCOURSE.

Colchicine is an alkaloid drug obtained from the roots of the autumn crocus. It is used to treat gout. A side effect is diarrhea.

Cold. *See* COMMON COLD.

Cold abscess is an abscess that commonly accompanies tuberculosis. It develops so slowly that there is little inflammation and becomes painful only when there is pressure on the surrounding area. A cold abscess may appear anywhere on the body, but is most commonly found on the spine, hips, lymph glands, or in the genitourinary region.

See also ABSCESS.

Coldsore, or fever sore, is a small blister that appears, becomes an ulcer, and then heals with a scab. Coldsores usually occur around the lips and nose, but they are also common in the genital region, and tend to recur.

Coldsores, known medically as herpes simplex, are caused by the virus *Herpesvirus hominis*. This virus is present in many people and produces no symptoms when the person is in good health, but causes coldsores when another infection, such as the common cold, occurs. In some women, coldsores appear with the menstrual period.

Colectomy is an operation to remove part or all of the large intestine (COLON). It is usually performed to treat cancer of the colon or severe colitis. After a total colectomy or a partial colectomy close to the anus, an artificial opening is made in the wall of the abdomen (ileostomy or colostomy). When only a part of the colon is removed, the two ends are joined, but a temporary colostomy may be done to help speed healing.

Colic is acute pain in the abdominal cavity. The pain is usually localized in one of the ducts or hollow organs in the abdomen.

Q: *What causes colic?*

A: Colic in infants is usually related to diet, feeding methods, or emotional upset. An attack of infant colic is usually mild, although it may look severe and be accompanied by prolonged crying, abdominal distention, reddening of the face, and legs drawn toward the abdomen.

Colic in adults is in most cases severe. When its cause is an obstruction, such as a gallstone in the bile duct, the person may vomit and double up with pain. Colic may also accompany menstruation.

Q: *How is colic diagnosed and treated?*

A: Infant colic is usually diagnosed by observing the signs. The infant should be comforted until the pain subsides, and special attention paid to diet and feeding methods. Adult colic is usually diagnosed using special X-ray techniques and treated by eliminating the cause, such as removal of a gallstone.

Colitis is inflammation of the COLON. The commonest forms of the disorder are mucous colitis and ulcerative colitis.

Q: *What is mucous colitis and how is it treated?*

A: Mucous colitis is more common and usually milder than ulcerative colitis. It is thought to be brought about by psychological or emotional distress. Diagnosis of mucous colitis is often made when a person under stress has symptoms, such as abdominal pain, insomnia, headache, fatigue, and diarrhea, interspersed with constipation.

Treatment is primarily psychological, but the person's diet may need to be altered to correct irregular bowel movements, and sedatives may help the person to relax. In some severe cases, regular psychiatric help may be needed.

Q: *What is ulcerative colitis?*

A: Most cases of ulcerative colitis are severe and potentially life threatening. The exact cause of the disorder is not known, but the commonest of its symptoms is explosive, and sometimes bloody, diarrhea. Other symptoms may include severe abdominal pain, loss of weight, high fever, abdominal tenderness, toxemia, and peritonitis.

Q: *How is ulcerative colitis diagnosed and treated?*

A: Examination of the rectum, with an instrument called a proctoscope, and X rays of the colon usually detect this disorder. Treatment should be aimed at stopping the diarrhea before dehydration and severe malnutrition occur. The attacks of diarrhea must in any case be halted before a proctoscopic examination can be done or X rays taken. When a positive diagnosis has been made, additional treatment may include rest, psychiatric counseling, antibiotics, blood transfusions, intravenous transfusions, a special diet, steroid therapy, and even surgery to repair or to remove a part of the colon.

Collapsed lung is a condition in which a section of lung contains no air. It may occur if there is an obstruction by a tumor or foreign

body in the main bronchus (*see* ATELECTASIS), or if air enters the pleural cavity that surrounds the lung (pneumothorax), and compresses the lung.

Collarbone. *See* CLAVICLE.

Colles' fracture is a fracture of the radius bone in the forearm, just above the wrist, in which part of the radius shifts and causes the wrist to be unnaturally positioned upward. A general anesthetic is normally given while an orthopedist restores the bone to its original position. The forearm is immobilized in a cast for about six weeks, after which physiotherapy is needed to restore normal movement to the wrist. A bad repair may leave the wrist permanently weak, and the tendons in the wrist may tear from rubbing against the fracture site.

Coloboma is a congenital eye defect that may appear as a white swelling or as a gap. Or it may appear as a groove or cleft in the iris, the lens, or the choroid. Sometimes the eyelid is also involved. Vision may be impaired, and there is no treatment for the condition.

Colon is the part of the large intestine that extends from the cecum to the rectum. ("Large" refers to diameter, not to length.) Sections of the colon have different names. For example, the ileum of the small intestine joins with the cecum of the colon. Where the colon extends upward, it is called the ascending colon; where it crosses the abdomen, it is called the transverse colon; and where it moves downward toward the pelvis, it is called the descending colon. The last part is the sigmoid colon, which meets the rectum.

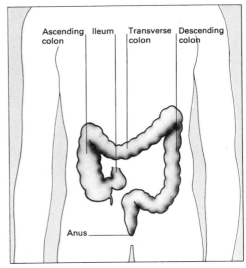

Colon receives indigestible fiber from the ileum and passes it along to the anus by peristalsis.

Colonic irrigation

Q: *What is the function of the colon?*

A: Although most of the digestive process occurs in the small intestine, the colon absorbs excess water and salts to be taken into the blood. This function of conserving and recycling is an important one: without it, dehydration can take place. After the excess water and salts have been absorbed by the blood, the remaining contents of the colon take on the consistency of feces, which are stored in the rectum until passed through the anus.

Colonic irrigation. *See* ENEMA.

Color blindness is an inherited defect of vision resulting in a person's inability to distinguish between specific colors. Partial color blindness is more common than total color blindness, in which a person sees everything as shades of gray. The most common form of partial color blindness leads to an inability to distinguish between red and green; rarely, the difficulty is between blue and yellow.

Color vision depends on the stimulation of the 10 million cone cells in the light-sensitive membrane at the back of the eye (retina). The three colors distinguished by the eye – red, green, and blue – cause three different pigments in the cone cells to react. Absence of one or more of these pigments at birth results in defects of color vision.

Q: *How common is color blindness?*

A: The defect is genetically determined, and is passed on to about ten percent of the male population. Only about one percent of all women have some form of color blindness. Total color blindness is rare.

Q: *How is color blindness diagnosed?*

A: Ishihara's test is used. This is composed of a series of colored cards on which numbers or lines of equal shade can be read by a person with normal color vision but not by someone with defective color vision.

Colostomy is an artificial connection between the large intestine (COLON) and the surface of the body at the abdominal wall, which is produced by means of surgery. A special bag over the opening in the abdominal wall is usually necessary to collect stools.

Q: *Why might a patient need a colostomy?*

A: A diseased area of colon may have to be removed (partial COLECTOMY). Then the two new ends each side of the removed portion may be brought to the surface. This type of colostomy may be temporary, until the two ends can themselves be joined surgically. But if the whole of the lower part of the colon is diseased and has to be removed, the upper part alone may be brought to the surface. This type of colostomy is permanent.

Q: *What adjustments might a colostomy patient have to make?*

A: Usually, a colostomy is no great inconvenience, once the patient has learned how to deal with it. The diet should be regulated to avoid constipation or diarrhea. Some patients find that a morning ENEMA via the colostomy clears the colon for the day, and the bag may not be required.

The patient gains confidence from the emotional support of other colostomy patients. This can come from the many colostomy societies, which offer help and mutual advice.

Colostrum is the yellow fluid secreted by a woman's breasts for a few days before and after childbirth. It contains about twenty percent protein, including the mother's antibodies to the diseases that she has had (*see* ANTIBODY). Colostrum has a higher concentration of salts but less fat and carbohydrates than normal breast milk.

Coma is a deep and sometimes prolonged unconsciousness state (for EMERGENCY, *see* First Aid, p.579). It may result from a head injury, stroke, reaction to drugs or alcohol, or an epileptic seizure. Or it may be caused by a disease such as diabetes or uremia (retention in the blood of substances usually excreted by the kidneys).

Treatment is to place the patient in the recovery position and to keep the airway open (*see* p.550). Breathing and pulse rate should be monitored. The patient should be hospitalized at once.

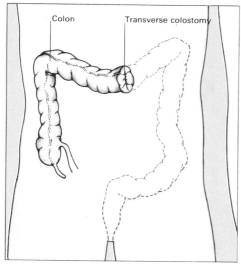

Colostomy performed on the transverse colon is managed post-operatively with a bag.

134

Comedo. *See* BLACKHEAD.

Comminuted fracture is a bone fracture in which the bone is splintered.

Common cold, known medically as coryza and often called merely a cold, is a contagious virus disease of the respiratory tract. It is a droplet infection, that is, people catch a cold by inhaling airborne water droplets sneezed out by a patient with the disorder. Symptoms appear about forty-eight hours after exposure to the virus, which may be any one of (or a combination of) more than one hundred different types. Colds are more frequent among the young and are more likely to occur during the winter months.

Q: What are the typical symptoms of a cold?

A: Early symptoms of a cold include a runny nose, watering eyes, a headache, and a sore throat. Later, there may be a stuffy nose, a slight cough, and aching muscles. The patient may also have a chill and a slight fever.

Q: Can a cold be serious?

A: A cold, although extremely annoying, is seldom serious. But babies and young children and patients with asthma, bronchitis, a heart disorder, or kidney disease who have symptoms of a cold may be at risk and should have medical advice.

Q: Can a cold be cured?

A: There is no cure for a cold. Home treatment to relieve the symptoms includes regular doses of a mild painkiller such as aspirin or acetaminophen, an antihistamine drug to help to dry up the nasal discharge, a cough medicine, and throat lozenges for the sore throat. Contrary to popular belief, antibiotics do not cure a cold (or any other virus infection). The patient should drink plenty of fluids, and avoid contact with others to prevent spreading the infection.

Communicable disease is one that is transmitted from one person to another. *See* CONTAGIOUS DISEASES.

Complex is a psychological term, introduced by Carl Jung, for an idea or group of ideas repressed into the unconscious. It is because these ideas have a strong emotional charge, that complexes may influence a person's behavior. Examples of complexes include the Electra complex, the sexual love of a daughter for her father; Oedipus complex, the sexual love of a son for his mother; and inferiority complex, a state of mind in which a person feels inferior to others.

The term complex is often loosely used to mean an obsession. Complex also refers to the lines traced by an electrocardiograph that represent the beating of the heart. A collection of symptoms may also be called a complex, but such a collection is more usually termed a syndrome.

Compound fracture is a bone fracture in which the broken bone causes a surface wound. The bone may or may not be visible. A compound fracture is more serious than an ordinary fracture because of the risk of infection. For EMERGENCY, *see* First Aid, pp.552–557.

Compress is a pad of material by means of which heat or cold can be applied to the body.

Computerized axial tomography. *See* CAT SCANNER.

Conception is the moment in the reproduction cycle when a sperm fertilizes an ovum. This usually takes place in a woman's fallopian tube. The fertilized egg then passes into the womb (uterus), where it becomes implanted in the wall and develops first into an embryo and then into a fetus. *See* PREGNANCY AND CHILDBIRTH.

Concussion is an injury to a part of the body resulting from a blow or from violent shaking. Concussion usually refers to an injury to the brain. Brain concussion is commonly caused by a head injury, but it may also result from a fall on to the lower end of the spine.

Q: What are the symptoms of brain concussion?

A: The symptoms of brain concussion vary according to the site and extent of the injury. Brain concussion usually, but not always, produces unconsciousness. The

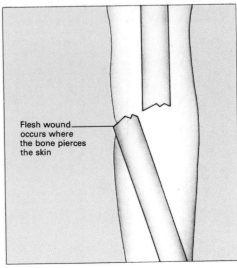

Flesh wound occurs where the bone pierces the skin

Compound fracture is susceptible to infection because an external wound contacts the break.

return to consciousness often occurs gradually. Following the initial injury, there may be headache; difficulty in concentrating; nausea; vomiting; difficulty in focusing; and a feeling of depression and irritability. Events immediately before the injury may be forgotten at first (retrograde amnesia), but the memory of them usually returns.

Q: *How is brain concussion treated?*

A: A physician should be consulted in all cases of concussion because there may be more serious brain damage. Bed rest is essential for at least a day after the injury. Painkillers may be given to relieve the headache. Alcohol, sedatives, and tranquilizers may aggravate the symptoms. The patient should avoid sports and work requiring concentration or skill until he or she is completely recovered.

Conditioned reflex is either a modification of an inborn reflex or a completely new automatic response that is developed as a result of an individual's experience. Conditioned reflexes were first demonstrated by Ivan Pavlov in the 19th century. He taught a dog to salivate at the sound of a bell by first teaching the dog to associate the ringing of a bell with the appearance of food.

See also REFLEX.

Condom. *See* CONTRACEPTION.

Condyloma is an infectious wartlike growth on the genitals or near the anus. *See* SYPHILIS; WART.

Congenital refers to any characteristic or condition that is present at birth.

Approximate incidences of some congenital anomalies		
Defect	Ratio M:F	Incidence per 1,000
Congenital heart disease	1:1	🧍🧍🧍🧍🧍
Pyloric stenosis	4:1	🧍🧍🧍🧍
Clubfoot	2:1	🧍🧍
Down's syndrome	1:1	🧍🧍
Spina bifida	1:1	🧍🧍
Hydrocephalus	1:1	🧍🧍
Encephaly	1:2	🧍
Congenital dislocated hip	1:6	🧍
Harelip and cleft palate	2:1	🧍
Klinefelter's syndrome	1:0	🧍

Congenital anomalies are defects that occur in only a few of every 1,000 newborn children.

A talk about Congenital anomalies

Congenital anomalies are mental or physical abnormalities that are present at, and usually before, birth. Some anomalies may be medically insignificant and may not appear for some time. In other cases, the anomaly may pose a direct threat to life and require immediate attention. There are, however, some anomalies that cannot be treated.

Q: *What are examples of congenital anomalies?*

A: Congenital anomalies include BLINDNESS, BONE DISORDERS, CATARACT, cleft palate, CRETINISM, DEAFNESS, DOWN'S SYNDROME, endocrine gland disorders, CONGENITAL HEART DISEASE, HEMOPHILIA, HYDROCEPHALUS, jaundice, JOINT DISORDERS, PYLORIC STENOSIS, and SPINA BIFIDA.

Limbs or organs may be malformed, duplicated, or entirely absent. Organs may fail to move to the correct place, as in CRYPTORCHIDISM, fail to open correctly, as in IMPERFORATE ANUS, or fail to close at the correct time, as in PATENT DUCTUS ARTERIOSUS. Congenital anomalies often occur together. For example, forty percent of babies born with Down's syndrome also have heart disease.

Q: *What may cause the development of congenital anomalies?*

A: Congenital anomalies arise from the faulty development of a fetus, caused either by genetic disorders or other factors. Some anomalies arise from a combination of factors, and the underlying cause is far from clear in all cases.

Q: *How are genetic disorders responsible for congenital anomalies?*

A: Inherited congenital anomalies generally result from the presence of abnormal GENES or CHROMOSOMES. Heredity is determined by corresponding pairs of genes, called alleles. One of these paired genes is dominant and the other recessive, and it is the dominant gene that governs the transmitted trait or characteristic. Thus, if the abnormal gene of a pair is dominant, the abnormal or anomalous trait will be conveyed to the embryo. If the abnormal gene is recessive, then both genes in the pair have to be recessive for an abnormality to occur.

Some congenital anomalies, such as hemophilia, are linked to a defect of one of the sex chromosomes. Many genetic disorders, however, are neither wholly dominant, recessive, nor sex-linked, but may be caused by more than one abnormal pair of genes.

Q: *What other factors may cause congenital anomalies?*

A: Infection in the mother is a common cause of abnormality in a baby. For example, an attack of RUBELLA during the first three months of pregnancy may cause her child to be born deaf or have cataracts, heart disease, jaundice, or other anomalies. Infectious HEPATITIS, MUMPS, and TOXOPLASMOSIS also cause congenital anomalies.

Certain drugs taken by a woman during pregnancy are often responsible for abnormalities in the child. For example, corticosteroid drugs may cause cleft palate, and drugs used in the treatment of thyroid disorders may result in GOITER or cretinism in the baby. Other drugs may cause gross abnormalities, such as the defects arising from thalidomide.

Injury to a pregnant woman or to a fetus is another cause of congenital anomalies. For example, limbs may be malformed if an intrauterine device (IUD) is not removed early in the pregnancy. Smoking during pregnancy is implicated as one factor in the incidence of abnormally low birth weight in babies, and malnutrition seems to be related to a high incidence of congenital anomalies. The age of the woman at the time she conceives can also be a factor. For example, Down's syndrome occurs more frequently when conception occurs after the age of about forty.

Congenital anomalies have also been attributed to the effects of X-ray examination made early in a pregnancy.

Q: *It is possible to diagnose congenital anomalies in a fetus?*

A: Yes. The most reliable method of diagnosis is to examine a sample of fluid from the amniotic sac at about the fourteenth week of pregnancy. The sample is obtained by AMNIOCENTESIS, and microscopic examination of the cells in the fluid reveals possible abnormalities in the chromosomes. Congenital anomalies that can be diagnosed in this way include Down's syndrome, spina bifida, and anencephaly. Sometimes the diagnostic use of ultrasound can detect abnormalities of the skull or spine.

Q: *Can congenital anomalies be treated?*

A: Treatment depends entirely on the nature and severity of the condition. Many anomalies can be treated, but for some there is no treatment.

Q: *In what circumstances might abortion be considered?*

A: Abortion might be considered if serious fetal disorders are found early in a pregnancy. The decision to abort rests with the parents, and is taken after considering the advice of the physician and specialists on the nature of the disorder and the consequences of abortion.

Q: *Are congenital anomalies more likely to occur in first-born babies?*

A: No. Statistics disprove this commonly held belief.

Q: *Does a congenital anomaly in a baby indicate that subsequent babies will be similarly affected?*

A: The branch of medicine that deals with such questions is GENETIC COUNSELING. In many cases it is possible to state risks numerically. For example, a baby with congenital heart disease is likely to be followed by a similarly affected child in two percent of pregnancies instead of the ordinary risk of one percent. Spina bifida occurs in about one child in every 3,000 but if a previous child was born with the condition, there is about a one-in-forty chance that it will occur in a later child.

Congenital heart disease

Congenital heart disease is any heart disorder that is present at birth, although the condition may not be diagnosed until later in life. The most common problems are a narrowing of the aorta (the main artery from the heart); the wrong positioning of the aorta or the artery that leads to the lungs; and constriction of the valves in the left side of the heart, with weakness of the heart muscle. Many defects are complex and some involve a hole

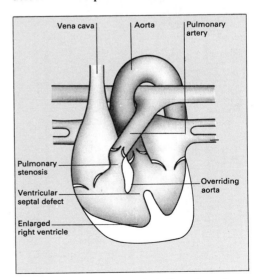

Congenital heart disease that affects four sites in the heart is known as Fallot's tetralogy.

137

Congestion

in the central portion of the heart, through which blood passes from one side to the other.

Q: *What are the symptoms of congenital heart disease?*

A: The symptoms, if present at all, depend on the nature of the disorder. For example, ventricular septal defect may be detected by a heart murmur. Breathing difficulty and a bluish color to the skin may also be symptoms in a baby (*see* BLUE BABY; FALLOT'S TETRALOGY). An infant with congenital heart disease who survives is likely to have frequent respiratory infections.

Q: *What are the causes of congenital heart disease?*

A: Often the cause is unknown, although genetic factors are thought to be important. Some forms of congenital heart disease may be caused by a virus infection in the mother during the first three months of pregnancy, such as rubella.

Q: *How is congenital heart disease treated?*

A: Successful treatment depends on a speedy diagnosis. If possible, the appropriate type of heart surgery is then undertaken.

Q: *Are some babies more susceptible to congenital heart disease than others?*

A: Yes. Although less than one percent of first-born babies have a congenital heart disease, the likelihood of it occurring in a subsequent baby is increased to one in fifty. There is a one in twenty-five chance that a baby born to parents who themselves have a congenital heart disorder will also have a heart problem.

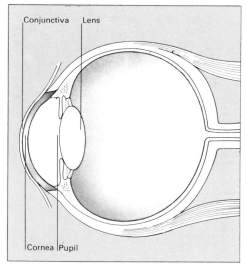

Conjunctiva lines the inside of the eyelids and covers the front portion of the eyeball.

Congestion is the swelling of body tissues due to the accumulation of blood or tissue fluid. It may be a reaction to infection or injury, or it may be caused by a blockage in veins returning blood to the heart.

Congestive heart failure is a condition in which the heart is unable to maintain the normal circulation of the blood. The blood in the veins increases in volume, and the veins become dilated. The lungs, liver, and intestines become congested with blood. There are various causes of congestive heart failure, including weakness of the heart muscle; high blood pressure; hardening of the arteries; and rheumatic or syphilitic disease of the heart valves. Untreated, the condition can be fatal.

Q: *What are the symptoms of congestive heart failure?*

A: The symptoms include breathlessness, swollen ankles (a form of edema), and weakness.

Q: *How is congestive heart failure treated?*

A: A physician may prescribe a diuretic drug, which helps to relieve any swelling (edema) in the body tissues and reduces some strain from the heart. A salt-free diet is sometimes recommended, to help to prevent any further retention of fluids. In addition, digitalis may be used to improve the strength of the heartbeat. Bed rest, with hospitalization if necessary, is advised for acute congestive heart failure. Oxygen may be required, and a source of oxygen should be kept available.

Conjunctiva is the thin, mucous membrane that lines the eyelid and covers the white of the eyeball, or sclera.

Conjunctivitis (also called "pink eye") is inflammation of the membrane covering the eye (the conjunctiva). Acute conjunctivitis frequently occurs with viral respiratory illnesses, such as the common cold or influenza. More severe attacks are usually caused by bacterial infections. Conjunctivitis that is not associated with respiratory disorders may be caused by irritants such as dust, cosmetics, or smoke, or by an allergic reaction to a specific substance, such as pollen or penicillin. Conjunctivitis may also result from the tropical eye disorder trachoma, and from a number of other rare afflictions or conditions.

Q: *What are the symptoms of conjunctivitis?*

A: The eye tends to water profusely and the white of the eye is bloodshot or pink. The eye is painful when moved, and may be oversensitive to bright light. Sometimes there is a discharge of pus from the eyelids.

Q: *How is conjunctivitis treated?*

A: A physician usually prescribes an antibiotic drug and other treatments such as eye drops. Prolonged use of drops, however, may aggravate the inflammation. Conjunctivitis known to be caused by an allergy may be treated with corticosteroid drugs. Dark glasses give protection against bright light, but a patch over the eye may increase the inflammation. If the eye is painful, a mild painkiller such as aspirin gives relief. It is important not to rub the eye, because this may transmit the conjunctivitis to the other eye.

Connective tissue is any tissue that connects and supports other tissues or organs — for example, the fibrous tissue of ligaments. Dense connective tissue includes CARTILAGE and bone. Scars are formed from connective tissue.

A talk about Constipation

Constipation is the difficult or infrequent excretion of feces. The frequency of bowel movements considered to be normal depends on the individual: "normal" may range from movements three times a day to three times a week. Greater intervals of time between movements than is customary for a particular person are a sign of constipation. The condition is not an illness in itself, but it may be a symptom of one, and a person should consult a physician if it persists.

Q: *What causes constipation?*

A: Constipation is most often caused by insufficient bulk in the diet or the habit of ignoring the desire to defecate. This gradually makes the rectum tight as the feces accumulate there, especially if a person's diet contains little vegetable fiber and a lot of highly processed food. Some effects of hormones produced during pregnancy may aggravate the problem. A marked change in diet, for example, as a weight-losing measure, may cause constipation. Painkilling drugs taken regularly are often a cause. A person taking drugs that are used as treatment for hypertension, rheumatic disorders, or depression may suffer from constipation.

Q: *Why are babies often constipated?*

A: Hot weather, insufficient fluid in the diet, or a fever may cause slight dehydration in babies. This means that most of the fluid in the colon is absorbed into the bloodstream, leaving the feces hard and difficult to pass. If a baby is constipated from birth, it may be a sign of a developmental failure in the intestine called HIRSCHSPRUNG'S DISEASE.

Q: *Are laxatives an effective treatment for constipation?*

A: Laxatives are sometimes used for immediate relief from constipation, but they should be used sparingly and never taken if other symptoms indicate that the patient may have APPENDICITIS. The regular use of strong laxatives that contain chemicals and vegetable irritants (for example, senna or cascara), far from preventing constipation, actually maintain it.

Q: *How else can constipation be treated?*

A: Treatment must be aimed at removing the cause, such as depression. Nonirritant purgatives help to return the bowel to its normal rhythm; if the feces are hard, special softening laxatives may be recommended. An attempt should be made to establish some regularity in bowel movements and eating habits. A diet containing vegetable fiber, bran, cellulose, or other bulk produces large soft feces, which are easily passed.

Q: *Does constipation affect certain groups of people more than others?*

A: Constipation tends to affect twice as many women as men, and it occurs more frequently with advancing age. Those who spend many hours sitting down are more susceptible to constipation than those who are physically active.

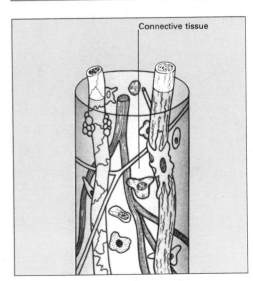

Connective tissue is a substance that supports cells and fibers in the body.

Consumption

Consumption. *See* TUBERCULOSIS.

Contact lens is a glass or plastic lens that fits over the cornea of the eye to correct a vision defect. Contact lenses adhere to the cornea and move with the eyeball, providing greater peripheral vision than conventional EYEGLASSES. The soft, hydrophilic plastic lenses, which allow fluids to pass through, are more comfortable to wear than the older, harder types. And unlike hard lenses, soft lenses do not require a special solution to lubricate the cornea when they are put in.

Q: What are the advantages and disadvantages of contact lenses?

A: Apart from good general vision, contact lenses can provide the means of keeping medication in contact with the eyeball for persons with keratitis (inflammation of the cornea). They may also retard the progress of myopia and conical corneas (keratoconus).

But contact lenses may require skilful fitting, and be expensive. In the time needed for the eye to become used to a lens, conjunctivitis may occur: lenses must not be worn when the eye is inflamed, even with the mild conjunctivitis that occurs with a cold. The lenses must be removed and sterilized every night. They can also cause an allergic reaction.

Yet to most people they are more convenient than conventional eyeglasses, when they have been worn for a time.

Contagious diseases are infectious diseases that are transmitted from one person to another. The following is a list of contagious diseases, each of which has a separate entry in the A-Z section of this book.

BRONCHIAL PNEUMONIA	PERTUSSIS (whooping cough)
CHICKENPOX	PLAGUE
CHOLERA	PLEURODYNIA
COMMON COLD	PNEUMONIA
CONJUNCTIVITIS	POLIOMYELITIS
DIPHTHERIA	PUERPERAL FEVER
GONORRHEA	RINGWORM
HAND-FOOT-AND-MOUTH DISEASE	ROSEOLA
INFLUENZA	RUBELLA (German measles)
LEPROSY	SCARLET FEVER
MEASLES	SMALLPOX
MENINGITIS	SYPHILIS
MONILIASIS (thrush)	TRACHOMA
MONONUCLEOSIS (glandular fever)	TUBERCULOSIS
MUMPS	TYPHOID FEVER
PARATYPHOID	VACCINIA
	VENEREAL DISEASES
	YAWS

A talk about Contraception

Contraception, or birth control, is the prevention of pregnancy. There are various contraceptive methods. Some are designed to prevent the male sperm from fertilizing the female egg (ovum), and others to prevent the already fertilized egg from developing. The most suitable method is a matter of personal choice and medical advice, and often involves some experimentation. The failure rate of each method is expressed as the number of pregnancies per 100 that occur in women using the method each year.

Q: What forms of contraception require no artificial aids?

A: There are two common "natural" methods. (1) Coitus interruptus is the withdrawal of the penis from the vagina before ejaculation. Although it is a widely practiced method, it is unreliable, because some sperm nearly always escape before orgasm. The technique also induces stress during intercourse, and many couples find this method frustrating. The failure rate is about 30-40 per 100.

(2) In the rhythm method or safe period, intercourse is avoided on the days before and following ovulation, when an egg is released from an ovary and travels along a fallopian tube to the womb. These so-called "safe" days are calculated using the date of ovulation, with the knowledge that the egg survives for a maximum of one day and the sperm

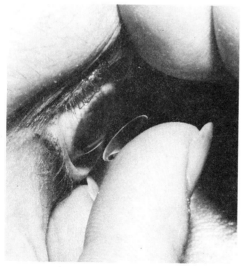

Contact lens is a cosmetic alternative to eyeglasses. It is shaped to fit over the cornea.

for not more than three days. Ovulation usually occurs between 12 and 16 days before a menstrual period is due. A woman can calculate her own ovulation time using either the calendar method or the temperature method, although neither method is totally reliable.

Q: *What is the calendar method?*

A: For this method, a record of menstruation must be kept for at least six months. The first "unsafe" day is found by subtracting 19 from the shortest recorded cycle, and the last by subtracting 10 from the longest cycle. Thus, if a woman's shortest cycle was 27 days and her longest 32, she must avoid intercourse from days 8 to 22, counting the first day of menstruation as day 1.

Q: *How does the temperature method work?*

A: Each month a woman's body temperature rises slightly at the time of ovulation. She can record this rise if she takes her temperature every morning before (and not after) getting out of bed. The "safe" period is usually from three days after until five days before the next rise in temperature. The failure rate is about 20–30 per 100.

Q: *What are the artificial aids to contraception?*

A: Two methods use simple physical barriers between the sperm and the egg. (1) The condom, worn by the man, is a sheath of thin rubber or plastic, and often has a small teat at the end to collect the ejaculated sperm. The condom is rolled onto the erect penis just before intercourse. After orgasm the penis must be withdrawn from the vagina before it becomes flaccid, or the condom may fall off in the vagina. For added protection the woman should use a spermicide.

The condom is probably the most widely used form of artificial contraceptive, and has a failure rate of about 10–20 per 100.

(2) The diaphragm, or Dutch cap, is a dome-shaped piece of rubber or plastic attached to a flexible wire ring. It is placed across the upper end of the vagina covering the cervix to prevent sperm from entering the womb.

Q: *How does a woman choose the correct size of diaphragm?*

A: The first fitting must be made by a gynecologist. After an examination, a woman is given the correct size of diaphragm and taught how to fit it herself. She should fit it each night as a matter of habit, whether or not she has intercourse. For maximum effectiveness,

the diaphragm should be used with a spermicide and left in place for at least six hours after intercourse. The failure rate is about 5 per 100, but is higher if the diaphragm does not fit well or is not used properly.

Q: *How do spermicides work?*

A: Spermicides are chemicals available as jellies, foams, or pessaries that kill sperm in the vagina. They are inserted high into the vagina with an applicator, at least five minutes before intercourse and must be reapplied before further intercourse. Spermicides should never be used alone.

Q: *How does an IUD work?*

A: The intrauterine device (IUD) is a small, flexible piece of plastic that is inserted into the womb through the vagina. It is usually shaped as a coil, loop, or ring, and may contain copper, zinc, or progesterone. The copper, zinc, or progesterone is believed to increase the effectiveness of the plastic, but exactly how an IUD works is not known.

Q: *Can any woman use an IUD?*

A: Some forms of IUD, such as the loop and the coil, are best suited to women who have borne children. Also, women who suffer particularly heavy periods are advised against using an IUD, since it tends to increase the menstrual flow.

Q: *How is an IUD fitted?*

A: A woman must consult a gynecologist, who first examines her carefully for infection or pregnancy. A thin plunger containing the IUD is then inserted through the cervix into the womb, where

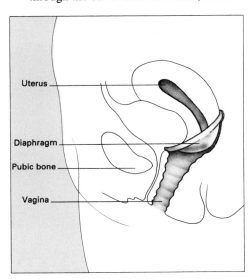

Diaphragm has a springy outer rim that holds it in position over the entrance to the uterus.

Contraception

it is released. Insertion is easiest during a period, when the cervix expands a little.

Q: *What are the side effects of an IUD?*

A: After insertion there may be intermittent bleeding and some abdominal cramp, as the womb tries to expel the IUD, but these symptoms should disappear after a few weeks. Another side effect is that the first few periods may be heavier and cause more backache than usual.

Q: *What happens if the side effects of the IUD persist?*

A: A woman should consult her gynecologist, in case she is not suited to an IUD. If side effects are accompanied by irritation and a heavy vaginal discharge, they may be caused by an infection. This infection can spread from the womb to the fallopian tubes and may lead to infertility if left untreated.

Any woman with an IUD should have regular gynecological checkups.

Q: *Is the IUD a safe and effective contraceptive?*

A: Yes. Although about ten percent of users expel the device, serious complications are unusual and fewer than those from the contraceptive pill. An IUD does not need a spermicide and is less bother than a condom or a diaphragm. The failure rate is about 2 in 100.

Q: *What is the birth control pill?*

A: Oral contraceptives, or the pill, were introduced in the 1950's as hormone preparations used to prevent pregnancy. The pill must be prescribed by a physician. It is by far the most reliable

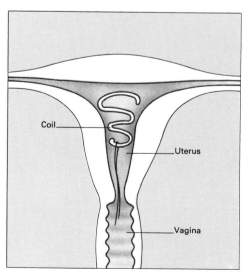

Coil is thought to work as a contraceptive by preventing the implantation of a fertilized egg.

contraceptive, and possible side effects are its only drawback. Recently, side effects have been greatly reduced by using the lowest dosage of hormone capable of preventing pregnancy.

Q: *How does the pill work?*

A: There are many different types of birth control pills, but they all contain synthetic preparations of one or both of the hormones known as estrogen and progesterone. The estrogen works by preventing ovulation each month in the same way as the natural hormones do during pregnancy. As a result, there is no egg to be fertilized by the sperm. The progesterone has three functions: (1) it helps to prevent ovulation; (2) it thickens the cervical mucus, thus presenting a barrier to the sperm; and (3) it affects the lining of the womb, making it unreceptive to a fertilized egg.

Q: *What is the combined pill?*

A: This pill has both estrogen and progesterone hormones. One pill is taken each day for three weeks in the menstrual cycle, thus allowing menstruation to occur in the fourth week, when no pills are taken. The withdrawal of hormones usually produces a lighter and shorter period. The first course of pills is started on the fifth day after menstruation starts, but additional contraceptive precautions must be taken for at least two weeks during the first course. The failure rate is about 0.025 in 100.

Q: *How does the progesterone-only pill work?*

A: This so-called "minipill" relies solely on the effects of progesterone. The dosage is continual and low, and menstruation occurs irregularly, sometimes with breakthrough bleeding between periods. It is essential that the pill be taken each day, preferably at the same time. If two consecutive pills are missed, the woman must use an additional means of contraception until her next period. Even when used correctly, the minipill incurs a higher risk of pregnancy than the combined pill. The failure rate is about 1 in 100.

Q: *What are the side effects of the pill?*

A: Common side effects of the pill are: (1) occasional nausea and weight gain, which may occur in the early weeks of use; (2) an increase in tenderness of the breasts and in vaginal discharge; (3) variable effect on the skin, with either an improvement in, or worsening of, acne, and occasionally a brownish discoloration of the face (chloasma); (4) slight fatigue or weariness in muscles, loss of sexual drive, and mild depression; (5) increase or decrease in headaches and migraine; and (6) spotting and breakthrough bleeding. (Spotting is slight blood loss from the womb, and the pill should be continued for the rest of the cycle. Breakthrough bleeding is like normal menstruation, and the pill should be stopped and a new cycle started after a week.)

If adverse symptoms persist for more than two or three months, a gynecologist should be consulted, because a different preparation may be needed.

Q: *What are the more serious complications associated with the pill?*

A: (1) A woman's fertility may be affected temporarily after she stops taking the pill and before the return of normal menstruation. This happens more often to women whose periods have previously been irregular. (2) Although diabetes is not caused by the pill, mild diabetes may be made worse by it. (3) Hypertension may occur in some women, particularly in those who have had high blood pressure in pregnancy. (4) Recent studies have shown that thrombosis has slightly increased in women taking a pill containing estrogen. The risk of thrombosis increases in those over the age of thirty-five, but the risk is much less than that associated with pregnancy and childbirth.

Q: *Is it true that the pill can cause cancer?*

A: Research is still continuing, but there is no conclusive evidence yet that the pill causes cancer of the breast or the womb.

Q: *Can any woman take the pill?*

A: The pill should be prescribed only after a gynecologist has made a thorough examination and selected the type of pill most suited to the woman. Any woman using the pill should have regular pelvic examinations and cervical smear (Pap) tests.

Q: *Is there a surgical form of contraception?*

A: Yes. Surgical sterilization may be performed on men or women to make them infertile. It is a minor operation for either, but one that is difficult to reverse. Sterilization of men is known as vasectomy; sterilization of women is known as tubal ligation.

Q: *How should a woman decide which contraceptive to use?*

A: In a younger woman, the combined pill is the safest and most convenient form of contraception, unless there are reasons why she cannot use it. Women often express anxieties about continuing it for possibly fifteen or twenty years. In this case, they may use the IUD, which offers

convenience and safety, provided it does not cause side effects. If an IUD is uncomfortable, a woman may try the diaphragm or return to the pill.

The increasing awareness of the hazards of pregnancy after the age of forty leads many women at this age to choose sterilization. It is important that, before selecting a contraceptive, a woman consult her gynecologist, consult the nearest branch of Planned Parenthood, and talk to other women friends to learn about each method and its hazards.

Contrecoup injury is an injury to one side of the brain as a result of a blow to the head on the opposite side. For example, a blow on the back of the head can cause the front parts of the brain to be rotated and bruised.

Contusion is a superficial injury in which the skin is not broken, often producing a bruise. There may be pain, swelling, and a discoloration of the skin.

Convalescence is the period of recovery from the end of an acute stage of an illness or operation to the return of a normal level of health and activity. During this period, a person may be weak and in need of both physical and psychological help.

Q: *What practical measures should be provided during convalescence?*

A: Most of the specific measures provided during convalescence are, of course, determined by the person's physician. There are, however, some general measures that are applicable to

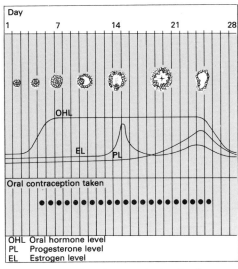

Oral contraception changes the levels of hormones in the blood and stops ovulation.

Convulsion

most people during convalescence. For example, conditions favoring rest should be provided. Meals should be small in quantity but more frequent than normal to help encourage the return of a healthy appetite. As the person's strength returns, regular exercise such as walking should be encouraged to help restore normal muscle tone. The person's morale will benefit from companionship, especially during a long convalescence.

Convulsion (for EMERGENCY treatment, *see* First Aid, p.534) is a series of sudden muscular spasms, activated by the brain and involving contortions as muscles alternately contract and relax. Loss of consciousness is also usual. A convulsion (also called a seizure or fit) may occur as a symptom of various disorders: epilepsy; infection in the brain (for example, encephalitis or meningitis); drug withdrawal; diabetes; high fever, particularly in children; brain tumor; arteriosclerosis (in elderly people); toxemia of pregnancy; and poisoning.

Q: What immediate treatment should be given?

A: Most importantly, the patient should be protected against injuring himself or herself. No spoons, pencils, or other hard objects should be placed in the mouth. An unconscious patient should be turned on his side, which will have the effect of keeping the airway open and prevent choking. A convulsion in a feverish child may be prevented by sponging with cool or tepid water, so that heat is lost by evaporation. A diabetic should be given

sweets or sugar because the convulsions may be caused by excess insulin.

Extra sugar is not harmful to a diabetic in such circumstances.

Cooley's anemia. *See* THALASSEMIA.

Cordotomy is an operation to cut some of the nerves in the spinal cord. It is a method sometimes used by surgeons for relieving chronic severe pain.

Corn is the thickening of the skin on or between the toes. It is usually produced by friction or pressure caused by tight or ill-fitting shoes. If present on exposed surfaces, a corn is hard; if it occurs between the toes, it is soft and may become inflamed.

See also First Aid, p.585.

Cornea is the clear transparent layer on the front of the eyeball. Its curvature is greater than that of the other layers of the eyeball, and so it acts (with the lens) to bend light rays and focus them onto the retina at the back of the eye.

Corneal graft is a form of eye surgery in which a damaged cornea is replaced by a healthy cornea, usually taken from a deceased donor. A cornea removed from the eye of a deceased donor within six hours of death can be preserved in special frozen solutions before it is needed for a corneal graft.

Q: How might the cornea be damaged?

A: Scarring of the cornea from injury or disease often renders it useless. If the damage is severe, a graft may not be possible. In such cases it may be possible to replace the cornea with one made from plastic.

Coronary generally refers to the heart. The term "coronary" is also sometimes used to mean a HEART ATTACK, in which case it is actually an abbreviation of "coronary thrombosis."

See also CORONARY HEART DISEASE.

A talk about Coronary heart disease

Coronary heart disease is any damage to the heart muscle resulting from reduced blood supply from the two coronary arteries, which encircle the heart. Normal blood supply is reduced by the narrowing of any section of an artery. The type of ARTERIOSCLEROSIS known as atherosclerosis, a build-up of fatty deposits in the arterial walls, is the most common cause, and the artery most commonly affected is the first descending branch of the left coronary artery.

Q: What are the symptoms of coronary artery disorders?

A: Sometimes a pain in the center of the chest (angina pectoris) occurs during

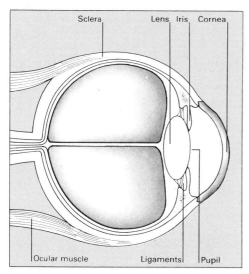

Labels: Sclera, Lens, Iris, Cornea, Ocular muscle, Ligaments, Pupil

Cornea is the transparent front portion of the sclera, the fibrous coat that surrounds the eye.

exercise. Such pain usually vanishes when the exercise ceases. Often there are no symptoms at all until thrombosis (occlusion) shuts off the blood supply completely. This causes death of part of the heart muscle, a condition known medically as myocardial infarction. In popular usage it is called a "coronary," "heart attack," or "infarct." For EMERGENCY, *see* First Aid pp.562–565.

See also HEART DISEASE.

Q: *What are the symptoms of a heart attack?*

A: The patient usually complains of severe, tight, constricting pain in the chest. This may extend to the shoulders, arms, hands, into the neck and jaw, and sometimes down into the upper abdomen. The pain may be accompanied by shortness of breath, nausea, and sweating. A patient with these symptoms should be hospitalized as soon as possible. It is also possible to have a "silent" heart attack, with no symptoms, which may only be discovered much later on an electrocardiogram (EKG).

Q: *How long does the pain last?*

A: The pain may last for a few minutes to several hours, after which the patient is exhausted.

Q: *Does the heart stop beating?*

A: If the condition is severe, it is possible for the heart to stop beating, which causes death if the heartbeat is not restored immediately.

Q: *How is a heart attack diagnosed?*

A: The diagnosis of a heart attack is made using several factors: (1) by studying the patient's history of pain; (2) by observing characteristic changes in the electrocardiogram; (3) by detecting the presence of various enzymes in the blood.

Q: *What is the treatment for a heart attack?*

A: The patient may be admitted to a coronary care unit, where electrocardiographic monitoring is done to detect any irregularities in the pulse. Such irregularities may indicate that the heart may be about to stop. Pulse irregularities can be treated with drugs. Injections of painkilling drugs can be given if needed. Some patients may be given anticoagulant drugs (for example, heparin or warfarin) to prevent thrombosis. After two to three days, the most dangerous period is over and the patient is usually permitted to get out of bed. This reduces the chance of deep vein thrombosis in the legs.

Q: *For how long may a coronary heart disease patient be hospitalized?*

A: It depends on the severity of the

Coronary heart disease

obstruction to the blood supply of the heart, and any complications. But a patient may be hospitalized for about ten days to three weeks.

Q: *What advice can be given about convalescence?*

A: The patient should live a quiet and relaxed life, without stress, and gradually take a little exercise. The taking of anticoagulant drugs may be continued at home for several weeks. Sexual intercourse may be resumed after the first month. Heavy lifting and strains should be avoided for two months following the attack. After six weeks, the dead muscle in the heart will have been replaced by scar tissue. To strengthen the heart, the physician may recommend increasing amounts of exercise.

Q: *Does a heart attack alter the life style of a patient?*

A: There are a number of precautions that a patient must observe for life. Most physicians advise physical exercise for 10–15 minutes a day. Initially, exercises may be taught at a coronary rehabilitation center, where monitoring equipment shows up any signs of heart strain in the patient.

A person who has had a heart attack must never smoke, but can drink alcohol in reasonable quantities if it does not interfere with a weight-reducing, low cholesterol diet. If the patient suffers from hypertension (high blood pressure), this must be treated and kept well under control.

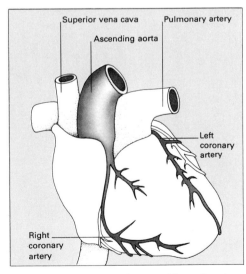

Coronary heart disease is caused by reduced blood supply in the two coronary arteries.

Corpuscle

Q: *What are the complications of coronary heart disease?*

A: Damage to the electrical conducting mechanism of the heart may cause atrial FIBRILLATION, with the symptom of an irregular, rapid pulse. Congestive heart failure (due to inadequate pumping by the heart) may occur at times, and if the heart muscle has been damaged, ANGINA PECTORIS may be a complication. Angina pectoris may also precede a heart attack.

Q: *Are certain groups more prone to coronary heart disease than others?*

A: Four times as many men as women have coronary heart disease; also it tends to affect more men earlier in life than women. Coronary heart disease is more common in women after menopause. There is a high incidence of the disorder in the following groups: smokers; those with hypertension; the overweight; those with high blood cholesterol levels; those with physically inactive jobs; and those with anxious or aggressive dispositions. The possibility of a heart attack is greatly increased in those who have had one already, those who have a family history of them, and those who are diabetic.

Q: *Is it possible to prevent coronary heart disease?*

A: Patients who are overweight, who are hypertensive, who smoke, or who are inactive with a high cholesterol level can reduce the chances of heart attacks by changing their habits appropriately.

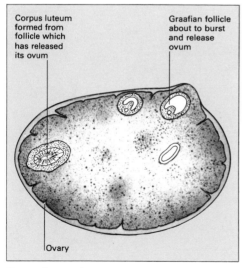

Corpus luteum formed from follicle which has released its ovum

Graafian follicle about to burst and release ovum

Ovary

Corpus luteum is a structure that develops in an ovary and secretes progesterone.

Corpuscle is the medical term for any small, rounded body. It is usually applied to blood cells: red blood corpuscles (erythrocytes) and white blood corpuscles (leukocytes).

Corpus luteum is a small, yellow hormone-producing structure that develops in an ovary at the site of a released egg (ovum). In addition to the hormone called estrogen, also being produced by the ovaries and the adrenal glands, the corpus luteum produces progesterone. These hormones prepare the lining of the womb (endometrium) for the implantation of a fertilized ovum. If conception takes place, and an ovum becomes fertilized, the corpus luteum remains; if not, it degenerates and shrinks when menstruation starts.

Cortex is the outer layer of an organ, as distinct from the inner portion (medulla). For example, the CEREBRAL CORTEX is the layer of nerve cells (gray matter) on the surface of the brain, and the adrenal cortex is the outer layer of an adrenal gland.

Corticosteroid drugs are synthetic derivatives of CORTICOSTEROIDS used to treat Addison's disease, allergies, rheumatic disorders, and inflammation. They must be used with particular care in the presence of infection.

See also ALDOSTERONE; CORTISOL.

Corticosteroids (corticoids) are various steroid hormones produced in the outer layer (cortex) of the adrenal glands. The term is also used for a number of synthetic derivatives (corticosteroid drugs) that have similar properties to the natural hormones.

There are three main groups of naturally-occurring corticosteroids: (1) ALDOSTERONE, which regulates the excretion of sodium and potassium salts through the kidney; (2) CORTISOL (hydrocortisone), which promotes the synthesis and storage of glucose and regulates fat distribution within the body; and (3) sex hormones, which have only a minor effect on the body of an adult. Aldosterone and cortisol are essential to life, and they affect many chemical processes within the body. They work together to maintain a constant internal environment, despite the fact that the body is continually subjected to changes.

Corticotropin. *See* ACTH.

Cortisol (hydrocortisone) is the most important naturally occurring of the CORTICOSTEROIDS. It controls the level of glucose, fats, and water in the body. Several synthetic cortisol drugs are available. They all work by preventing the body's normal reaction to disease or damage. This effect can be useful in treating such conditions as allergy or inflammation, but cortisol drugs must never be used if infection is present.

Q: *What are the medical uses of cortisol?*

A: It is given in small daily doses to treat ADDISON'S DISEASE, in which there is a lack of natural cortisol. In tablet form it is used to treat some types of asthma, muscle pains, acute allergies, and some forms of cancer. As an injection it is used to treat some rheumatic conditions (for example, rheumatoid arthritis) and shock. Cortisol is also available in cream, lotion, and ointment forms, which are used to treat localized inflammation of the skin and eyes. A recent use of cortisol is in the suppression of organ rejection following transplant operations.

Q: *Can cortisol produce any adverse effects?*

A: Yes. Although the level of naturally-produced cortisol is carefully regulated by the body, excessive use of cortisol as a drug can lead to serious complications. It may cause diabetes, calcium loss from bones (osteoporosis), weight increase, and muscle weakness. Wounds heal slowly and the onset of infections and internal abscesses may be overlooked, because cortisol prevents the body from reacting normally. Prolonged use of cortisol may cause acne and red stripes on the skin because of changes in metabolism; the adrenal glands may also stop working. This may cause problems when trying to reduce the dosage, which must be done gradually to allow the adrenal glands to recover.

People taking cortisol should carry a card stating they do so, in case they are involved in a traffic accident or similar emergency.

Cortisone is one of the CORTICOSTEROID hormones. It is inactive until changed into CORTISOL by the liver.

Coryza. *See* COMMON COLD.

A talk about Cosmetic surgery

Cosmetic surgery is a form of surgery done to improve a person's appearance. It is a branch of PLASTIC SURGERY.

Q: *Why do people have cosmetic surgery?*

A: Usually because they are distressed or dissatisfied by their natural face or figure, or because they have been involved in a disfiguring accident. Skillful surgery can alleviate mental as well as physical anguish, giving or restoring confidence to those who would otherwise avoid normal contacts.

Q: *What kinds of cosmetic repairs can be made?*

A: Almost any kind that is required. A cleft lip may be closed; a hand made immobile by scars can be restored to function; injuries to the face, from car accidents or industrial accidents, can be repaired by sculpting and realigning the delicate bones. In such cases, wires and splints are used to reconstruct facial features, and flaps of muscle fill the vacant spaces left by bone that has been destroyed or removed. Bone grafts may also be used.

Women who are dissatisfied with the shape or size of their breasts can have them altered by MAMMOPLASTY. Some physicians, however, question the safeness of such techniques.

Q: *What other methods of cosmetic surgery are there?*

A: Skin GRAFTS are sometimes made to cover large raw areas, as in severe burns, and to serve as an efficient dressing to protect the raw area from infection and loss of body fluid. A thin layer of skin is surgically removed from one part of the body and laid over the injured area, where the skin cells are soon nourished by the tiny blood vessels of the injured area.

Pitting of the skin, caused by acne or smallpox for example, may be treated by a dermatologist with surgical planing, often called dermabrasion. In this method, a local anesthetic is given, and the doctor uses a rapidly rotating wire brush to remove the pitted surface of the skin. Healing takes place beneath a scab in a little more than a week. The new skin that forms is usually a great

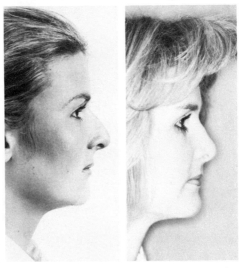

Cosmetic surgery performed on the nose (left) results in a smaller nose with a better shape.

Cough

improvement over the scarred and pitted one. Wrinkles, if they are not deep, may also be removed or made less conspicuous in this way.

Another method used is cryotherapy, in which the skin is frozen with solid carbon dioxide. This produces peeling of old, scarred, or wrinkled skin.

Q: Can scars result from cosmetic surgery operations?

A: Every surgical operation leaves a scar, but its size depends partly on the skill of the surgeon and partly on the healing properties of the individual.

Cough is an action that clears an irritated area of the lungs or throat. It is a common symptom of a number of disorders, such as a common cold, influenza, or a minor respiratory illness. A cough may also accompany a serious lung disorder or heart disease.

Any cough that lasts for more than a few days should be discussed with a physician.

Q: Should medicine be taken to stop a cough?

A: Coughing is a useful and protective mechanism, and treatment that completely suppresses it could do more harm than good. When a person coughs, a deep breath is taken in, the vocal cords close, and pressure builds up within the lungs. When the cords open, a violent expulsion of air takes place as the body attempts to expel any foreign material in the throat or lower respiratory tract.

Cough syrups that help the person to bring up phlegm are called EXPECTORANTS,

and many kinds are available without prescription from a drugstore. Other preparations containing ANTIHISTAMINES may help to dry up secretions. A cough suppressant, sometimes prescribed by a physician, contains a drug such as codeine or dextromethorphan.

Q: Apart from infection, what else can cause a cough?

A: Smoking can produce a cough, especially in the morning, because in people who smoke the lining of the air passages to the lungs (the bronchi) is damaged and the lungs fail to empty themselves naturally during the night.

Q: What can be done for a dry cough?

A: Eating something dry, a soda cracker or a cookie, may help to stop the irritating tickle. In a dry, overheated room, a vaporizer can relieve congestion of the nose and throat membranes.

Sometimes a dry cough, especially in a child, can be exhausting and debilitating, as in PERTUSSIS (whooping cough) or some of the virus illnesses that commonly occur during the winter months. In such cases, a medicine that suppresses the cough to some extent is helpful, but should be used only on medical advice.

Cowpox, medical name vaccinia, is an infection of cattle that can cause a mild illness in human beings. It is the virus originally used by Edward Jenner in 1796 for vaccinating human beings against SMALLPOX. In the milk cow, the udder and teats are affected by a slight eruption. Similar, pus-filled blisters appear on the skin of human beings who have either been inoculated with cowpox vaccine or been in contact with infected cows.

Coxalgia is the medical name for pain in the hip.

Coxa vara is a deformity of the thighbone (femur). The angle of the neck of the bone, where it joins the part leading to the hip joint, is reduced. This makes the knee move inward. Coxa vara is much more common than the associated condition coxa valga, in which the bone angle is increased.

There are various possible reasons for coxa vara: it may be congenital; caused by a fracture; or caused by a softening of the bone from rickets, osteomalacia, or parathyroid disease. The condition may also result from any injury during childhood that causes the head of the thighbone to slip or move out of position. The patient has a limp because one of the legs acts as if it were shorter than the other. There is often pain in the hip (coxalgia).

Treatment depends upon the cause, which should be diagnosed by a bone specialist.

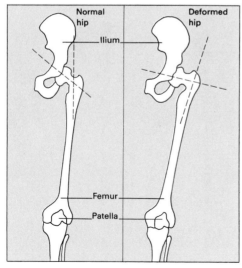

Normal hip	Deformed hip
Ilium	
Femur	
Patella	

Coxa vara is a deformity of the hip that may occur as a result of injury, or rickets.

Coxsackie infection is caused by a family of viruses that can produce a number of serious disorders, including a severe, influenzalike illness (Bornholm disease) and a virus form of meningitis. It is named for a city in New York State where it was first isolated in 1948. Diagnosis is usually made by means of blood tests after the patient has recovered, and treatment is with painkilling drugs and rest.

Cramp is a sudden, involuntary, and often painful contraction of a muscle or a group of muscles. The affected muscles may become hard and knotted. Cramp in the abdomen is sometimes called colic, and cramp in the leg is popularly called a charleyhorse. Cramp may occur after prolonged exercise, such as swimming; at night, especially in the elderly and usually affecting the leg muscles; or at the start of menstruation. The causes of cramp are not fully understood, but in some cases cramp may be caused by salt loss from excessive sweating or diarrhea, or from poor blood circulation.

Q: How can cramp be treated?
A: Because the causes of cramp are so little understood, there is no single treatment for all types of cramp. Stretching and warming the affected muscle may help. Drinking water to which salt has been added may relieve cramp caused by salt loss. If cramp occurs frequently, especially in the calf muscles after walking (intermittent claudication), a physician should be consulted because there may be a more serious underlying cause, such as a disorder of the blood circulation.

Craniotomy is an operation to make an opening in the skull, as a preliminary to brain surgery.

Cranium is the anatomical name for the skull. It usually refers to the part that surrounds the brain, but excludes the bones of the face and the jaw.

Cretinism is a condition of stunted body growth and impaired mental development. The symptoms, which appear during early infancy, are the gradual development of a characteristic coarse, dry skin, a slightly swollen face and tongue, and an open mouth that drools. The baby is usually listless, slow moving, constipated, and a slow feeder. Cretinism is the result of a congenital deficiency in the secretion of the hormone thyroxine from the thyroid gland. In some cases this is thought to be caused by an insufficient amount of iodine in the diet of the child's mother during pregnancy.

Q: How is cretinism treated?
A: After the condition has been diagnosed with the help of blood tests, treatment with thyroid hormone promotes normal physical and mental development. It is essential that treatment be started during the first six weeks of life, or irreversible changes may take place.

Crib death. *See* SIDS.

Crohn's disease (regional ileitis or regional enteritis) is a chronic inflammatory condition of the intestine. There is no known cause for the disease, although it may be hereditary. It is usually confined to the lower end of the small intestine (ileum), but may involve the large intestine (colon). The symptoms of Crohn's disease include intermittent attacks of diarrhea and abdominal pain, weight loss, and fever. Rarely, the intestine may burst (causing PERITONITIS) or become blocked, or ulcerate into adjacent areas. Treatment involves a nutritious diet, painkilling drugs, antibiotics, and sometimes corticosteroids. If complications occur, the physican usually recommends surgery to remove the diseased section of intestine.

Cross-eye. *See* STRABISMUS.

Cross infection is the infection of one patient by another. This is a serious problem in hospitals, especially if the disease-producing organism is resistant to most antibiotics.

Croup is an acute breathing disorder, most often occurring in young children. The mucous membrane of the larynx, trachea, and bronchial tubes becomes inflamed and swollen, and produces excessive mucus.

Q: What causes croup?
A: Respiratory infections caused by various kinds of virus can often result in croup.

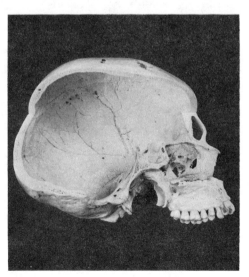

Cranium is that portion of the skull that encloses the brain.

Crush syndrome

However, a more serious but less common kind of croup, called membranous croup, occurs most often as a symptom of diphtheria.

Q: *What are the symptoms of croup?*

A: For most cases of croup, there is loss of appetite, high fever, difficulty in breathing, and a barking cough that ends with a whistle upon inhalation. Only in the most severe cases of croup do certain other symptoms occur, such as cyanosis (blue-tinged skin) due to insufficient oxygen. This condition is a medical emergency.

Q: *How are most cases of croup treated?*

A: The mildly ill child may be cared for at home. He or she should be made comfortable and be given plenty of liquids. Rest is important. A vaporizer may be used to aid breathing.

Crush syndrome is the failure of the kidneys and liver to function after severe injuries, especially a crushed leg. It occurs because large amounts of proteins from damaged muscles have been released into the circulation system, and the kidneys cannot cope with them; shock is another factor. Treatment of this very serious condition requires hospitalization. KIDNEY DIALYSIS may be necessary until the kidneys recover.

Cryosurgery is a surgical technique in which tissues are exposed to extreme cold, usually below −4°F (−20°C). It is used to remove cataracts and malignant tumors. Cryosurgery is also used in brain surgery, in the treatment of cervical erosion and warts, and to reduce bleeding.

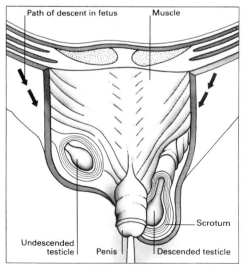

Cryptorchidism is the failure of a testis to descend from the abdomen to the scrotum.

Cryptorchidism (cryptorchism), commonly known as undescended testicles, is the condition in which one or both of the testicles have not descended into the scrotum. It is often accompanied by a hernia in the groin.

Q: *Why does cryptorchidism occur?*

A: The reason is not known. The testicles develop in the abdomen of a fetus, and before birth they descend through the abdominal wall into the scrotum. If this fails to happen, cryptorchidism results. In many boy babies the testicles appear to be absent, because the attached muscles pull them up to the abdominal wall. This is perfectly normal and should not be confused with cryptorchidism.

Q: *How is cryptorchidism treated?*

A: If the testicle can be located outside the abdomen an operation may be performed to fix the testicle in the scrotum. If the testicle is in the abdomen, major surgery is involved. It may still not be possible to find the testicle. An alternative, but less certain, method is the administration of human chorionic gonadotrophic hormone, which may stimulate the testicle to descend.

Curare is the general name for a wide variety of chemical extracts derived from several South American trees. Curare causes rapid paralysis of the muscles throughout the body and was originally used on poisonous arrows by the South American Indians. A refined preparation of curare called d-tubocurarine may be used as a muscle relaxant drug during generel anesthesia.

Curettage is the scraping clean of the interior of a body cavity with a spoon-shaped instrument called a curette. *See* D AND C.

Cushing's syndrome is a rare glandular disorder in which there is excessive production of cortisol and similar corticosteroids by the adrenal glands. Cushing's syndrome may occur spontaneously or it may be caused by a tumor of the adrenal glands, or a tumor of the pituitary gland, causing an excessive amount of corticotropin to be produced and overstimulation of the adrenal glands. Cushing's syndrome may also result after prolonged medication with large doses of corticosteroid drugs.

Q: *What are the symptoms of Cushing's syndrome?*

A: The symptoms of Cushing's syndrome include fatty swellings on the back of the neck; a characteristic "moon face"; fatigue; weakness; obesity of the trunk, while the limbs remain thin; and skin discoloration with pink streaks. There may also be excessive hair growth, reduced sex drive in men, and the cessation of menstruation in women. In cases where the cause is cancer, Cushing's syndrome may be fatal.

Q: How can Cushing's syndrome be treated?

A: There are drugs available that may temporarily control the symptoms, but surgical removal of either the tumor or the overproductive tissue is the most common treatment. Radiation therapy is also sometimes used. If an adrenal gland is surgically removed, there will be a lack of the hormones that it normally produces. Such a lack may be compensated for by taking corticosteroid drugs.

Cut. For treatment of cuts, *see* First Aid, p.588.
See also HEMORRHAGE.

Cutaneous refers to the skin. For example, cutaneous nerves are sensory nerves that are situated in the skin.

Cuticle is a layer covering the free surface of epithelial cells. It may be horny or calcified, as in tooth enamel. The term is also used for the thin outer layer of the skin, often that adjacent to a fingernail.

Cyanosis is a bluish discoloration of the skin, most easily seen in the lips. It is caused by a lack of oxygen in the blood. This, in turn, may be caused by sluggish surface circulation in cold environments, failure of the lungs to oxygenate the blood fully, pneumonia, heart failure, asphyxiation, or overdose of certain drugs. It also occurs in children with some forms of congenital heart disease (*see* BLUE BABY). Treatment depends on the cause.

Cyclamate is any salt of cyclamic acid. In the United States cyclamates are not generally available because they were implicated as cancer-forming agents (carcinogens) in experiments on animals.

Cyclopropane is a colorless gas that is used as a general anesthetic. *See* ANESTHETICS.

Cyst is an abnormal swelling or sac that usually contains fluid. Cysts can occur in almost any body tissue, but they are most frequently found in the skin and ovaries, where they may grow to a large size. There are several kinds of cysts: (1) nonmalignant tumors with cells producing liquids that cannot escape; (2) cysts containing cells of tissues that are normally found elsewhere in the body (for example, a DERMOID CYST may contain elements of skin and hair); (3) cysts caused by parasitic infection (for example, *see* HYDATID CYST); and (4) ordinary glands that have become blocked (for example, a sebaceous gland in the skin blocked by a plug of fat forms a sebaceous cyst). Treatment, if any, depends on the type of cyst.
See also TUMOR.

Cysticercosis is a disorder caused by infection with the pork tapeworm (*Taenia solium*). The tapeworm eggs penetrate the intestinal wall and spread throughout the body, causing small cysts in the muscles, eye, heart, liver, or tissue of the central nervous system. During the first weeks of infestation, there may be no symptoms, but later fever, headache, and aching muscles usually occur. Other symptoms may take many years to appear: epilepsy, heart disease, nerve damage, or even personality changes. A physician may diagnose cysticercosis by means of X rays, blood tests, and biopsy. The usual treatment is the removal of any cyst that causes specific problems, or the drug quinacrine.
See also TAPEWORMS.

Cystic fibrosis is a noncontagious, inherited disorder in which mucus secretions from several parts of the body become thick and sticky and interfere with normal functioning. Commonly affected are the lungs, liver, and pancreas. Mucus in the lungs can block the bronchi, making breathing difficult. Thick mucus can also block the ducts of the liver and the pancreas, causing improper digestion.

Q: What are the symptoms of cystic fibrosis?

A: In most cases, persons with cystic fibrosis seem to be born healthy, but begin showing signs of this disorder between infancy and adolescence. Such signs may include greasy, foul-smelling stool; chronic cough; persistent wheezing; recurrent respiratory problems; and decreased growth rate.

Q: How is cystic fibrosis diagnosed?

A: Along with observation of symptoms common to this disorder, special tests often help in the diagnosis. It seems that the sweat glands are also affected by

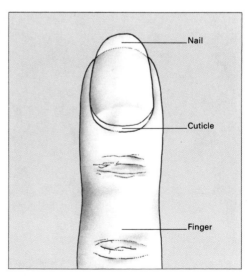

Cuticle is the hard skin around a fingernail or toenail. If it is injured, a hangnail may form.

Cystitis

this disorder and produce excessive amounts of salt, which can be detected by testing perspiration samples.

Q: How is cystic fibrosis treated?

A: There is no known cure for this disorder, which is often fatal during childhood. Treatment usually involves alleviating symptoms. For example, antibiotics to fight infections and special diets to combat malnutrition may be prescribed. Sometimes digestion can be improved by taking missing digestive enzymes. Bronchial drainage is done repeatedly to loosen and remove mucus in the lungs.

A talk about Cystitis

Cystitis is the acute or chronic inflammation of the bladder. It causes frequent, painful, cloudy urination. Milder symptoms may be only a slight increase in the frequency of urination, which is accompanied by a burning sensation. Fever and backache may occur, particularly if infection has spread to the kidneys (pyelonephritis). The pain during urination may be so severe that children refuse to pass urine.

Q: What causes cystitis?

A: Cystitis is usually caused by infection of the bladder, usually from the urethra. Causes other than infection may be the aftereffects of radiotherapy for bladder tumors.

Q: Can other disorders increase the chances of getting cystitis?

A: Yes. The presence of any abnormality

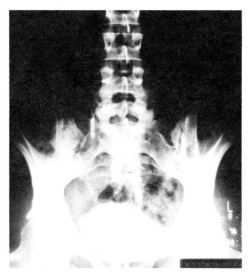

Cystogram is an X ray of the bladder after a radiopaque die has been injected into it.

that affects the bladder may make cystitis more likely: an obstruction that affects the normal flow of urine (for example, an enlarged prostate gland); pouches in the bladder resulting from a birth defect; the presence in the bladder of stones or a tumor; or, in tropical countries, schistosomiasis. A distended womb during pregnancy may obstruct the normal flow of urine and cause cystitis.

Q: How is cystitis diagnosed and treated?

A: Cystitis is usually diagnosed by testing a urine sample for the presence of infection. The disorder can be treated effectively by simple methods. Large quantities of fluids (at least one glass of water every hour) should be drunk. Potassium citrate mixture, an old-fashioned remedy, often brings relief from the burning pain that accompanies urination. A short course of an antibiotic drug may be prescribed by a physician. After an attack of cystitis, a physician may test a urine specimen again to make sure that the infection has disappeared.

Q: Does treatment differ if another attack of cystitis occurs?

A: No, but the disorder should be more fully investigated. This may involve blood tests; examination of the prostate gland; and X rays with intravenous pyelography (IVP) and a cystogram. Sometimes the physician examines the bladder with a special instrument (cystoscope), to make sure that stones or other abnormalities are not present. Urine specimens may have to be examined on several occasions to make sure that a low-grade infection is not present all the time, and to rule out the rare possibility of tuberculosis. Recurrent (chronic) cystitis commonly affects women.

Q: Why is chronic cystitis a common problem in women?

A: In women, the urethra is short, and this makes it easy for bacteria to reach the bladder. Sexual intercourse may move more bacteria into the urethra (honeymoon cystitis).

Q: What precautions might prevent honeymoon cystitis?

A: Simple measures such as emptying the bladder immediately after intercourse remove any bacteria that may have passed up the urethra. Hygiene is important, and the anus should be wiped from front to back to prevent intestinal bacteria from entering the vaginal area. Washing from the groin to the anus should take place twice a day. If these simple measures are not successful, an antiseptic cream should be applied around the vaginal entrance and urinary exit before intercourse. A physician may prescribe a single dose of an antibiotic to be taken after intercourse, so that the first urine that enters the bladder kills the infection before it has time to grow. Most attacks of honeymoon cystitis improve spontaneously with these measures. Sometimes, however, a CYSTOSCOPY is done to make certain there is no anatomical reason for the cystitis.

Cystogram is a special X ray taken after a radiopaque dye has been placed in the urinary bladder, usually after the bladder has been emptied by means of a catheter. X rays can be taken before and during urination to detect the presence of stones in the bladder.
See also CALCULUS.

Cystoscopy is the examination of the inside of the bladder using a special instrument that is equipped with a lens (cystoscope) and a light. The cystoscope is introduced through the urethra, the tube that carries urine from the bladder to the outside of the body. Long, thin instruments can be passed into the bladder to take a biopsy of a tumor, to crush stones, or to treat the bladder tissue.

Cytology is the study of the structure, function, and formation of cells. It is now widely used, for example, in the early diagnosis of cancer, especially cancer of the cervix. *See* CERVICAL SMEAR.

Cytotoxic drugs are drugs that destroy cells or prevent their multiplication. They are mainly used in the treatment of cancer, but are occasionally used to treat other disorders, such as psoriasis. The administration of cytotoxic drugs must be carefully controlled, because excessive doses may cause serious blood disorders, hair loss (alopecia), and reduced resistance to infection.

D

Dacryocystitis is inflammation of the tear sac, caused by a blockage of the duct or by infection from the nose. The symptoms are pain, swelling, and tenderness in the corner of the eye, with the discharge of pus, and tears that cannot drain normally. To treat the condition, a physician may wash the sac with an antibiotic solution, prescribe antibiotic tablets, or resort to surgery.

Dalmane (Trademark) is a preparation of flurazepam hydrochloride, a drug of the benzodia-zepine group. Dalmane is used primarily as a sleep-inducing agent.

D and C is the abbreviation commonly used for dilatation and curettage. Specifically the expression refers to dilatation (stretching) of the cervix, the neck of the uterus, and curettage (scraping with an instrument called a curette) of the inside of the uterus. D and C is a surgical procedure, performed while the patient is under anesthetic. Because pieces of tissue removed by a D and C can be microscopically examined in a laboratory, the technique is valuable for the diagnosis of gynecological disorders. It is also used to remove any placental tissue remaining after an abortion or after childbirth, to clean the inside of the uterus, or as a method of producing an abortion or removing polyps.

Dandruff is a minor condition in which the scalp is dry and scaling, often caused by surface skin glands that do not secrete enough moisture. Dandruff tends to get worse when it occurs with seborrhea (a disorder of the sebaceous glands) or atopic eczema. To treat dandruff the hair should be washed well two or three times a week. A physician may prescribe a preparation containing corticosteroid hormones to be applied at night.

Dapsone is a drug that is used to treat LEPROSY. It is taken by mouth in increasing doses to a maximum of 300 mg a week for three or four years. Side effects may include anemia, fever, and dermatitis.

Daraprim (Trademark) is a commercial preparation of the drug pyrimethamine. It is taken by mouth once a week as protection against MALARIA.

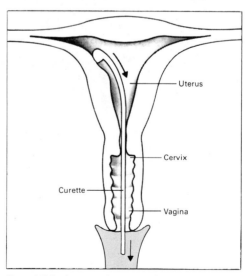

D and C is done under general anesthetic. A curette is used to scrape the uterus lining.

153

Darvocet-N

Darvocet-N (Trademark) is a drug prepared from propoxyphene napsylate and acetaminophen, a combination of a narcotic painkiller and a nonnarcotic painkiller. Its use may produce adverse effects such as dizziness, insomnia, skin rashes, abdominal pain, and constipation. Persons with respiratory disorders should use Darvocet-N with caution. Because Darvocet-N contains a narcotic component, persons taking the drug for a long period may develop a tolerance to it or even a dependence on it.

Darvon (Trademark) is a preparation of the drug propoxyphene hydrochloride. Darvon is a painkiller, available in a number of forms. Its uses and effects are similar to those of DARVOCET-N.

DDT is a common abbreviation of dichlorodiphenyltrichloroethane, now known also as chlorophenothane. DDT was once an extremely effective odorless insecticide, but many pests have now developed an immunity to it. DDT is no longer used when substitutes are available because its presence in foodstuffs is thought to be harmful to animals and human beings. DDT taken through the mouth causes acute poisoning.

Deaf-mute is a person who can neither hear nor speak. The condition exists in a person born totally deaf, who is therefore unable to imitate the sounds of speech. It is possible, using specialized methods, to teach some totally deaf persons how to speak, but those who never learn to speak may instead learn to lip-read and to communicate by fingerspelling, sign language, and body language.

See also DEAFNESS.

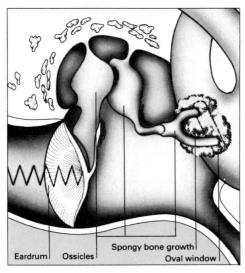

Deafness may be conductive as in otosclerosis when a growth of bone stiffens an ossicle.

Eardrum | Ossicles | Spongy bone growth | Oval window

Deafness is the inability to hear. It may affect both ears or only one, either totally or only partially. Deafness may be present at birth (congenital deafness) or it may occur at any age, suddenly or gradually.

Q: Are there any obvious signs that a person may be deaf?

A: Yes. Deafness may be suspected if a person fails to react to sounds at various levels or speaks more loudly than is necessary. A child who is partially deaf may give the impression of being bored or disinterested and will have difficulty in learning to speak. Such a child may not progress well at school, and it is often a teacher's report that first leads a parent to suspect that the child may have impaired hearing. Deafness in an older person can lead to a sense of isolation and make the person bad-tempered. The degree of hearing loss, however, depends on the kind of deafness involved.

Q: What different kinds of deafness are there?

A: It is usual to categorize deafness as being either conductive deafness or perceptive deafness. Some persons, however, suffer from a combination of the two.

Q: What is conductive deafness?

A: Conductive deafness is hearing loss resulting from interference with the transmission of sound waves through either the outer or the middle ear. Conductive deafness may be either a temporary or a permanent condition.

Q: What causes conductive deafness?

A: Conductive deafness can have many causes, perhaps the most common of which is earwax (cerumen) that obstructs the ear canal and prevents sound waves from reaching the inner ear. Another common cause of conductive deafness is infection of the middle ear (otitis media), which often arises from various childhood diseases, particularly those involving the upper respiratory tract. Infections of the upper respiratory tract often cause swelling in or around a Eustachian tube. This tube connects the middle ear with the nasopharynx and helps equalize air pressure on both sides of the eardrum. When the pressures are unequal, as often happens during upper respiratory tract infections, deafness can result. Flying in aircraft, or deep-sea diving, can also change pressure within the ear and cause conductive deafness. *See* BAROTRAUMA.

Q: How is conductive deafness diagnosed?

A: In addition to direct observation of the signs, otologists and audiologists (specialists in problems of the ears and of hearing) use various tests to diagnose this kind of hearing impairment. One such test involves the use of a tuning fork. If the sound of a vibrating tuning fork is heard more clearly when the fork is placed against the skull than when it is placed close to the ear, the deafness is likely to be conductive. Specialists may then use an audiometer to determine the degree of deafness and X-ray photographs of the skull to pinpoint obstructions that may be causing the deafness.

Q: *How is conductive deafness treated?*

A: Treatment depends on the cause. For example, if earwax is the cause, removal of the wax often restores hearing. This removal should be done only by a trained person, however, because an untrained person may force the wax deeper into the ear or puncture the eardrum.

Other forms of treatment for conductive deafness may also include antibiotics, as in the case of otitis media; draining the fluid build-up from the middle ear; and surgery, in the case of a punctured eardrum or an immobile stapes. Surgery in cases of otosclerosis, called stapes mobilization, is a common and highly successful procedure.

Q: *What is perceptive deafness?*

A: Perceptive, or nerve, deafness arises from the inability of nerve impulses to reach the auditory center of the brain because of nerve damage either to the inner ear or to the brain. For example, nerve damage to the cochlea, which contains the sense organ for hearing (the organ of Corti), can result in perceptive deafness, as can damage to the ear's auditory nerve and nerve damage to the cerebral cortex of the brain.

Q: *What causes perceptive deafness?*

A: Diseases are a common cause of perceptive deafness. The diseases include ANEMIA, ARTERIOSCLEROSIS, INFLUENZA, LEUKEMIA, MÉNIÈRE'S DISEASE, MENINGITIS, MUMPS, RH DISEASE, and SYPHILIS.

Many children born with perceptive deafness have mothers who contracted RUBELLA (German measles) during the first three months of pregnancy. Such a child is called a DEAF-MUTE.

Other causes of perceptive deafness include tumors of the brain or the middle ear, concussion, blows to the ear, and repeated loud sounds. The toxic effects of certain drugs may also cause perceptive deafness in some persons.

Q: *How is perceptive deafness diagnosed and treated?*

A: Together with observation of the obvious signs of deafness, audiologists and otologists use electronic equipment to detect and diagnose perceptive deafness. Such equipment, which includes various types of audiometer, can also help specialists to determine if tumors or other problems are involved in causing the deafness. Perceptive deafness is irreversible and cannot be treated.

Q: *Can hearing aids help all deaf persons?*

A: No. Hearing aids amplify sound, but such devices are helpful only to persons who retain some hearing.

A talk about Death

Death occurs when all activity of the brain ceases and life is completely extinct (*see* DYING). It may come at the end of a long illness, or be sudden and unexpected as the result of an accident or a heart attack. But in every case, every individual person can spare his or her loved ones a great deal of unnecessary anguish by thinking out clearly, in advance, all the details and instructions surrounding arrangements for his or her own death. The funeral will have to be organized; the family must be comforted and cared for; and any other special circumstances, such as a part of the body left for medical research, must be taken into account.

Q: *What is the first thing to think about when death has occurred?*

A: A death certificate will be issued and signed by a physician familiar with the deceased or the physician who was in

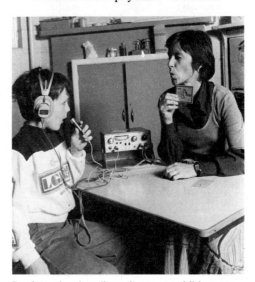

Deafness is a handicap that many children can overcome with the help of specialized training.

155

Debility

attendance at the time of death. When a person dies in a hospital, the certificate will be signed by an attending physician and is obtained from the hospital business office along with any personal effects belonging to the deceased. Receipt of these is usually acknowledged by signature. Copies of the certificate are made available from the health department. In the event of an accidental or unexplained death, the certificate will be issued by the Medical Examiner's office, who may not be able to state the cause of death without performing an autopsy.

Q: *Isn't an autopsy too harrowing for the relatives to bear at this time?*

A: It is as distasteful to the hospital staff as it is to the bereaved to have to face the decision to perform an autopsy at this most grievous time. But so much has been learned from autopsy studies that the request should never be resented.

Q: *How are the arrangements made for the funeral?*

A: The services of a capable funeral director can considerably ease the administrative burden of death arrangements. On notification by the family, the funeral director obtains permission to remove the body to the funeral home, consults with a responsible relative on details of casket, service, burial or cremation, hours of visiting so that people can pay their respects, whether the head and shoulders are to be on view or the coffin closed, and so on. The director should also take care of press obituaries.

Q: *Who takes care of medical bequests by the deceased?*

A: If the deceased has left his or her body to a medical school, the funeral director will usually convey the body there for a small fee. In cases of sudden, accidental death in young, fit people, consideration must be given to kidney, heart, and liver donation, if facilities are available. If the deceased has bequeathed his or her corneas for transplant or experimental use, the local eye bank (which works closely with the Lions Clubs) will send a technician immediately upon notification. Speed is essential, and it is important to know about such bequests ahead of time.

Q: *What is the best way to help the bereaved relatives?*

A: Somebody must take charge of affairs, and most families look to one or two members to do this. Often it will be the eldest child of the deceased, or an old and trusted friend who may be executor of the estate. It is usually better that the individual concerned be able to be fairly detached, in order to take the burden off the most grieving survivor (usually the deceased's spouse), especially in the choice of a funeral director. The telephone will be in frequent use for a time, and it is advised that the family member who is in charge use a phone nearby, leaving the home phone clear for calls of sympathy and help from other relatives and friends. The family lawyer should be told immediately, particularly if the deceased had left any special instructions. The family priest, minister, or rabbi should also be informed at the earliest opportunity.

Death is a test of a family's strength: it can bring out the best or the worst in family and friends. Perhaps the best guide to conduct is to try to act in a manner that would have been approved of by the deceased.

Average annual death rates for the U.S.

	1	2	3	4	5	6	7	8	9	10	11	12	13	14	15	16
per 1,000 population

1975
1970
1965
1960
1955
1941–1950
1931–1940
1921–1930
1911–1920
1901–1910

Death rate in the U.S. is decreasing because of better nutrition and medical care.

Debility. See WEAKNESS.

Débridement is the cleansing of a wound by the surgical removal of foreign matter and dead or damaged tissue or bone.

Decalcification is the loss of calcium salts from the bones. This condition may occur in persons who are confined to bed for long periods of time, and in persons who are subjected to long periods of weightlessness. Decalcification may result from various disorders: overactive parathyroid glands, causing osteitis fibrosa; rickets and osteomalacia, caused by vitamin D deficiency; and osteoporosis. Local decalcification may be caused by bone tumors (osteosarcomas), or the spread of cancer from other parts of the body. Decalcification may lead to the formation of stones in the kidneys and bladder (*see* CALCULUS).

Decompression sickness. *See* BENDS.

Decongestant is a drug or other agent that reduces any congestion of mucus produced by various mucous membranes, particularly those in the nose. Decongestants should be used strictly according to the prescribed dosage, and for no longer than two or three weeks, or the chemical effects of the drugs may further irritate the mucous membranes and prolong the presence of mucus.

Decubitus ulcer. *See* BEDSORE.

Defecate is the medical term for having a bowel movement. It also applies to the release of feces from an artificial opening that has been made in the intestines, such as a colostomy or an ileostomy.

Defibrillation is the term used for stopping the trembling, or fibrillation, of the heart muscle by means of drugs or an electric shock. In certain conditions, for example, coronary heart disease, the heart may stop beating while the heart muscle continues to fibrillate. Sometimes, normal heart contractions can be restored by electric shocks from a machine called a cardiac defibrillator.

Deficiency diseases are disorders that are caused by a lack or deficiency of a substance that is essential to the proper functioning of the body, such as various vitamins, minerals, and proteins. Deficiency diseases often result from an inadequate diet, but they can also be caused by metabolic disorders such as pernicious anemia (which is caused by inadequate absorption of vitamin B_{12}); intestinal disorders; overexcretion of the substance in the urine, feces, or by vomiting; the presence of a parasite, for example, a hookworm or tapeworm; or by a prolonged illness.

Q: What are the most common deficiency diseases?

A: The most common deficiency diseases are those caused by a lack of vitamins or minerals. They include anemia (lack of iron); scurvy (lack of vitamin C); beriberi (lack of vitamin B_1); night blindness (lack of vitamin A); rickets and osteomalacia (lack of vitamin D); and goiter (lack of iodine).

Q: How are deficiency diseases treated?

A: In most cases the disorder is treated by a special diet that is rich in foods that restore the deficient substance. The diet is sometimes supplemented with vitamin tablets or specific drugs.

See also VITAMINS.

Dehydration is the excessive loss of water from the body. In normal conditions an adult needs about 5 pints (2.4 liters) of water each day to replace that lost by breathing, sweating, urinating, and defecating. If this fluid loss is not replaced, dehydration results.

The major symptom of dehydration in adults is thirst, and muscle cramps may occur if dehydration is combined with fatigue. Dehydration is potentially serious, especially in babies and young children. Danger signs are drowsiness, constipation, wrinkled skin, and a depressed "soft spot" (fontanel) in a young baby's skull. The major causes of dehydration include diarrhea, vomiting, excessive water loss through sweating caused by fever or high air temperatures, illness such as diabetes, and a reaction following surgery.

Q: How is dehydration treated?

A: A seriously dehydrated baby should be hospitalized immediately. A lesser degree of dehydration can be treated with small and frequent drinks of water or milk and water. In adults, dehydration can usually be treated with water to which a little salt has been added. If the cause is a disorder such as cholera or diabetes, hospital treatment is required.

Delhi boil. *See* LEISHMANIASIS.

Delirium is a state of mental confusion and extreme excitement, commonly accompanied by hallucinations and continual but aimless physical activity. Delirium is the immediate result of a disturbance in brain function, but the disturbance itself can be caused by any, or by a combination of several, generally serious, conditions. High fever, particularly

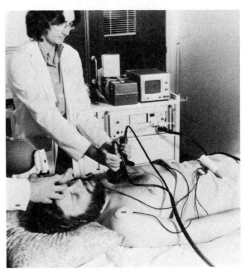

Defibrillation is used either to stop the heart for surgery, or to restart it beating.

Delirium tremens

from pneumonia, may cause delirium, as may malaria, meningitis, encephalitis, or heart failure. Another cause is alcoholism, which can lead to DELIRIUM TREMENS, a dangerous psychiatric disorder that involves both visual and auditory hallucinations. Drug overdoses and some mental disorders, such as schizophrenia, may also cause delirium.

Delirium may be reduced with sedatives or tranquilizers, but hospitalization is generally necessary for treatment of the underlying serious condition.

Delirium tremens (DTs) is a form of DELIRIUM that occurs in severe ALCOHOLISM and in opium addiction. It is a potentially fatal condition, and hospitalization is urgently necessary. Delirium tremens may be acccompanied by epilepsy, pneumonia, and heart and liver failure.

Q: What are the symptoms of delirium tremens?

A: The symptoms of delirium tremens include sleeplessness, anxiety, and nausea, and there is often an aversion to food. Persons with delirium tremens may suffer delusions and hallucinations and become extremely agitated. For example, such persons may experience strange skin sensations, see monstrous creatures, and make wild gestures with the hands.

Q: What is the treatment for delirium tremens?

A: Treatment usually consists, initially, of bed rest, sedation, and a controlled diet. Long-term treatment aims at helping patients to overcome their addiction to alcohol or opium.

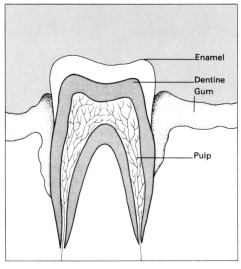

Dentin is a bonelike substance surrounding the tooth pulp and protected by enamel.

Delivery is the final stage of childbirth. The term also includes the expulsion of the placenta. *See* PREGNANCY AND CHILDBIRTH.

Delusion is a false and unshakable belief that is inconsistent with reality. There is no clear distinction between mild, harmless delusions and simple mistakes. Such delusions are thought to be part of a person's normal defense mechanisms, and help to maintain an individual's self-image. But in a serious mental disorder, such as SCHIZOPHRENIA, a person's delusions may be both extreme and harmful. Delusions in such cases are often an integral part of the person's loss of contact with reality. For example, persistent delusions of persecution and grandeur are characteristic of PARANOIA.

Q: How are serious delusions treated?

A: Serious delusions are often difficult to treat because they are usually part of a mental disorder that affects many aspects of the personality. Treatment of the underlying disorder may overcome the delusions, and such treatment may include regular psychiatric consultations and some form of drug therapy. However, hospitalization may become necessary if patients are a danger to themselves or to others.

Dementia is a form of mental deterioration that is often associated with loss of physical control of the body. The progress of dementia is gradual, and it often begins with memory loss, particularly of recent events. This forgetfulness may be accompanied by childish and unreasonable behavior. As deterioration progresses, there may be disturbances of the patient's speech, which may become disconnected and incomprehensible. In the final stages, the patient may be incontinent, unable to perform simple tasks, and unresponsive to his or her surroundings.

There are various causes of dementia, including old age (senile dementia); Alzheimer's disease (presenile dementia); general paralysis of the insane (GPI), a form of syphilis; arteriosclerosis of the arteries serving the brain; alcoholism; schizophrenia; and, rarely, brain tumor.

Dengue (also known as breakbone fever) is an acute tropical disease, caused by a virus infection transmitted by the mosquito *Aedes aegypti*. The disease is rarely fatal. Symptoms include fever, vomiting, skin rash, headache, and severe pains in the muscles and joints. The symptoms often subside after the fifth or sixth day, but then return for another three or four days.

There is no specific treatment, although painkilling drugs and plenty of fluids may ease the symptoms. An attack of dengue is often followed by a period of depression and severe debility before normal health returns.

Dental caries. *See* TOOTH DECAY.

Dental disorders. The following table lists some common disorders of the teeth and gums. These disorders come within the competence of a dentist or an orthodontist. Most disorders have a separate article in the A-Z section of this book.

Symptom	Possible disorder
Teeth	
Decay	PLAQUE (saliva and food sugar containing harmful bacterial enzymes)
Sharp pain	ABSCESS
	TOOTH DECAY affecting the dentin
Temperature sensitive	TOOTH DECAY affecting the enamel and dentin
Dull, throbbing pain	ABSCESS
	TOOTH DECAY affecting the tooth pulp (soft inner part of tooth containing nerves and blood vessels)
	Impacted or emerging tooth
Acute pain	ABSCESS at base of tooth
Loose tooth	Infected GINGIVITIS
	PLAQUE (saliva and food sugar containing harmful bacterial enzymes)
	Deciduous teeth (in young children only)
Overcrowded teeth	MALOCCLUSION
Speckled enamel	Excessive amount of FLUORIDE
Gums	
Irritation	PLAQUE (saliva and food sugar containing harmful bacterial enzymes)
An open sore	CANKER SORE (ulceration of the mouth or lips)
	Badly fitting DENTURES
Pus-filled swelling	ABSCESS due to badly fitting DENTURES
	PYORRHEA

Dentifrice. *See* TOOTHPASTE.

Dentin is the hard substance that makes up a tooth. It surrounds the central pulp, and is itself covered by harder external enamel.

Dentures are artificial teeth. The term may refer to any number of teeth attached to a plastic or metal appliance (plate), which is fitted to the upper or lower jaw. The appliance may be removable or permanently fixed. Dentures should be cleaned at least once a day.

Deodorants are agents used to destroy or disguise odors of the body or the breath. Most body odors arise from the decomposition of bacteria in a mixture of dead skin cells and sweat, usually because a person does not wash often enough (*see* BROMHIDROSIS). Most commercial skin deodorants contain an antiperspirant, such as aluminum chloride, which reduces sweating; usually perfumes are also added. However, care should be taken in the use of deodorants because some can cause skin reactions in those people who are allergic to them.

Bad breath is often caused by food decomposing between the teeth (*see* BAD BREATH). Commercial mouthwashes and deodorants disguise the smell of bad breath but do not treat the cause.

Depersonalization is a term used in psychiatry to describe a loss of personal identity. An individual may seem to ignore or forget about the body, be unaware of pain, or be concerned about a nonexistent disfigurement. Depersonalization is usually associated with mental illness.

Depilatory is a substance or device that removes hair. Chemical depilatories are alkaline creams that remove the hair painlessly without damaging the root. ELECTROLYSIS is a method of removing hair permanently. It destroys each hair root by an electric current. Electrolysis is particularly useful on sensitive areas of the body, but it is impractical for areas of dense hair growth, and may cause inflammation and pain.

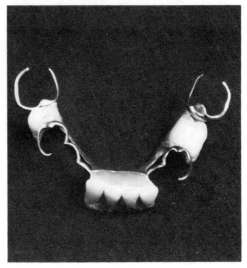

Dentures convincingly replace missing teeth, but need to clip firmly onto those remaining.

159

Depression

A talk about Depression

Depression is a mental state that is characterized by feelings of guilt, lack of hope, melancholy, dejection, and the general feeling that life is not worth living. There may also be an impairment of mental and physical functions, such as appetite, sleep, work, and libido.

Q: What are the signs and symptoms of depression?

A: Boredom, overeating, quietness, inhibitedness, insomnia, pessimism, irritability, an inability to concentrate, and general listlessness may all indicate mild, or normal, depression.

When these signs and symptoms become persistent, however, a more serious type of depression should be suspected. Other indications of serious depression include loss of appetite, loss of weight, constant fatigue, chest pains, and headaches that may become chronic. The abuse of alcohol or other drugs may also indicate a serious depression, and there may be a tendency for seriously depressed persons to offer violence to others or even to harm themselves.

Q: Can depression be normal?

A: Yes, to some degree. Many women, for example, feel depressed prior to menstruation (*see* PREMENSTRUAL TENSION), and the onset of middle age might cause an ordinarily healthy person to feel depressed.

Almost everyone suffers from periods of sadness, grief, loneliness, or discouragement under certain circumstances. It is normal for a person to be depressed by the terminal illness or death of a relative or friend, for example. But this type of depression is generally soon overcome and does not usually cause the person to lose touch with reality.

Q: What is endogenous depression?

A: Endogenous depression is a mental disorder that stems from factors within the person. The depression may affect the victim's personality, and may be so immobilizing that hospitalization is necessary. There are two main types of endogenous depression: manic-depressive psychosis and involutional melancholia.

Manic-depressive psychosis is characterized by alternating periods of high elation (the manic phase) and periods of severe depression with feelings of persecution and a distorted sense of bodily appearance (the depressive phase).

Involutional melancholia occurs in late middle age and is characterized by despondency, possibly suicidal tendencies, and often feelings of personal unworthiness.

Q: What causes depression?

A: The precise underlying causes of depression are not known. Almost anybody can become depressed if subjected to enough emotional stress, but some persons seem to become depressed more easily than others. A personal trauma or stressful event may trigger a depressive episode, and depression frequently occurs with withdrawal from drugs or following a surgical operation. Some types of depression, such as PREMENSTRUAL TENSION and MENOPAUSAL DEPRESSION, are apparently related to a person's metabolism and age.

Many psychiatrists believe that depression may have its roots in the experiences of a person's childhood, and studies undertaken by researchers indicate that some types of depression may run in families. For example, hereditary origins of depression may be suspected in persons who persistently become depressed for no apparent reason. Such persons display many of the common signs of depression for weeks or even months at a time, and then appear to make a gradual and complete recovery, but their depression usually recurs.

Q: What are the dangers of depression?

A: In all types of depression, the main danger is that of suicide. The risk

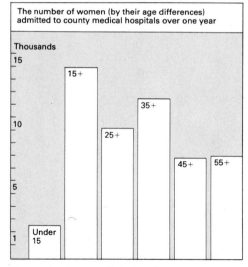

The number of women (by their age differences) admitted to county medical hospitals over one year

Thousands

Depression is most likely to affect a woman during early adulthood and early middle age.

of suicide is always present and cannot be judged by the apparent depth of the depression. Making light of a person's depression, or trying to cheer the person up, is likely to increase the feeling of isolation. And it should not be assumed that the more a person talks of committing suicide the less chance there is of that person actually attempting it.

Q: How is depression treated?

A: Treatment for depression depends on the type of depression and its severity. For example, the so-called normal depression that stems from the death of a relative or friend usually needs no medical treatment. But both persistent mild depression and endogenous depression usually require medical intervention.

Medical treatment for such cases may include psychiatric counseling; drug therapy (such as tranquilizers, sedatives, and antidepressants); and hospital confinement. Hospitalization is imperative for suicidal patients.

In persons who are so ill that their condition constitutes an emergency, electroconvulsive therapy may be necessary (*see* ELECTROCONVULSIVE THERAPY). How this method works is not fully understood.

Above all, persons suffering from depression should be treated with care and consideration, and every effort should be made to reestablish their sense of personal worth.

Dermatitis is inflammation of the skin. There are many different causes, and treatment depends on the diagnosis by a dermatologist. Most forms of dermatitis respond to skin preparations containing corticosteroid drugs. If infections are present, the physician may also prescribe antibiotics and, sometimes, antifungal agents.
See also ECZEMA.

Dermatographia is a form of urticaria (hives). It is a sensitive condition of the skin, in which scratching or rubbing produces raised red areas. The term literally means "skin writing," and gentle drawing of a blunt point over the skin causes visible lines to appear and remain for a time. Usually, dermatographia is not a serious condition and does not require medical treatment.

Dermatology is the branch of medical science concerned with diseases of the skin and the treatment of skin disorders.

Dermoid cyst is a nonmalignant CYST formed from surface skin cells. The cyst may contain elements of skin, hair, sweat glands, and

bone, and forms a small, hard swelling in the body. A dermoid cyst is caused by a fault in the folding of tissues during embryonic development or by a wound that forces surface skin cells under the skin. The usual treatment is surgical removal of the cyst.

DES (diethylstilbestrol) is a synthetic female hormone used primarily to treat postmenopausal symptoms. DES was once used to prevent miscarriages. However, it is no longer so prescribed because it was implicated in the development of vaginal cancer in the offspring of some of the women that had taken DES during pregnancy.

Desensitization is a method of treating an ALLERGY. Tests on the patient identify the substance causing an allergy. Sensitivity is reduced by regular injections of the specific allergen in solutions of increasing strength.

Detached retina is the separation of the retina in the eye from its vascular base, the choroid. It causes partial loss of vision. The symptoms include "floating" specks and transient flashes of light, followed later by a shadow in front of the eye.

Q: How is detachment caused?

A: Detachment results from a hole in the retina that allows fluid to leak through and separate the retina from the choroid. The hole is usually a result of degenerative changes in the retina, most common in nearsighted people, or from a blow on the eye. Detachment may also be caused by a tumor or disease in the eye.

Q: What is the treatment?

A: Various surgical techniques, including the use of laser beams, are used to reseal the

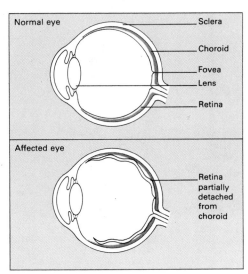

Detached retina is the partial or total separation of the retina from the choroid of the eye.

Deviated nasal septum

retina to the choroid.

Deviated nasal septum is a condition in which the partition in the nose (the septum) is bent, so that it partly blocks one or both nasal passages. Deviation is usually caused by a broken nose, but it may be congenital, or occur for no obvious reason. One nostril may be smaller than the other, with symptoms of snoring, difficulty in breathing, mucus, and recurrent sinusitis.

When a deviated septum causes chronic or acute symptoms, a physician may recommend an operation called a submucosal resection. The deformed part of the septum is removed, and the nose firmly filled with gauze for a few days while it heals. Or, an operation called a septoplasty may be required, to rebuild the septum.

Devil's grip. *See* PLEURODYNIA.

Dexedrine (Trademark) is a preparation of dextroamphetamine sulfate, an amphetamine stimulant. It is used to treat NARCOLEPSY. It can also be used in the treatment of HYPERKINESIS in children.

Like most other amphetamines, Dexedrine increases blood pressure, elevates blood sugar level, dilates the pupils of the eyes, increases respiration rate, and suppresses appetite. Because it suppresses the appetite, Dexedrine was once widely prescribed as a weight reducing drug. However, it is inadvisable to use Dexedrine as an appetite suppressant primarily because it is addictive. The drug has been widely abused so physicians tend to be cautious about prescribing it.

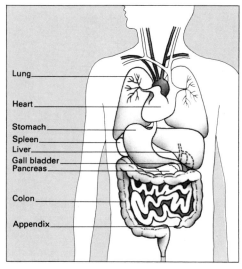

Dextrocardia may be part of a condition in which organs are located abnormally.

Dextrocardia is a congenital abnormality in which the heart is located in the right side of the chest instead of the left. Dextrocardia is often associated with reverse positioning of all the organs, known as situs inversus. In the absence of other associated abnormalities, this condition produces no real problems, although it may cause some confusion in diagnosis of other conditions.

Diabetes is the name of two metabolic disorders that are generally serious. The term by itself is commonly used as an abbreviation of DIABETES MELLITUS, which is one of the two major forms; the other is DIABETES INSIPIDUS.

Diabetes insipidus is a disorder that arises from a hormonal imbalance that makes the kidneys overactive or renders them unable to reabsorb the water passed to them from the blood. A person who has the disorder urinates excessively (polyuria) and has a raging thirst (polydipsia) and a decreased appetite (anorexia). These are symptoms also of DIABETES MELLITUS, but the two disorders are otherwise unrelated.

Q: What are the causes of diabetes insipidus?

A: Diabetes insipidus generally occurs because of a lack of vasopressin, an antidiuretic hormone (ADH) that controls the body's urine output. The hormone is produced in the hypothalamus (a part of the brain) and is stored in and secreted by the pituitary gland. The normal secretion of vasopressin can be disturbed by any disease or injury to either the pituitary gland or the hypothalamus. Other causes of diabetes insipidus include diseases such as encephalitis, meningitis, and syphilis. In extremely rare cases, the cause may be the impaired ability of the kidneys themselves to hold water.

Q: How is diabetes insipidus treated?

A: Following diagnosis by skull X rays and special tests, a physician may advise an injection of ADH to correct the hormone deficiency. Recent treatment involves synthetic ADH used as a nasal spray. If the cause of the disease is a kidney disorder, treatment with a diuretic is sometimes effective. Diabetes insipidus cannot be cured, but treatment greatly improves a patient's condition.

A talk about Diabetes mellitus

Diabetes mellitus, or sugar diabetes, is a disorder in which the body cannot make use of sugars and starches in a normal way. A key element in the proper use of sugar and starches is the hormone INSULIN, which is secreted by special cells (beta cells) in an area of the pancreas known as the ISLETS OF LANGERHANS. Diabetes results from either a lack of insulin or an inability of the body to use the insulin properly, but the cause of diabetes is not known. Damage to the pancreas arising from viral diseases such as measles or mumps may be a cause, and persons may inherit a tendency toward diabetes. Obesity may also be a factor in the onset of diabetes.

There are two major forms of diabetes mellitus, Type I, sometimes called insulin-dependent, or juvenile-type and Type II, sometimes called non-insulin dependent, maturity-onset, or adult-type diabetes. One is usually found in persons under age twenty; the other, in persons over thirty-five.

Diabetes is a serious, sometimes fatal disorder. There are about six million known diabetics in the United States and at least four million estimated unknown diabetics. According to the U.S. National Commission on diabetes, the disease and its complications cause more than 300,000 deaths a year in the United States, making it a leading cause of death.

Q: What causes the imbalance in blood-sugar levels?

A: Normally, food digested in the body releases a form of sugar called glucose into the blood. This increase in blood-sugar level causes beta cells in the pancreas to release insulin, which aids in transporting glucose from the blood to storage in such tissues as the liver and muscle.

In victims of Type 1 diabetes, the pancreas is unable to produce insulin. In Type II diabetes, the pancreas produces some insulin, but the tissues do not respond to it properly. As a result, in both cases, high concentrations of sugar build up in the blood after eating (hyperglycemia). A vicious circle then begins.

The fatty acids released from tissue throughout the body are converted by the liver into biochemicals called ketone bodies. These also pour into the bloodstream, causing a condition in which the blood becomes dangerously acidic (ketoacidosis). This can lead to a diabetic coma and, if untreated, to death.

Q: What are the symptoms of diabetes?

A: The general symptoms of diabetes include increased frequency of urination and persistent thirst. In Type I diabetes these symptoms are often accompanied by weakness and increased appetite.

A physician can diagnose diabetes by testing for sugar in the urine and blood. A GLUCOSE TOLERANCE TEST determines how well the body uses and stores sugar.

Q: What is the treatment for diabetes mellitus?

A: Any diabetic who has lapsed into a coma requires immediate emergency medical attention and must be hospitalized.

Type I diabetics need daily injections of insulin. A physician determines the correct dosage, and patients are taught how to prepare and administer the insulin themselves. The technique is simple, even for children. Most diabetics also test their urine daily for sugar.

A strict diet is important in controlling diabetes to keep the levels of insulin and sugar in the blood from fluctuating too widely. Careful regulation of activity, food intake, and insulin is also necessary to prevent insulin shock (hypoglycemia), in which the insulin level rises too high and blood sugar drops too low.

The first signs of insulin shock are mild hunger, dizziness, sweating, and heart palpitations; then follows mental confusion and coma. Diabetics can stop insulin shock by consuming some substance high in sugar, and should always carry sugar or candy. It is advisable for diabetics to have an identification card, tag, or bracelet so that they will receive emergency care.

Type II diabetes is much easier to control. Some cases are treated with diet

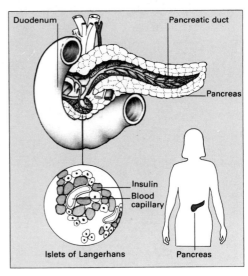

Duodenum — Pancreatic duct — Pancreas — Insulin — Blood capillary — Islets of Langerhans — Pancreas

Diabetes mellitus results when insulin, made by the pancreas, is missing or ineffectual.

Diagnosis

alone, others with diet plus oral antidiabetic drugs. Some cases are treated with insulin.

Most Type II diabetes can be controlled with diet alone, at least at the onset of the illness, if the patient maintains proper body weight. Ninety percent of all adult-type diabetics are overweight at the time of diagnosis.

Q: What complications arise from diabetes mellitus?

A: Diabetics have increased fatty acids in their blood. This predisposes diabetics to atherosclerosis, a type of arteriosclerosis, which may lead to heart disorder and damage to small and large blood vessels. Nerve tissue degeneration resulting in loss of sensation is another complication of diabetes. Generally, the longer the diabetic condition exists, the more prone the patient is to complications.

Q: Is it safe for a diabetic woman to have a baby?

A: Although there is some risk involved, most diabetic women who have not suffered from the disease for a long period of time have perfectly healthy children, but there is definitely a need for special care during pregnancy, childbirth, and just after. During pregnancy, a diabetic woman's blood sugar level may vary widely, which means that if she needs insulin, her insulin requirement will vary also. Usually, the physician takes regular blood-sugar tests and instructs the woman about testing her urine to be sure she has the proper insulin dosage.

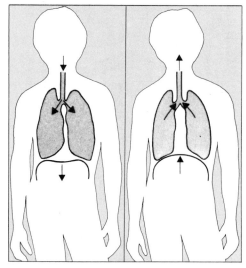

Diaphragm contracts and flattens during inhalation, then relaxes during exhalation.

The fetus carried by a diabetic woman is usually larger than normal. The newborn infant of a diabetic mother may be particularly prone to respiratory disorders for the first twenty-four hours of life, and lose a considerable amount of weight for the first week. After that time, however, the progress of the baby should be the same as that of other children.

Most medical experts recommend that diabetic women have no more than two pregnancies, because pregnancy tends to aggravate the disease.

Q: Can diabetes be prevented?

A: Maintaining proper body weight is the best precaution for an individual with a family history of diabetes, especially if a glucose tolerance test reveals that the person's sugar-processing mechanism is not normal.

Diagnosis is the process by which a physician identifies a disease or disorder from its symptoms, causes, and signs. In order to get information for making a diagnosis, the physician may ask the patient to undergo an X-ray examination or various medical tests.

Dialysis. *See* KIDNEY DIALYSIS.

Diamorphine, or diacetylmorphine, is the medical term for HEROIN.

Diaper rash is inflammation of a baby's skin in the area covered by the diaper. The red inflamed area round the buttocks and genitalia may ooze and crust. Diaper rash is usually caused by bacteria in the feces reacting with the urine to produce ammonia. The longer a baby lies in a wet, dirty diaper the stronger the ammonia becomes. The rash may be aggravated by the diaper's moisture, and the chemical effect of any detergents or soaps left in a diaper that has not been properly rinsed after washing.

Q: What is the treatment for diaper rash?

A: Frequent changing of the diaper is essential. Exposure to the air without any covering is the surest way to heal the skin. The urine in the diaper must be able to evaporate, so plastic pants should not be worn until the rash has disappeared. Various soothing applications, such as calamine lotion, zinc compound cream, or petroleum jelly, are effective and should be applied frequently after careful washing of the inflamed area. If the area becomes infected, a physician may prescribe antibiotic or antifungal creams.

See also BABY CARE.

Diaphoretic is a substance that increases sweating, e.g., camphor, opium, and pilocarpine.

See also PERSPIRATION.

Diaphragm is any thin tissue that separates one structure from another. The term is most commonly applied to the large sheet of muscle between the abdominal cavity and the chest cavity. Diaphragm is also the name of a device used in CONTRACEPTION.

Diarrhea is a condition characterized by frequent bowel movements and feces that are soft or watery, and that may contain blood, pus, or mucus. The condition can prevent the body from absorbing necessary water and salts into the bloodstream, which may lead to DEHYDRATION. Diarrhea can be acute or chronic.

Q: *What can cause acute diarrhea?*

A: Attacks of mild acute diarrhea can often be traced to a simple dietary cause, such as eating rich food, or to an emotional upset. But serious acute diarrhea may be caused by CHOLERA, DYSENTERY, FOOD POISONING, or OTITIS MEDIA. Among other causes of serious acute diarrhea are chemical poisoning and certain respiratory infections.

Q: *How is acute diarrhea treated?*

A: All persons with acute diarrhea should drink plenty of fluids, to prevent dehydration. Most persons with mild acute diarrhea benefit from a diet of bland foods, such as boiled or poached eggs, crackers, custards, gelatins, and rice. In some cases physicians may prescribe antidiarrheal or antispasm preparations to help ease the symptoms.

Persons with serious acute diarrhea usually need immediate medical help, because of the high risk of dehydration. Signs that dehydration is taking place include a decrease in urine output, dark or light brown urine, sunken eyeballs, rapid pulse rate, vomiting, constant thirst, and drowsiness or even unconsciousness. Dehydration is a serious condition that may prove fatal, especially to infants and young children.

Q: *What can cause chronic diarrhea?*

A: Chronic diarrhea may be a symptom of various serious disorders. Among such disorders are infections of the colon, intestinal cancer, sprue, and infestation of the intestines with worms.

Q: *How is chronic diarrhea treated?*

A: All persons with chronic diarrhea should drink plenty of fluids, to avoid dehydration. Treatment for chronic diarrhea depends partly on the cause, which may be determined by diagnosis of the symptoms and by the results of certain tests. These tests may include sigmoidoscopy, barium enema, and stool-sample examination.

Diastole is the normal period of relaxation of the heart muscle; it alternates with the period of contraction (SYSTOLE). During the diastole, the heart cavities fill with blood; the diastole of the atria (upper chambers) occurs momentarily before that of the ventricles. The diastolic blood pressure is the point of least pressure in the arteries, because blood is not being pumped by the heart during this phase.
See also p.8.

Diathermy is the painless production of heat within the body tissues by means of a high-frequency electric current. Physiotherapists use shortwave diathermy to relieve the symptoms of inflammation and stiff, painful joints and muscles. Surgical diathermy is a method of sealing blood vessels using an electrically heated probe (*see* CAUTERY).

Diathesis is a constitutional or hereditary tendency to develop a particular disease or disorder. With some disorders that apparently run in families, it is the diathesis that is inherited, not the actual disorder. It may be possible to avoid developing such a disorder by taking appropriate preventive measures.

Diazepam is the chemical name for the tranquilizing drug commonly known as Valium. *See* VALIUM.

A talk about Diet

Diet refers to the types of food a person eats regularly. Diet also refers to a set of practices to control the types and amounts of food eaten in an effort to promote health.

A normal diet should provide the body

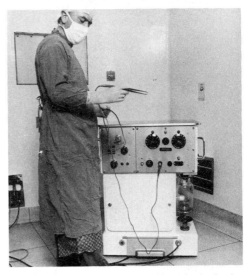

Diathermy is the production of heat in the body using a high frequency electric current.

Diet

with all the substances necessary to maintain growth, keep in good health, and repair damaged tissues. These substances come from a balanced diet that contains proteins, fats, carbohydrates, vitamins, minerals, and water. A normal diet should also contain the exact amount of food to satisfy the body's energy needs and no more. When a body takes in more food than it can use for energy, the excess may be stored as fat (*see* WEIGHT PROBLEMS).

Q: *How is the energy content of foods measured?*

A: Foods are measured for their heat energy value in metric units called calories. One calorie is the energy needed to raise the temperature of one gram of water one degree centigrade. Nutritionists use the kilocalorie (1,000 calories), properly written Calorie (with a capital C), to express the energy content of foods. But by convention, in this context, the kilocalorie is written calorie.

The daily number of calories needed depends on a person's age, size, and occupation. Generally, men need more calories than women, and youngsters more than older persons.

Carbohydrates and fats are the chief source of calories in a balanced diet.

Q: *What foods make up a balanced diet?*

A: Nutritionists classify foods for a balanced diet in various categories. One such system uses seven basic food groups.

Meat, poultry, fish, eggs, beans, peas, and nuts make up the first group. They are rich sources of protein, vitamin B,

iron, niacin, phosphorus, and some carbohydrates. A balanced diet requires one or two servings of these foods a day.

Leafy, green, and yellow vegetables provide folic acid, vitamin A, the B vitamins, vitamin C, calcium, iron, and nonnutritive fiber. A person should have at least one serving from this group each day.

Citrus fruits, green vegetables and tomatoes supply vitamins A and C, calcium, and iron. At least one daily serving is recommended.

Potatoes, other vegetables, and noncitrus fruits provide carbohydrates, minerals, and small amounts of most vitamins. One potato and another food from this group is recommended in the daily diet.

Whole-grain bread, breakfast cereal, and enriched flour are rich sources of carbohydrates, vitamins, and minerals. Some, such as bran, also supply fiber. Nutritionists recommend at least four daily servings.

Butter and fortified margarine supply vitamin A and fats.

Milk and such milk products as ice cream and cheese provide vitamin A, vitamin B_2, calcium, protein, and fats.

Q: *Why are proteins important?*

A: Proteins are body-building foods. They are essential for growth and maintenance of tissue. Skin, hair, muscle, blood, and other parts of the body are made up largely of proteins. *See* PROTEINS.

Q: *Why are carbohydrates important?*

A: Carbohydrates are starches and sugars. They are the main source of energy in the diet. Before the body can use carbohydrates as fuel, the food has to be broken down by the digestive system into the simple sugar, glucose. In a well-balanced diet, carbohydrates make up about 45 percent of the calorie intake. A diet too high in carbohydrates, however, leads to overweight. *See* CARBOHYDRATES.

Q: *Why are fats important?*

A: Fats are another major source of body energy. They provide about twice as much energy as does an equal weight of carbohydrate or protein. Fats make up about 40 percent of the calories in a balanced diet. Because fats give off a great deal of heat when they are "burned" by the body, a person needs more fat in the diet during winter and less during summer. Fats are also needed by body cells and to transport fat-soluble vitamins. High intakes of saturated fats, derived mainly from animals, have been

Percentage composition of some common foods						
Food	Fat	Protein	Carbo-hydrate	Vitamins and minerals	Water	Fiber
Bread	3	13.5	70	2	10	1.5
Chicken	16	20	0	1	63	0
Meat	17	18	0	1	64	0
White fish	0.25	17.5	0	1.25	81	0
Egg	12	12	1	1	74	0
Milk	4	3.5	4.5	1	87	0
Cheese	29	25	2	4	40	0
Tomato	0	0.5	3	0.5	95	1
Potato	0	2	17	0.5	80	0.5
Apple	0.25	0.50	13	0.25	84	2

Diet can be controlled so that a person can achieve a well-balanced food intake.

correlated with coronary heart disease. Therefore, most physicians believe that unsaturated fats, derived mainly from vegetables, pose less of a risk. *See* FATS.

Q: What roles do vitamins play?

A: The body cannot make most vitamins, and some it makes in only small quantities. Therefore, the body must get vitamins from food. Vitamins are not a source of energy, but they are indispensable to good health and the effective functioning of the body. Scientists have identified about twenty-five vitamins.

Vitamin A is essential for healthy skin, eyes, teeth, and bones.

Vitamin B (thiamin) aids the body in releasing energy from sugars and starches.

Vitamin B_2 (riboflavin) helps cells to use oxygen and aids in tissue repair.

Vitamin B_6 is necessary for healthy blood vessels and nerves.

Vitamin B_{12} and folic acid are needed by red blood cells and nerves.

Vitamin C (ascorbic acid) maintains supportive tissue, such as ligaments and tendons, and is needed for healthy gums and bones.

Vitamin D aids the body's use of calcium and phosphorus.

Vitamin E is needed by the heart and skeletal muscles.

Vitamin K is essential for proper blood clotting.

Niacin is necessary for healthy skin, cell metabolism, and the absorption of carbohydrates.

See also VITAMINS.

Q: What are the roles of minerals?

A: Minerals, like vitamins, do not provide energy but are needed for the growth and maintenance of body structure.

Important minerals include iron, which is essential for red blood cells; iodine, which is used by the thyroid gland; and calcium, magnesium, and phosphorus, which are necessary for healthy teeth and bones. Potassium, sodium, sulfur and other minerals are essential components of digestive juices and body fluids in and around cells.

Q: Why is fiber important in the diet?

A: The indigestible fiber found in fruits, vegetables, and cereals aids in eliminating solid waste from the body. Adequate fiber in the diet helps to prevent constipation, and may reduce the likelihood of hemorrhoids or diverticular disease.

See also DIGESTIVE SYSTEM.

Q: Can eating the wrong foods cause illness?

A: Good nutrition is definitely essential for general good health. But lack of specific elements in the diet can cause serious diseases. *See* DEFICIENCY DISEASES.

Too much of a certain type of food can also contribute to disease.

Digestive system

Digestive system is the series of organs that process and convert food into simpler substances that the body uses for nourishment. Starch and complex sugars are digested to simple sugars; fats to fatty acids and glycerine; and proteins to amino acids. These simpler substances consist of small molecules that can then pass through the intestinal wall and into the bloodstream for distribution to all parts of the body. The digestive system consists of the alimentary canal – mouth, pharynx, esophagus, stomach, and small and large intestines – aided by secretions from the liver and pancreas.

Q: What happens to food in the mouth?

A: The teeth break up food by chopping and grinding it into fine particles. Glands in the mouth lubricate and moisten food with saliva, which also contains a digestive enzyme. The tongue conveys food to the throat, and the pharynx muscles push it down the esophagus (gullet), a muscular tube about 10 inches (25 cm) long that leads to the stomach.

Q: What happens to food in the stomach?

A: The stomach both stores and helps to digest food. The stomach of an average adult can hold about 1 quart (0.9 liters). The muscular stomach churns food around and mixes it with gastric juice,

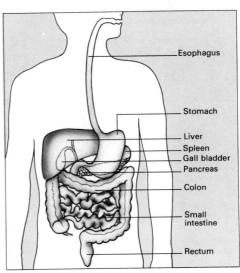

Digestive system processes food by means of many individual organs, from mouth to anus.

167

Digitalis

which includes hydrochloric acid to provide the acid medium needed for the enzyme pepsin to break down protein. The partly digested food (chyme) passes from the stomach to the small intestine, usually after two to five hours.

Q: How does the small intestine function?

A: The digestive process is completed in the small intestine, a narrow muscular tube about 20 feet (6 meters) long. Enzymes from the pancreas mix with enzymes from the duodenum. Bile, made by the liver and stored in the gall bladder, also enters the small intestine. Bile helps in the digestion of fats.

The digested food particles are then absorbed by lymph or blood vessels in the intestinal wall. Tiny fingerlike projections (villi) on the walls of the small intestine increase the surface area that can absorb the food. The digested particles are then carried by the bloodstream to the liver, which converts them into substances needed by the body.

Q: What is the role of the large intestine?

A: Eaten material that cannot be digested as food, such as plant fiber, passes into the large intestine, which is about 5 feet (1.5 meters) long. There water is removed from the liquid waste and bacteria convert it to its final form, feces. The waste material is excreted from the body through the end of the large intestine (rectum).

Q: How does food move through the digestive system?

A: Food is propelled along by wavelike contractions of muscles in the stomach and intestines. This is called peristalsis. The food moves in one direction only. Sphincters, circular muscles that close tightly, prevent the food from moving backward. There are sphincters at the lower end of the esophagus, at the exit from the stomach, at the lower end of the small intestine, and at the exit from the rectum.

Q: What are common diseases or disorders of the digestive system?

A: One fairly common disorder is ulcers of the stomach or duodenum, the first part of the small intestine. If bile stagnates in the gall bladder because of a blocked bile duct, gallstones can form and must be removed surgically. Disorders of the intestinal tract include colitis, diverticular disease, and enteritis.

Digitalis is a drug made from the dried leaves of the foxglove (*Digitalis purpurea*). Prescribed as tablets, capsules, or liquid, digitalis is important in the treatment of congestive heart failure, and some forms of heart palpitation. Treatment is normally continued for some time after the heart failure has been corrected.

Digitalis makes a failing heart more efficient by strengthening the contractions of the tired muscle, and making the heart beat more slowly. Digitalis indirectly reduces blood congestion in veins and the accumulation of fluids in the body, as well as increasing urine production by the kidneys. Great care has to be taken when prescribing digitalis, particularly in the elderly, or in those suffering from vomiting and diarrhea. The drug is eliminated from the body so slowly that doses may accumulate with correspondingly harmful effects.

Digitoxin is a heart stimulant drug prepared from the plant *Digitalis purpurea*. Its effects are similar to those of the related drugs DIGITALIS AND DIGOXIN.

Digoxin is a heart stimulant drug prepared from the plant *Digitalis lanata*. Its effects are similar to those of the related drugs DIGITALIS and DIGITOXIN.

Dilantin (Trademark) is an anticonvulsant drug and is a preparation of the generic drug phenytoin sodium. It is used to treat grand mal and focal EPILEPSY, but is not always effective against petit mal epilepsy. It may take several months to control the epileptic attacks, and it must be taken strictly as directed by a physician.

Dilatation and curettage. See D AND C.

Dimetapp (Trademark) is an antiallergy drug that is also used as a nasal decongestant. It is a preparation of the antihistamine drug

Action of the digestive system			
Site	Secretion	Food content	Action
Mouth	Saliva, alkaline	Starch	Water to aid lubrication of food
Stomach	Gastric juice, acid	Proteins	Provides acid medium for pepsin and kills most bacteria. Absorbs only alcohol
Duodenum	Pancreatic juice, bile	Fats Starch Proteins	Bile emulsifies fat for absorption
Ileum	Succus entericus	Fats Starch Proteins	Most absorption of food occurs here
Colon			Absorption of water

Digestive system breaks down food into elements that can be absorbed by the body.

brompheniramine maleate and two chemicals that stimulate the sympathetic nervous system, namely phenylephrine hydrochloride and phenylpropanolamine hydrochloride.

Dimetapp should be prescribed with caution for patients with an overactive thyroid gland, high blood pressure (hypertension), or coronary heart disease. The drug should not be taken during pregnancy. Dimetapp tablets are not suitable for patients with celiac disease and other persons requiring a gluten-free diet.

Diopter is the unit of measurement of the focusing power of a lens. *See* EYEGLASSES.

Diphtheria is an acute infectious disease caused by the bacillus *Corynebacterium diphtheriae*. This bacterium usually grows on the membranes of the nose and throat, but can affect other mucous membranes and occasionally infects the skin. Diphtheria is now a rare disease, because of widespread vaccination against it. It occurs most often in children under the age of ten.

Q: How is diphtheria spread?

A: The disease is usually spread by minute airborne droplets that are breathed out by an infected person. As a result, it can spread extremely rapidly. The diphtheria bacillus can be transmitted by a carrier, a person who is immune to the disease, who does not exhibit any symptoms, and who may be unaware of the infection.

Q: What are the symptoms of diphtheria?

A: Before any symptoms become apparent, there is an incubation period of up to five days; this period varies and symptoms may appear after only one day. There is a sudden onset of a sore throat and fever, accompanied by rapidly increasing feelings of ill health and weakness. A typical symptom is a thick, white, crustlike membrane at the back of the throat. The inflamed tissues are painful, and the lymph nodes in the neck often become swollen, but the infection rarely spreads any further.

Q: Are there any complications associated with diphtheria?

A: Yes. The crustlike membrane may obstruct breathing. In severe cases, this complication may need urgent treatment to prevent suffocation. Another complication is that the toxin produced by the infection may cause nerve damage (neuritis), heart muscle damage (myocarditis), and kidney damage. There may also be localized paralysis resembling poliomyelitis.

Q: How may diphtheria be treated?

A: A patient with diphtheria requires hospital treatment in isolation. This usually involves the administration of diphtheria antitoxin and antibiotics. The antitoxin counteracts the effects of the toxin, and the antibiotics kill the bacteria. Complete bed rest is essential during the acute stage of the disease, with a gradual return to normal activity afterward.

Q: Can diphtheria be prevented?

A: Yes. Diphtheria immunization is usually carried out in the first year of life. A SCHICK TEST determines whether or not a person is susceptible to diphtheria. If an individual is susceptible, he or she can be immunized with specially-treated toxin (toxoid). In practice, however, the Schick test is not much used today.

Diphyllobothrium latum is the largest of the parasitic tapeworms that infest human beings. The adult worm lives in the intestine, and may grow to about 30 feet (9 meters) long. Most cases of infestation arise from eating raw or undercooked fish. The first sign of infestation is often worm segments in the feces. Treatment is usually with drugs that kill the worm.

Diplegia is paralysis of like parts on both sides of the body, for example, both arms or both legs. *See* PARALYSIS.

Diplopia. *See* DOUBLE VISION.

Dipsomania. *See* ALCOHOLISM.

Disarticulation is an amputation through a joint. *See* AMPUTATION.

Discharge is the loss of a substance through a body opening. It may be the result of a normal body process, for example, urination, or it may be abnormal, for example, bloody mucus from the ear.

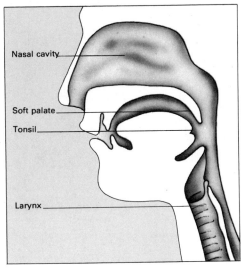

Diphtheria most commonly affects the mucous membranes of the nose, mouth, and throat.

Disinfectant

Disinfectant is a substance that destroys infection-causing organisms. The term is generally applied to chemicals used for treating such things as surgical instruments and sickroom floors.

See also ANTISEPTICS.

Disk is any flat, round, platelike structure. In medicine, the term commonly has two meanings. The optic disk is the point at which the optic nerve enters the back of the eye. An intervertebral disk is a fibroelastic ring with a soft, gelatinous center, which lies between each pair of vertebrae of the backbone. The intervertebral disks act as shock absorbers and enable the backbone to flex. Occasionally an intervertebral disk ruptures, causing the condition known as SLIPPED DISK.

Dislocation (luxation) is the displacement of a structure from its normal position in the body. In most joints, dislocations of bones are rare, except as a complication of a fracture or as a result of weakened joint ligaments. Dislocations most commonly occur in the shoulder, where there may be a congenital weakness of the surrounding ligaments. A dislocation always involves torn ligaments, and it may take several weeks for the tears to heal. Various surgical operations have been devised to strengthen or replace weak ligaments, and so overcome the problem. Occasionally, one or both hips may be dislocated from birth (congenital hip dislocation), and early diagnosis and treatment are required to prevent permanent disability.

Disorientation is a loss of normal awareness of place or time. Such mental confusion may occur in serious physical illnesses, with fever, as a result of certain drug treatments, or as a symptom of a mental illness.

Diuretics are agents that act on the kidneys to increase the output of urine. This is accompanied by a loss of sodium or, sometimes, potassium salts. Alcohol, tea, and coffee are mild, but nonmedical, diuretics.

Q: Which disorders may diuretics be used to treat?

A: Diuretics are used to treat virtually any disorder in which there is an excessive build-up of fluid in the body (edema). These include disorders of the heart, liver, and kidneys. Some weak diuretics are used to decrease excessive fluid pressure within the eyeball (glaucoma). Diuretics are used to treat certain lung disorders in which fluid accumulates in the lung tissue (pulmonary edema). They may also be used to decrease high blood pressure (hypertension) and to treat overdosage of certain drugs.

Q: Can diuretics produce any adverse effects?

A: Yes. The adverse effects of diuretics vary according to the specific drug used. The commonly prescribed diuretics may cause nausea, weakness, skin rashes, and allergic reactions. All diuretics should be used with care by diabetics and by those with impaired liver or kidney function.

Diuril (Trademark) is a diuretic drug, a preparation of chlorothiazide. Its main function is to increase the production of urine. Diuril causes sodium and potassium salts to be excreted, and if prolonged use of the drug is necessary, a high potassium diet or potassium supplements may be required. Unlike some other DIURETICS, Diuril seldom loses its effectiveness over time, but it may cause the adverse effects common to diuretic agents. Diuril may cause blood disorders in some persons, and should be used with caution by those taking DIGITALIS.

Diverticulitis and diverticulosis (diverticular disease) are common, related diseases of the colon, the main part of the large intestine. Diverticulitis develops from diverticulosis, which involves the formation of pouches (diverticula) on the outside of the colon. Diverticulitis results if one of these diverticula becomes inflamed. Bacteria may then infect the outside of the colon. If the infection spreads to the lining of the abdominal cavity (peritoneum), this can cause a potentially fatal illness (peritonitis). Sometimes inflamed diverticula can cause narrowing of the bowel, leading to an obstruction. Also, the affected part of the colon could adhere to the bladder or other organ in the pelvic area. These diverticular disorders most often affect middle-aged and elderly persons.

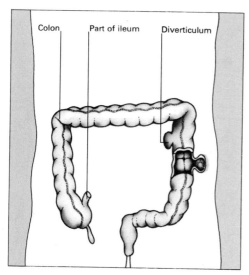

Colon   Part of ileum   Diverticulum

Diverticulitis occurs when a small pocket in the bowel becomes inflamed.

170

Q: What are the symptoms of diverticular disease?

A: Usually there are no symptoms accompanying diverticulosis. However, if diverticulitis develops, some patients experience abdominal pain and rectal bleeding. This occurs when an ulcer on a diverticulum erodes a blood vessel. A barium enema X-ray examination reveals the presence of diverticula.

The symptoms of diverticulitis include localized abdominal pain and tenderness, loose bowel movements, and fever. A blood test shows an increased number of white blood cells.

Q: What is the treatment for diverticular disease?

A: Persons with diverticulosis are put on a high-fiber diet, which aids in passing waste through the colon and thus reduces intestinal pressure. This could help to prevent diverticulitis from developing. However, in cases of severe bleeding, surgery is necessary.

An acute attack of diverticulitis is usually treated with antibiotics. When the infection has been controlled, patients suffering from such an attack are also placed on a high-fiber diet. However, recurring acute attacks or complications, such as peritonitis, require surgical treatment.

See also DIET; DIGESTIVE SYSTEM.

Diverticulum (plural: diverticula) is a small, fingerlike pouch, most often found in the intestinal wall but also occurring in other parts of the body. Diverticula may occur normally or they may result from a rupture of intestinal mucous membrane. Meckel's diverticulum, however, is present at birth. It is a pouch that protrudes from the ileum, and represents the yolk stalk of the embryo. In most persons, the stalk structure disappears at birth, but Meckel's diverticulum is fairly common, and does not require treatment.

See also DIVERTICULITIS AND DIVERTICULOSIS.

Dizziness is a sensation of unsteadiness or lightheadedness; the term is synonymous with giddiness. Dizziness should not be confused with vertigo, which is a feeling of movement, either of the external world rotating about the person, or of the person spinning.

See also BALANCE.

Dominant is a term used in the study of HEREDITY to describe a gene that affects the physical characteristics (phenotype) of an individual in preference to another gene of the same type. For example, the gene for brown eyes is dominant over the gene for blue eyes (which is said to be RECESSIVE).

The term dominant is also used by psychiatrists to describe persons with strong, overpowering personalities.

Donnatal (Trademark) is the name of four preparations, all of which contain hyoscyamine sulfate, atropine sulfate, and hyoscine hydrobromide, along with phenobarbital. It is used to treat spasms of involuntary (smooth) muscle, such as those that occur in intestinal colic and pyloric stenosis. It can also be used to treat cystitis, diverticulitis, colitis, ulcers, and diarrhea.

Q: What are the possible side effects of Donnatal?

A: It may produce drowsiness and lack of coordination; persons taking Donnatal should avoid driving, drinking alcohol, or operating machinery. Donnatal should not be used during or immediately following pregnancy unless the physician considers it essential. It should also be avoided in those suffering from glaucoma, obstruction of the intestinal or urinary tract, or impaired liver function.

Dorsal means relating to the back (dorsum) of a structure or the body. The opposite of dorsal is ventral.

Double vision (known medically as diplopia) is the perception of two images of a single object. Diplopia is a symptom rather than a disorder. The most common cause of double vision is a sudden imbalance in the power of the eye muscles. It may also result from incipient cataract, astigmatism, a displaced lens, or several disorders that affect nerves and muscles.

See also STRABISMUS.

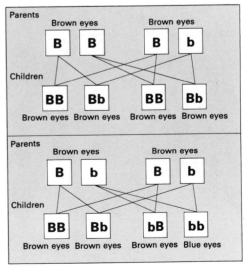

The dominant gene for brown eyes (B) prevails unless two recessive genes (bb) coincide.

Douche

Douche is a stream of vapor, water, or antiseptic fluid directed against a part of the body. It may be used either for personal hygiene or to treat a local disorder. The term is usually used to describe the washing of the vagina. The vagina cleanses itself naturally and is also cleansed in the normal bathing process, so there is little reason for a healthy woman to use a vaginal douche. Despite popular belief, there is no evidence that a vaginal douche following sexual intercourse is an effective method of contraception.

A talk about Down's syndrome

Down's syndrome, or Trisomy 21, is the medical name for mongolism, a congenital defect of mental and physical development. It is caused by an extra chromosome. There are forty-seven chromosomes instead of the normal forty-six. The defect is usually caused by an extra number twenty-one chromosome. The syndrome is associated with increasing age of the mother, and not with the number of pregnancies. A mother between the age of thirty-five and thirty-nine has a one-and-a-half percent chance of having a mongoloid child; a woman over the age of forty has a five percent chance of having a mongol. The physical characteristics include a flat, round head, which is also smaller than normal; small, low-set ears; a flattened nose; skin folds over the inner corner of the eyes; a large tongue that protrudes from a small mouth; and a typical pattern of creases on the palm. However, the most important fea-ture is mental retardation; an affected child may have an intelligence quotient (IQ) of fifty or lower.

Q: Are there any other abnormalities associated with Down's syndrome?

A: Yes. Down's syndrome is often associated with other congenital disorders, such as heart disease, umbilical hernia, and Hirschsprung's disease (a bowel disorder that causes constipation). Leukemia may develop in childhood or later.

Q: What can be done to help children with Down's syndrome?

A: There is no medical treatment that can cure Down's syndrome. However, with specialized education, most affected children can learn to look after themselves and to lead useful lives. Parents of a child with Down's syndrome should discuss education with their physician and a pediatrician who has a special interest in the disorder.

Q: After the birth of one affected child, what is the likelihood of subsequent children having Down's syndrome?

A: Because Down's syndrome is rarely inherited, there is an extremely good chance that any subsequent children will be normal, unless the mother is over age 40. Rarely, however, Down's syndrome is inherited. In either case, it is advisable to seek expert medical advice, for example, to obtain GENETIC COUNSELING before embarking on another pregnancy.

Q: Can Down's syndrome be detected during pregnancy?

A: Yes. By testing a sample of the fluid from around the fetus in the womb (amniocentesis), a geneticist can predict whether a baby will be born with Down's syndrome, while there is still time to consider an abortion.

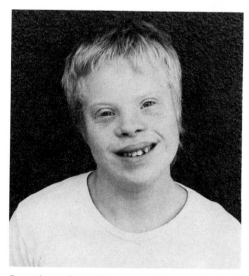

Down's syndrome is a congenital anomaly that produces typical facial characteristics.

DPT vaccine is a combination of diphtheria, pertussis (whooping cough), and tetanus vaccines, used in immunizing infants.

Dracunculiasis is infestation with the parasitic guinea worm. *See* GUINEA WORM.

Dreams are thoughts, emotions, and experiences that occur during sleep. Any of the senses may contribute to a dream, but most dreams are visual and are accompanied by rapid eye movements (REM). Everybody dreams, although not everybody can remember dreaming.

The purpose of dreams is not known. But persons who are deliberately deprived of dream sleep become irritable and restless. Dream deprivation may also cause emotional problems. Many psychiatrists believe that the events within dreams relate to the dreamer's life and that by studying a patient's dreams they can find clues to the underlying causes of the dreamer's problems.

See also NIGHTMARE; SLEEP.

Drop foot. *See* FOOT DROP.

Dropsy is an obsolete term for excessive fluid retention in the body; it is now called EDEMA.

Drop wrist. *See* WRIST DROP.

Drowning is death caused by smothering in liquid. *See* First Aid p.538.

A talk about Drug addiction

Drug addiction, or drug dependence, is the uncontrollable craving for a drug. Such craving may occur periodically or continuously, and is usually accompanied by an overwhelming compulsion to obtain the drug. The addict becomes preoccupied with thoughts about the anticipated effects of the drug.

The uncontrollable craving for a drug may be of physical origin, psychological origin, or both, and with some drugs the craving may develop in as short a time as twenty-four hours. In a person who is physically addicted to a drug, the body's chemical processes are altered so that the drug becomes essential for some of the normal metabolic functions. Psychological dependence on a drug does not involve a modification of the body's chemistry, but the addicted person believes that the drug is necessary in order to function normally.

Q: *Why do people take drugs for nonmedical reasons?*

A: There are many reasons for the nonmedical use of drugs. For example, some people with difficult problems, such as unemployment or large debts, become anxious, frustrated, and depressed. They feel trapped by problems that seem to have no solution and seek a release from reality in the effects of drugs.

Other people may take drugs out of boredom or curiosity, and some because their friends do and they feel the need to conform. This need to conform with friends is, perhaps, strongest among teenagers.

Q: *Are some people more likely than others to become dependent on drugs?*

A: Yes. In general, the likelihood of a person becoming dependent on a drug involves three interrelated factors; an individual's personality, the social environment, and the type of drug involved.

Some people are more sensitive than others to the effects of drugs and may

feel euphoric states more intensely. This may result in a relatively rapid attraction to and dependence on drugs. In others, feelings of tension or depression may be more acute, and the relief provided by drugs correspondingly greater, and so the dependence more probable.

A person's environment affects the likelihood of drug dependence in many ways. For example, poor housing and unemployment are known to cause depression and anxiety, two states that are common causes of drug addiction. It is also likely that dependence on a drug will be greater in a person who has to steal to get money for the drug than it will in a person who does not. There is for some people a special attraction in doing something illegal or merely antisocial, and this attraction may put people in danger of becoming drug dependent.

In some cases, the nature of the drug taken affects the likelihood of dependency. For example, a person taking heroin is more likely to become drug dependent than a person taking barbiturates.

Q: *Which drugs may cause dependency?*

A: There are many drugs on which people can become dependent. These drugs can be categorized as those that depress the central nervous system; those that stimulate the central nervous system; and those that produce hallucinations, and also affect the central nervous system. The main group of drugs that depress the

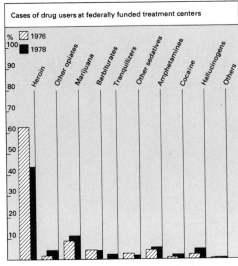

The people most in need of rehabilitation treatment are heroin users.

Drug addiction

central nervous system are the narcotics, such as codeine, Dilaudid, heroin, meperidine, methadone, morphine and paregoric. Other drugs in this category include alcohol, barbiturates, nicotine, tranquilizers, and some sleeping pills.

Drugs that stimulate the central nervous system include cocaine and the amphetamines, such as Benzedrine, Dexedrine, and Methedrine.

Drugs that produce hallucinations are known as hallucinogens or psychedelics. Some of the more common hallucinogens are DMT, DOM, LSD, MDA, psilocybin, mescaline, and THC.

Marijuana is classified as a mild hallucinogen, but it is much less powerful than other drugs in this category.

Q: *What effects do depressants produce?*
A: Depressants slow down the activities of the central nervous system. If this system slows down too much, the body's vital functions may stop, which could be fatal. Dependence on depressants usually takes the form of both physical and psychological dependence. The narcotic depressants can cause dependence much more quickly than other depressants.

The short-term effects of depressants include euphoria; relief of pain; and prevention of withdrawal symptoms. The long-term effects include depression; malnutrition; and constipation. The addict may also become infected with hepatitis or tetanus by using unsterile needles. If the drug is stopped, the addict will suffer withdrawal symptoms.

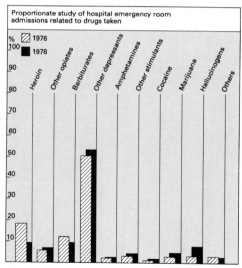

Proportionate study of hospital emergency room admissions related to drugs taken

% / 1976 / 1978

Heroin, Other opiates, Barbiturates, Other depressants, Amphetamines, Other stimulants, Cocaine, Marijuana, Hallucinogens, Others

Thousands are admitted to emergency rooms each year following drug abuse accidents.

Q: *What symptoms may be caused by withdrawal from a depressant?*
A: The symptoms of depressant withdrawal vary according to the drug involved, but are often extremely severe, and may be fatal. For example, within about eighteen hours of the sudden withdrawal of alcohol from an alcoholic there may be convulsions and delirium (delirium tremens). Delirium tremens (DTs) may also occur when an addict stops taking sleeping pills.

Other symptoms of depressant withdrawal include weakness; high blood pressure and pulse rate; profuse sweating; gooseflesh; diarrhea; vomiting; severe abdominal cramps; and, sometimes, cardiovascular collapse. The diarrhea and vomiting may cause dehydration.

Q: *What effects do stimulants produce?*
A: The short-term effects of stimulants include excitation; sleeplessness; hyperactivity; and euphoria. In the long-term, some heavy users of stimulants may also experience hallucinations, delusions, and toxic psychosis.

Dependence on stimulants is mainly psychological, although some degree of physical dependence may also develop. Amphetamines are perhaps the most dangerous of the stimulant drugs and many amphetamine addicts develop a high tolerance as part of their dependence on the drug. Tolerance usually occurs rapidly and the addict has to take larger dosages to achieve the desired effects. The larger amounts may cause the amphetamine addict to stay awake for several days, during which the addict may hallucinate, become disoriented, and suffer from paranoia. Following this ordeal the amphetamine addict may sleep for a day or more. On waking, the addict usually feels severely depressed and often takes another dose of the drug to relieve the depression, which begins the cycle all over again.

Q: *What symptoms may be caused by withdrawal from a stimulant?*
A: The symptoms of stimulant withdrawal include severe depression; muscle pains; apathy; and a strong desire to take more stimulants. These symptoms are felt most keenly by amphetamine addicts. Generally, however, the symptoms of stimulant withdrawal are milder because stimulants are less physically addictive than depressants.

Q: *What effects do hallucinogens produce?*
A: The effects of hallucinogens vary widely,

both between individuals and even in the same individual on different occasions. The main effects include exhilaration, sensory distortion, and illusions. But in some cases there may be feelings of paranoia and panic. Occasionally, "flashbacks" may occur. These are brief recurrences of a previous hallucinatory state that may occur weeks or months later without the person having taken a hallucinogen.

The hallucinogens do not seem to produce physical dependence, but they may produce psychological dependence. The long-term effects of these drugs are not known. But scientists are trying to determine whether long-term usage of hallucinogens can cause chromosome damage or genetic mutation.

Q: *Are babies of drug-dependent women born drug dependent?*

A: Yes, although the symptoms of drug dependence in babies vary according to the drug involved. For example, the newborn child of a heroin-addicted mother may be of small size and generally poor health. The baby may display withdrawal symptoms in the form of irritability, high-pitched crying, trembling, sweating, vomiting, and diarrhea. The withdrawal symptoms usually occur within about three days of birth, but withdrawal from barbiturate dependence usually takes longer. Methadone-dependent babies may exhibit breathing distress, convulsions, and fever.

Q: *What is the clinical treatment for drug dependence?*

A: The first stage of treatment is withdrawal of the drug (detoxification). In cases of physical dependence this usually involves a gradual reduction of the addict's intake over a period of about ten days. Sometimes a less harmful substitute with similar effects is administered, for example, methadone instead of heroin. The treatment of alcoholism may also include vitamin supplements and the administration of a deterrent drug, such as Antabuse. This drug produces nausea whenever alcohol is drunk. Withdrawal may be delayed if the person is in poor health.

In addition to withdrawal, treatment may also include a program of mental and social rehabilitation, which may involve psychiatric counseling. The treatment of drug dependence is often not completely successful, although the success rate varies from drug to drug.

The rehabilitation programs, such as therapeutic communities and Alcoholics Anonymous, greatly increase the chances of success.

See also ALCOHOLISM.

Drugs. The following table lists the major types of drugs and their medical usage. Most of these drugs have a separate article in the A–Z section of this book.

Drug	Medical usage
AMPHETAMINES	To treat narcolepsy and depression
ANALGESICS	To reduce pain
ANORECTICS	To reduce appetite
ANTACIDS	To counteract excess stomach acidity
ANTIBIOTICS	To treat micro-organismal infections
ANTICOAGULANTS	To treat thrombosis
ANTIDEPRESSANTS	To treat depression
ANTIHISTAMINES	To treat allergies
ANTINAUSEANTS	To treat nausea
ANTIPRURITICS	To relieve itching
ANTIPYRETICS	To reduce fever
BARBITURATES	To treat insomnia
BRONCHIAL DILATORS	To treat bronchial asthma
CHELATING AGENTS	To treat poisoning by heavy metals
CONTRACEPTIVES	To prevent conception
DIGITALIS	To treat heart failure
DIURETICS	To treat edema and high blood pressure
HEMATINICS	To treat anemia
INSULIN	To treat diabetes
MUSCLE RELAXANTS	To relax muscles especially during surgery
PEDICULICIDES	To destroy lice
RESPIRATORY STIMULANTS	To treat breathing stoppage
SCABICIDES	To destroy mites
SEDATIVES	To treat anxiety or insommia
THYROID PREPARATIONS	To treat goiter, hypothyroidism, hyperthyroidism, and thyroiditis
TRANQUILIZERS	To treat anxiety and various mental disorders
URICOSURIC AGENTS	To treat gout
URINARY ACIDIFIERS	To increase the effectiveness of certain drugs and to increase the elimination of drugs by the kidneys

Drunkenness. *See* ALCOHOLISM; INTOXICATION.

175

DTs. *See* DELIRIUM TREMENS.

Duct is any narrow tube in the body that carries secretions or fluids from one part of the body to another.

Ductless gland is another name for endocrine gland. It secretes substances directly into the bloodstream. *See* ENDOCRINE GLAND.

Ductus arteriosus is a blood vessel that joins the main artery leading to the lungs (the pulmonary artery) with the main artery that leads from the heart (the aorta). This link is present in a fetus so that the blood supply bypasses the lungs, which do not function until after birth. The ductus arteriosus closes off soon after birth. Failure to close is a common type of congenital heart disorder; the condition is corrected by tying off the vessel in a surgical operation.

Dumb. *See* MUTE.

Dumping syndrome is a digestion disorder that occurs in a patient who has had an operation for removing a large part of the stomach. Symptoms of sweating, dizziness, and weakness may be accompanied by pain and headache. The cause of dumping syndrome is not fully understood, but what happens is that the stomach absorbs and "dumps" its contents too quickly into the small intestine. The symptoms can be avoided by eating several small meals instead of one or two large ones.

Duodenal ulcer. *See* PEPTIC ULCER.

Duodenum is the first part of the small intestine, surrounding the head of the pancreas. It is about 10 inches (25 cm) long, and receives partially digested food from the stomach. The digestive process is continued in the

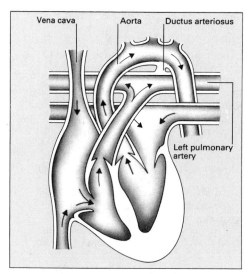

Ductus arteriosus is the blood vessel that bypasses the fetal lung; it closes after birth.

duodenum by the enzyme-containing fluids from the pancreas and the glands lining the duodenal wall, and the action of bile from the liver and gall bladder. When the digestive processes have been completed in the duodenum, the food passes into the jejunum.

Dupuytren's contracture is the inability to straighten the fingers, due to a thickening of the fibrous tissue lining the palm. Occasionally Dupuytren's contracture can involve the soles of the feet as well. The cause is not known, but it may be inherited. Treatment may involve a surgical operation to remove the thickened fibrous tissue and release the tendons.

Dutch cap. *See* CONTRACEPTION.

Dwarfism is the physical condition of being abnormally undersized. A dwarf may have normal body formations that are proportionally smaller throughout, or the condition may involve disproportionate stunting (achondroplasia). Dwarfism may be caused by abnormal fetal development (congenital), malnutrition, and other environmental factors, or hormone deficiency. Treatment of dwarfism depends on the cause.

Q: Which types of dwarfism are congenital?

A: The most common congenital disorder is achondroplasia, the form of dwarfism in which growth of the long bones is retarded. An achondroplastic dwarf has a normal sized head and trunk, but proportionally short arms and legs. If one parent has this condition, there is a 50 percent chance with each pregnancy of the couple having an affected child. There are other rare congenital disorders associated with dwarfism.

Q: What environmental factors may result in dwarfism?

A: Malnutrition deprives the body of food and vitamins essential to normal healthy growth. Stunted body growth in children with malnutrition can be offset by a normal diet, if treatment is started early enough. Chronic illness may retard or arrest growth during the childhood years. It has also been shown that the normal rate of growth may be affected by emotional deprivation, especially if the warm supportive environment that children need is lacking and replaced by hate and violence (*see* BATTERED CHILD SYNDROME). Malnutrition may also contribute to producing dwarfism from this cause.

Q: How do hormonal deficiencies cause dwarfism?

A: Growth hormone is produced by the pituitary gland at the base of the brain. If for any reason the pituitary gland of a child is underactive, dwarfism results. The body of a child with this deficiency remains small but is correctly proportioned. There is no mental impairment.

In cases where hormonal deficiencies are the cause of dwarfism, the treatment is to increase the output of the pituitary gland with injections of growth hormone.
See also CRETINISM.

Dyazide (Trademark) is a drug compounded of triamterene and hydrochlorothiazide. Dyazide is a diuretic (which increases the quantity of urine), and its main use is in the control of edema (retention of fluids) that occurs with heart failure, cirrhosis of the liver, and nephrotic syndrome of the kidney. Mild forms of high blood pressure (hypertension) may also be treated with Dyazide.
See also DIURETICS.

A talk about Dying

Dying is a natural process involving the progressive degeneration of those body functions essential to maintain life. To be dying of old age is the best example of this: the body's organs are worn out and eventually they cease to function. Drug treatment and other applications of medical knowledge have made it possible to postpone the dying process.

Q: *Should a dying person be made aware of the situation?*

A: Many patients prefer to know if they are to die from their illness and press the physician for a frank opinion. If direct questions are asked, it is generally because the patient wants honest answers. Close associates of the patient sometimes prefer that their friend or relative be spared the anguish of knowing, but the wishes of the patient must be the primary consideration. In other cases, the patient suspects the prognosis but prefers not to have it confirmed. It is unlikely that a physician will offer the information unless directly requested.

Q: *How strong does fear seem to be in people who are dying?*

A: It seems that most people dread that time in the future when they will know that death is imminent. However, people who are dying and know it usually manage to come to terms with the fact. It seems clear from experienced witnesses such as physicians and nurses that the dying process is not frightening in itself: as death draws near, the patient tends to become peaceful and accepting of a death which may well be desired by the final stages.

Q: *What is it about a drawn-out death that people think will be frightening?*

A: The fear of pain and suffering is probably the most common fear for those who contemplate their dying. This is why people often say that they would prefer to die instantaneously (for example, from accident or injury). Another fear is that approaching death will bring remorse or terrifying revelations.

Q: *What type of requests might a dying person make?*

A: It is natural for the patient to wish to be with close friends; such companions are of most comfort during this time and their understanding and concern may reduce the loneliness of the ordeal. The patient may feel the need to speak in confidence with certain people who are trusted, sympathetic, or admired. During such intimacies, it is likely that death will be discussed freely, and this can be a type of therapy. If other people can allay his or her alarm and fear, the dying person may more readily embrace what is natural and inevitable. Some patients cope with the thought of death by making sure that affairs consequent upon their death will cause as little inconvenience as possible to those who must attend to them. Matters of the will may be settled, funeral arrangements decided, and the patient may wish to participate in discussions about what everyday

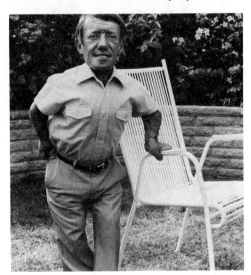

Dwarfism of the achondroplastic variety affects the growth of the long bones.

Dysarthria

adjustments may have to be made both short-term and long-term.

Q: *What practical care should be given the patient?*

A: The patient needs the regular, thorough care of home nursing. This requires patience in overcoming the initial difficulties of bed-bathing, feeding someone who has little or no appetite, and learning how to deal with possible involuntary urination and defecation. Prescribed medication has to be administered regularly and drugs have to be given as needed according to the advice of the physician. Measures to ensure maximum comfort for the patient should be taken such as propping up the pillows, regulating the amount of light entering the room, changing the bed linen, and ensuring adequate entertainment.

Q: *How can the family help?*

A: People who live in the patient's home cope best with the nursing requirements if the small everyday chores are shared. Intensive care of the patient means that regular daily activities may have to be curtailed. It is good to remember that in time of crisis, neighbors or friends are only too willing to be of assistance; if help is needed, there should be no hesitation in seeking it.

Q: *Might a person be conscious immediately before death?*

A: Yes. Sometimes a patient remains weak but alert until the moment of death. The presence of the family at this time must surely be of comfort. Often when a patient appears to be unconscious, the sense of hearing still remains; this should be considered at all times when discussing the illness in the presence of the patient.

Q: *Is it always obvious when a patient dies?*

A: No. Although a pallor and stillness typically occur with death, the exact moment of death is difficult to define even for physicians and nurses. Breathing prior to death may follow a cycle of being alternately shallow and deep for any length of time before death finally occurs during a shallow period (*see* CHEYNE-STOKES BREATHING). Within a few minutes of the event, the eyes become staring and the muscles of the face sag.

See also DEATH.

Dysarthria is the inability to speak clearly. The causes of the disorder include emotional stress, paralysis, and lack of coordination of the tongue and facial muscles, and of those supplying the voice box. Disease of the muscles or nerve disorders may also be causative factors.

Dysentery is an infectious disease characterized by severe diarrhea, with blood and mucus in the stools. It is accompanied by pain in the abdomen and, sometimes, contracting spasms of the anus with a persistent desire to empty the bowels (tenesmus).

There are two forms of dysentery: bacillary dysentery, caused by bacteria (*Shigella*); and amebic dysentery, caused by an ameba (*Entamoeba histolytica*). Both forms are transmitted by contaminated water or food. Dysentery is particularly common in tropical countries where standards of hygiene are poor.

Q: *What are the symptoms of bacillary dysentery?*

A: There are several forms of *Shigella* infection, which cause dysentery of varying severity. The symptoms start after about 48 hours with the acute onset of vomiting, diarrhea, and abdominal pains. A high fever may occur, and diarrhea continues for several days with blood and mucus in the stools. In babies and young children, life-threatening DEHYDRATION may occur rapidly.

Q: *What is the treatment for bacillary dysentery?*

A: It is most important to ensure that the patient drinks plenty of fluids. A physician may prescribe antispasmodic and antidiarrheal drugs to control the worst of the symptoms until the condition improves naturally. This may take up to ten days, although the patient is often

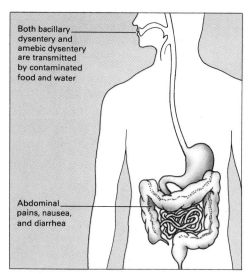

Both bacillary dysentery and amebic dysentery are transmitted by contaminated food and water

Abdominal pains, nausea, and diarrhea

Dysentery is an intestinal disorder that can be caused by bacteria, or the ingestion of amebas.

better within 48 hours. Babies and children may have to be admitted to a hospital for intravenous infusion, if serious dehydration occurs. Antibiotics are used only in the severest cases.

Q: *What are the complications of bacillary dysentery?*

A: Sometimes a patient develops an eye inflammation, such as conjunctivitis or iritis. Because the stools may remain infectious for some weeks, it is necessary for the patient to take great care with personal hygiene, washing the hands thoroughly after each bowel movement. The physician may culture the patient's feces on several occasions to check whether the infective organism has disappeared.

Q: *In what way does amebic dysentery differ from bacillary dysentery?*

A: Amebic dysentery may take some time to appear. Often some other minor intestinal disorder causes it to flare up, resulting in recurring attacks. The attacks are accompanied by colicky abdominal pain and, sometimes, fever. Intermittent attacks may already have gone on for several months, causing the patient to feel vaguely unwell, before a major attack necessitates consulting a physician.

Q: *How is amebic dysentery diagnosed?*

A: A physician diagnoses amebic dysentery by examining the feces for the infective organism, and by examining the inside of the colon with a lighted tube (sigmoidoscope). The physician can often see small ulcers in the colon; specimens from these ulcers contain the infection.

Q: *How is amebic dysentery treated?*

A: It can be treated with a variety of drugs. The drug metronidazole is usually effective in uncomplicated cases.

Q: *What are the complications of amebic dysentery?*

A: The infection may form a palpable mass inside the intestine to infect the liver, forming a liver abscess. It may also extend into the lung to produce a lung abscess. Both are serious conditions, and require specialized treatment.

Q: *What precautions can a person take to prevent catching dysentery?*

A: Because dysentery is more common in tropical countries, it is important in such localities to avoid eating uncooked foods and to ensure that all foods are prepared in the most hygienic way. It is essential not to drink unboiled water, because this may carry the infection. All foods must be kept covered to prevent flies from contaminating them with the disease.

Dysmenorrhea

Dyslexia is an imprecise term used to describe a variety of reading and writing disorders. It may be a disturbed understanding of what is read, ranging from a minor disability to a complete and permanent inability to read, which is inconsistent with the individual's intelligence. It is usually accompanied by an inability to spell correctly. The specific causes of dyslexia are disputed, but it may be due to congenital or acquired brain damage, probably affecting the speech centers. Dyslexia is not a sign of low intelligence, and some affected individuals may benefit from special teaching.

Dysmenorrhea is pain associated with menstruation. Primary dysmenorrhea occurs for no apparent cause. Secondary dysmenorrhea, usually happening later in life, has an underlying cause.

Q: *What are the symptoms of primary dysmenorrhea?*

A: The pain begins just before or at the onset of menstruation, and is centered in the lower abdomen. It may be cramplike, and lasts for the first day or two of the menstrual period. The abdominal pain is often accompanied by backache and, sometimes, vomiting.

Q: *How is primary dysmenorrhea treated?*

A: Painkilling and antispasmodic drugs may be prescribed. They should be started just before menstruation, and continued for the first two or three days of the period. The drugs should be taken regularly, not just when pain reappears. If these measures fail to control the symptoms, certain hormonal drugs, such as birth

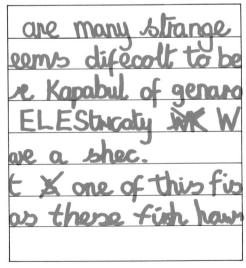

Dyslexia may be a cause of poor spelling but does not indicate lack of intelligence.

179

Dyspareunia

control pills, will prevent ovulation and stop the pain. Sometimes it is necessary to lie down with a heated pad over the lower abdominal area. Finally, the gynecologist may recommend D AND C.

Q: *Are the symptoms of secondary dysmenorrhea different from those of primary dysmenorrhea?*

A: Yes. The pain usually starts after the onset of menstruation, causing a dull ache deep in the pelvis, and it often continues throughout the period.

Q: *What are the causes of secondary dysmenorrhea?*

A: Secondary dysmenorrhea is usually caused by some gynecological disorder, such as inflammation of the womb (endometritis) or of the fallopian tubes (salpingitis), or by the spread of intestinal inflammation. In some cases the cause may be endometriosis, in which tissue resembling womb lining occurs in other parts of the pelvic cavity.

Q: *How can secondary dysmenorrhea be treated?*

A: The treatment must be directed at the cause. If there is infection, prolonged treatment with antibiotics may be necessary. Occasionally a cause such as an ovarian cyst has to be dealt with surgically.

Q: *Are there any other reasons for a woman to experience dysmenorrhea?*

A: Yes. It is common for menstruation to be accompanied by mild abdominal discomfort, a feeling of pressure in the pelvis, headache, and slight nausea.

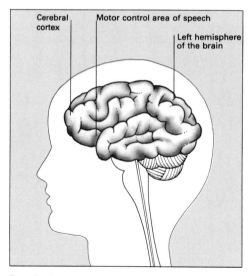

Dysphasia, a speech defect, is caused by a disorder of the left hemisphere of the brain.

These symptoms may be much worse if the woman is overtired or has been under emotional stress. Psychological factors, such as depression, may aggravate these symptoms enough for the woman to complain about them.

Dyspareunia is painful sexual intercourse. There are two forms of the condition, primary dyspareunia and secondary dyspareunia.

Q: *What causes primary dyspareunia, and how is it treated?*

A: The cause of primary dyspareunia is involuntary contraction of the muscle around the vagina, which makes sexual intercourse difficult, and sometimes impossible. The reason for the involuntary muscular contraction is usually psychological, for example, an excessive anxiety about the act of sexual intercourse or perhaps the fear of an unwanted pregnancy. Treatment for this form of dyspareunia is to remove the person's sexual fears and anxieties.

Q: *What causes secondary dyspareunia, and how is it treated?*

A: In secondary dyspareunia the pain arises from some other disorder, such as inflammation or a structural defect. It is the only form of dyspareunia experienced by men, the most common cause being inflammation of the foreskin. In women the causes of secondary dyspareunia include inflammation or infection of the vagina (vaginitis), the fallopian tubes (salpingitis), or the womb (endometriosis), or an unusually rigid hymen.

The pain can be expected to disappear after the underlying cause has been treated.

Dyspepsia. *See* INDIGESTION.

Dysphagia is difficulty in swallowing.

Dysphasia is the lack of coordination of speech and failure to arrange words in a comprehensible way. It is a less severe form of APHASIA. Dysphasia commonly follows brain damage caused by a stroke or injury involving the side of the brain that controls SPEECH. There is a tendency for the condition to improve naturally, and careful speech therapy can teach the patient how to talk, even though this may take many months.

Dyspnea is the medical term for breathlessness. The essential characteristic of dyspnea is that shortness of breath may occur without undue physical exertion. This is often a symptom of a disorder. *See* BREATHLESSNESS.

Dystrophy is a wasting condition.

Dysuria is painful or difficult urination. It is a symptom of various disorders, including

180

cystitis, prostatitis, and urethritis. Rarely, it is caused by cancer of the cervix in women or pelvic peritonitis. Any person with dysuria should consult a physician, so that the precise cause can be diagnosed and treated.

See also BLADDER DISORDERS.

E

Ear is the organ of hearing and balance. It consists of a series of sensitive structures that detect sounds and create impulses in the auditory nerve leading to the hearing center in the brain. There are three sections in the ear: (1) the outer ear; (2) the middle ear; and (3) the inner ear.

Q: What is the function of the outer ear?

A: The outer ear has two main parts: the visible flap, called the auricle or pinna, and the auditory canal. The funnel-shaped auricle picks up sound waves and passes them along the auditory canal to the middle ear. In the outer third of its length the auditory canal has a lining of fine hairs and a number of glands that secrete wax (cerumen). The hairs and the cerumen protect the ear's delicate structures by collecting much of the foreign matter that routinely enters the canal.

Q: How does the middle ear function?

A: The middle ear is separated from the outer ear by the eardrum, or tympanic membrane. As sound waves vibrate the eardrum, they set up vibrations in three tiny bones (ossicles) in the middle ear; the bones are called the hammer (malleus), anvil (incus), and stirrup (stapes). The auditory ossicles intensify and pass on the vibrations to a membrane of the inner ear called the oval window.

Pressure in the middle ear is kept the same as atmospheric pressure, allowing the eardrum to vibrate, by means of the Eustachian tube, which connects the middle ear with the back of the throat (pharynx). Two small muscles join the ossicles to the surrounding bone. These muscles contract in reaction to loud noises, and protect the inner ear by limiting its vibration.

Q: How does the inner ear function as an organ of hearing?

A: The inner ear, or cochlea, is a tube that is coiled like a snail's shell and is filled with fluid. It contains the organ of Corti. Vibrations of the oval window activate the nerve endings within the organ of Corti causing impulses to pass along the

auditory nerve to the hearing center in the brain, where sound is registered.

Q: How does the ear act as an organ of balance?

A: The inner ear also contains three fluid-filled loops, called semicircular canals, set at right angles to each other. Any movement of the head affects the fluid in one or more of them. The ends of the canals contain receptor cells that register movements of the fluid and pass the information to the brain. The whole system of canals and cavities in the inner ear is called the labyrinth.

Another organ in the inner ear contains sensitive cells with fine hairs that include small "stones" (otoliths) of calcium carbonate. When the head is held upright, the otoliths press on certain receptors. If the head is moved, the otoliths press on other receptors. In this way, receptors register any position of the head, and pass this information also to the brain. The sense of balance comes from a combination of movement and position of the head (*see* BALANCE).

See also EAR DISORDERS; p.17.

A talk about Earache

Earache is a variable and often intense throbbing pain deep inside the ear. Normally, atmospheric air pressure inside the middle ear is maintained by a channel (Eustachian tube) that connects with the back of the throat. If this tube becomes blocked during a

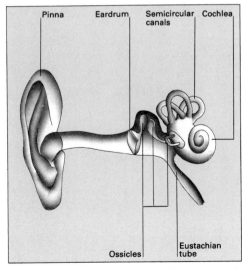

Ear has complex parts, some of which are used for hearing, and others for sensing balance.

Ear disorders

respiratory infection, a build-up of pressure in the middle ear affects the sensitive eardrum and causes pain. Sudden changes in atmospheric pressure (for example, when flying or diving) may cause a similar condition in the middle ear (*see* BAROTRAUMA).

Inflammation in the outer ear (for example, a boil) also causes pain because the lining adheres tightly to the underlying bone.

Pain may be referred to the ear from disorders elsewhere in the body, for example the neck, the pharynx, or the sinuses.

Q: Can infection spread to the ear from other parts of the body and cause earache?

A: Yes. Infection can spread from the throat along the Eustachian tube to the middle ear. The eardrum becomes inflamed from the inside, and pus forms. The pressure of the pus may be enough to burst the eardrum, in which case there is a discharge from the outer ear. The infection may also spread to the mastoid portion of the ear (temporal) bone just behind the outer ear or, in the most serious cases, through the bone to the brain.

Q: What conditions affecting the outer ear can cause earache?

A: Accumulated wax which becomes hardened and is manipulated against the ear-canal skin may irritate the auditory canal and cause earache. If particles lodge in the outer ear, interference with the auditory canal may cause pain. Skin infections such as boils, inflammations resulting from swimming, cuts, or bruises sometimes cause earache.

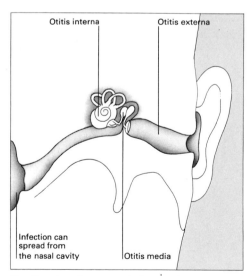

Ear disorders that cause inflammation can affect the outer, middle, or inner ears.

Q: How is earache treated?

A: Because of potential damage to the ear, a physician should be consulted. Until the cause is determined, little can be done other than to take painkilling drugs. Middle ear disorders are treated with antibiotics, decongestant nasal drops, or antihistamines. Occasionally surgical opening of the ear drum is necessary. Infections in the outer ear are treated with antibiotic eardrops. Any foreign object or lump of hardened wax in the outer ear should be removed by a physician.

Ear disorders. The following table lists some of the disorders that affect the ear and the basic characteristics of each disorder. Each disorder has a separate article in the A-Z section of this book.

Disorder	Basic characteristics
BOIL (inside and outside the ear)	Abscesses, causing pain and diminished hearing
DEAFNESS	Nearly complete or total loss of hearing
LABYRINTHITIS	Inflammation of inner ear, resulting in hearing loss and balance disturbances
MASTOIDITIS	Inflammation of the mastoid process
MÉNIÈRE'S DISEASE	Deafness, noises in the ear, and vertigo
OTITIS externa, media, or interna	Inflammation of external, middle, or inner ear
OTOMYCOSIS	Fungus infection of outer ear and/or auditory canal
OTORRHEA	Discharge from the ear
OTOSCLEROSIS	Hereditary condition characterized by bone changes in inner ear, resulting in hearing loss
TUMOR (in auditory canal, middle ear, or acoustic nerve)	Impaired hearing, deafness, balance disturbances and ear noises (tinnitus)
VERTIGO	Dizziness
WAX	Impaired hearing

The following table lists some general health disorders that may cause ear problems grouped according to symptom. The symptoms listed may also indicate other clinical disorders. A good medical history and physical examination by a physician are essential for adequate diagnosis of a problem.

Each disorder has a separate article in the A-Z section of this book.

Symptom	Disorder
Auditory hallucinations	DRUG ADDICTION SCHIZOPHRENIA (and other mental disturbances)
Earache	COMMON COLD GUMBOIL INFLUENZA PHARYNGITIS PIMPLE or foreign body in the outer ear SINUSITIS TONSILLITIS
Impaired hearing/deafness	HEMORRHAGE (into inner ear) INFLUENZA MENINGITIS MUMPS RUBELLA (in mother during pregnancy) SCARLET FEVER SYPHILIS
Outer ear skin problems	Aural IMPETIGO DERMATITIS ECZEMA RODENT ULCER Sebaceous CYST

Eardrum, known medically as the tympanic membrane, is a layer of skin, fibrous tissue, and mucous membrane at the end of the auditory canal that separates the outer ear from the middle ear.

See also EAR; EAR DISORDERS.

ECG. *See* ELECTROCARDIOGRAM.

Echocardiogram is a record of the echo produced when ultrasonic sound waves are reflected from the heart. Analysis of the echo pattern can aid diagnosis of heart disorders. *See* SONOGRAPHY.

Echogram is a record of the echo produced when ultrasonic sound waves are reflected from various body tissues. *See* SONOGRAPHY.

Eclampsia is a serious form of toxemia of pregnancy. It can occur in women during the final three months of pregnancy or, much less commonly, after the delivery of the baby. Eclampsia is an extremely grave – but rare – condition, characterized by convulsions, high blood pressure (hypertension), and finally coma that may be fatal. The cause of eclampsia is not known, but usually the condition follows preeclampsia. *See* PREECLAMPSIA.

Q: What is the treatment for eclampsia?
A: Urgent hospitalization is essential. Treatment varies but commonly sedatives are used to prevent further convulsions, and other drugs are given to reduce blood pressure. If treatment appears to be failing, labor is induced immediately or a Cesarean section is performed.

ECT. *See* ELECTROCONVULSIVE THERAPY.

Ecthyma is an ulcerative form of the skin infection impetigo in adults. *See* IMPETIGO.

Ectopic pregnancy occurs when a fertilized ovum, instead of passing along the fallopian tube from the ovary and implanting in the lining of the womb, implants in the tube or, rarely, on the ovary. Such a pregnancy seldom lasts more than two months; usually, the fallopian tube then bursts. Occasionally the embryo dies and is absorbed, although there have been cases in which a fetus has survived long enough to be born by Cesarean section. Ectopic pregnancy may be caused by infection of the fallopian tube (salpingitis).

Q: What are the symptoms of ectopic pregnancy?
A: In its early stages it may be impossible to distinguish between a normal and an ectopic pregnancy. Later there may be a sudden onset of severe abdominal pain with vaginal bleeding caused by bursting of the fallopian tube. This bleeding causes shock and collapse.

Q: How is an ectopic pregnancy treated?
A: If the embryo is detected before the tube ruptures, it may be removed surgically. When the fallopian tube ruptures, urgent hospitalization is necessary and the entire tube has to be removed.

Q: Can a woman conceive after having had an ectopic pregnancy?
A: Yes, further pregnancies are usually possible if one healthy fallopian tube remains. Expert medical advice should be sought.

See also PREGNANCY AND CHILDBIRTH.

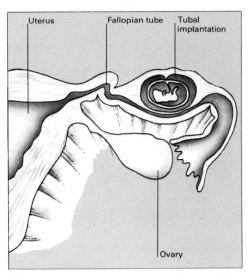

Uterus · Fallopian tube · Tubal implantation · Ovary

Ectopic pregnancy can occur anywhere outside the uterus – a common site is in the tube itself.

Ectropion

Ectropion is the turning inside out of an edge, commonly the edge of the eyelid. It may be caused by a relaxation of the lid muscles or, rarely, by damage to the facial nerve. The condition may also result from an infection of the eyelid. Ectropion is common among elderly persons.

Q: Can an ectropion be treated?

A: Yes, in most cases. The condition can be corrected either by a special surgical technique using a cautery needle, or by plastic surgery.

Q: Can ectropions affect any other parts of the body?

A: Yes. If the womb has been lacerated, during childbirth, for example, the edges of the necklike exit (cervix) may turn inside out.

See also ENTROPION.

Eczema is a red, itching, noncontagious inflammation of the skin. Eczema may be acute or chronic, with red skin patches, pimples, crusts, or scabs occurring either alone or in combination. The skin may be dry, or it may discharge a watery fluid, resulting in an itching or burning sensation.

The various causes of eczema are classified as either external (irritations, allergic reactions, exposure to certain microorganisms, and exposure to certain chemicals), or constitutional (eczema caused by an inherited predisposition).

Q: How is eczema treated?

A: The treatment depends on the cause. Oral antihistamine drugs help reduce the irritation, and ointment containing a corticosteroid may also lessen the

symptoms. If eczema is an allergic reaction, the allergen must be identified and removed.

Edema is a localized or general swelling caused by the build-up of fluid within body tissues. Excess fluid may be a result of (1) poor circulation of the blood; (2) a failure of the lymphatic system to disperse the fluid; (3) various diseases and disorders; or (4) a combination of factors.

Other causes of edema include salt retention caused by disease of the heart or kidneys, or a reduction in the amount of protein in the blood, which may occur as a result of cirrhosis, chronic nephritis, or toxemia of pregnancy (eclampsia). Localized edema may result from injury or infection.

Q: How is edema treated?

A: The treatment depends on the underlying cause of the edema. Diuretic drugs, which make the kidneys eliminate excess salt and water, often produce an immediate improvement. Edema caused by varicose veins and pregnancy can be prevented by wearing elastic stockings. Edema of the ankles, from any cause, may be helped by lying down with the feet raised.

EEG. *See* ELECTROENCEPHALOGRAM.

Effusion is the accumulation of fluid in a body space. The cause of effusion is generally inflammation or congestion.

See also EDEMA.

EKG. *See* ELECTROCARDIOGRAM.

Elavil (Trademark) is a preparation of amitriptyline hydrochloride, a drug that is used to treat depression. It also has a sedative effect, and for this reason Elavil is particularly useful for treating depressed patients with sleep disorders.

Elavil and similar antidepressants can produce unpleasant effects, including drowsiness, dry mouth, blurred vision, fatigue, and retention of urine. The adverse effects gradually disappear over a period of between two and five weeks. After this period, the drug has its desired effect. Elavil is not generally prescribed on an "as needed" basis.

Elbow is a hinge joint between the lower end of the upper arm bone (humerus) and the two bones of the lower arm (radius and ulna). Two muscles in the upper arm, the biceps and the triceps, control the action of the elbow. When the biceps contracts, the arm bends; when the triceps contracts, the arm straightens.

The funny bone is not a bone, but a nerve that lies on the inner side of the tip of the elbow, near the humerus.

Elbow injuries are disorders that affect the elbow as a result of trauma. The most common injuries are fractures, of which there

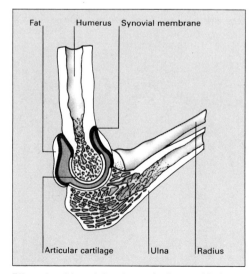

Fat   Humerus   Synovial membrane

Articular cartilage   Ulna   Radius

Elbow is a hinge joint that articulates with the larger of the two forearm bones, the ulna.

184

are many types. The elbow may be dislocated, especially following a fall on an outstretched hand. Like other joints, the elbow is vulnerable to sprains, twists, and torn ligaments. For EMERGENCY treatment, *see* First Aid, p.552.

Q: What complications might result from a fracture?

A: The chief risk with an elbow fracture is that the main artery supplying the forearm and hand may become blocked by pressure from the broken bone. This quickly causes death to the muscles the artery supplies. For this reason the pulse should always be checked at the wrist immediately after the accident. If the pulse is absent, urgent hospital attention is needed. Temporary paralysis may result if there is pressure on nerves.

If a fracture sets badly, friction of the ulnar nerve on the back of the bones of the elbow may cause tingling in the forearm and in the fourth (ring) and fifth (little) fingers of the hand. Muscles in the hand may also become weak. If the symptoms are severe, surgical repositioning of the nerve to the front of the elbow is necessary.

Q: What is a "locked elbow"?

A: The bones of the elbow or surrounding muscle fibers may join together, resulting in a stiffening of the joint. This condition is known medically as ANKYLOSIS. "Locked elbow" may occur after infection or inflammation of the tissues surrounding the elbow joint. It is a difficult condition to treat. Mobility in the joint is often restored by heat therapy, exercise, and manipulation.

Q: Why does an elbow become inflamed?

A: Inflammation of the elbow is a form of BURSITIS, in which the fluid-filled sac (bursa) surrounding the joint becomes swollen. This may be the result of injury, or it may be a symptom of such conditions as gout or rheumatoid arthritis. "Students' elbow" (olecranon bursitis) is inflammation of the bursa at the elbow caused by constant rubbing on a flat surface such as a desk or table. If the bursa becomes infected, a physician may prescribe antibiotic drugs.
See also TENNIS ELBOW.

Electric shock. For EMERGENCY treatment, *see* First Aid, p.544.

Electrocardiogram (EKG or ECG) is a record of the electric currents that occur in the heart muscle during every heartbeat. The electric currents are monitored by a highly sensitive machine known as an electrocardiograph.

Q: How is an electrocardiogram obtained?

A: Electrodes (metal strips) are attached to the skin on the patient's wrists and legs, and a fifth electrode can be placed on the chest over the heart. A combination of different impulses picked up by the electrodes produces the electrocardiogram.

Q: What is the purpose of an electrocardiogram?

A: A study of the recording assists a physician in the diagnosis of heart disorders. *See* HEART ATTACK; HEART DISEASE.

Electroconvulsive therapy (ECT), sometimes called shock therapy or electroshock therapy (EST), is the passage of an electric current through the brain to induce alterations in the brain's electrical activity. It is used in treating certain mental disorders, such as depression or schizophrenia, but ECT is increasingly being replaced by drug therapy.

Electroencephalogram (EEG) is a record of the electric currents that occur in the brain. It takes the form of an irregular line traced on a moving strip of paper. The instrument that monitors the brain's electrical activity is known as an electroencephalograph.

Q: How is an electroencephalogram obtained?

A: Electrodes are attached to the patient's scalp, and the difference in electrical potential between two sites on the skull is monitored. Changes in the usual brain rhythms are recorded during rest, sleep, and during mental concentration. It is a painless procedure.

Q: What is the purpose of an electroencephalogram?

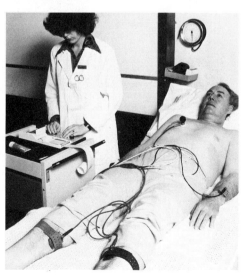

Electrocardiogram is obtained by placing electrodes on the outside of the body.

Electrolysis

A: The test assists physicians in the diagnosis of epilepsy and in the identification of sites of tumors or lesions in the brain. An EEG is also used in the definition of clinical death when a patient has been kept alive by artificial means. When no electrical activity is recorded, brain death is said to have occurred.

Electrolysis, in medicine, is the decomposition of certain body tissue by the passage of an electric current through it. It is possible to destroy hair follicles by this method, and electrolysis is often used to remove unwanted hair. *See also* DEPILATORY.

Electromyogram (EMG) is a record of the electrical impulses produced by the muscles. A physician uses an electromyogram in the diagnosis of muscle or nerve disorders.

Elephantiasis is a condition characterized by gross swelling of the skin and underlying tissues. Arms, legs, and feet are most commonly affected. In males, the genitals may also be affected; in females, the breasts. The first symptoms are attacks of dermatitis, before the affected part begins to swell, accompanied by fever; the skin surface may become ulcerated and discolored.

Q: What causes elephantiasis?

A: Elephantiasis, which occurs most commonly in tropical countries, is caused by an infestation of the lymph channels by the filarial worm *Wuchereria bancrofti.* The worm enters the body through the bite of an infected mosquito (*see* FILARIASIS). Eventually, the lymph vessels that normally drain fluid away from tissues become obstructed, and swollen.

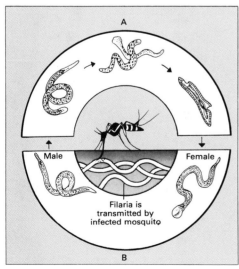

Elephantiasis is caused by worms from a mosquito (A), which infest humans (B).

Q: Is there any treatment for elephantiasis?

A: Drugs poisonous to the filarial worm are available, but may have uncomfortable side effects. Treatment for swelling of the lymph vessels (lymphedema) depends on severity. Mild cases of elephantiasis in the legs may require only rest with the legs raised, an elastic stocking, and scrupulous foot care to prevent further infections. But elephantiasis of other parts of the body may require surgery.

Embolism is an obstruction of an artery, or less commonly a vein, by material that has been carried there in the bloodstream. This material is called an embolus and may be a blood clot (thrombus), a clump of cancer cells, fat globules from the site of a broken bone (fat embolus), infected tissue from an abscess, or an air bubble (air embolus).

Q: What are the symptoms of an embolism?

A: If the embolus is small, there may be no immediate symptoms.

A large embolus can totally obstruct a blood vessel, and the area of tissue supplied by it dies (*see* INFARCTION). If this occurs in the heart the patient suffers acute ANGINA. An obstructed vessel in the brain causes a STROKE. If an embolus blocks the femoral artery, the patient experiences acute cramplike pain in the leg, which quickly goes white and cold. An embolus in the lung (pulmonary embolism) produces symptoms similar to those of coronary thrombosis; severe pain, shock, and collapse, and the coughing of bloodstained mucus. An embolus in the kidney causes HEMATURIA.

Q: How can an embolism be treated?

A: Severe symptoms, such as those occurring with pulmonary embolism, require emergency hospital treatment. The patient is treated for shock, and given oxygen and anticoagulant drugs. Sometimes, surgery (embolectomy) is performed.

Embryo is the developing organism from the moment of fertilization (conception) to the end of the second month of pregnancy.

See also PREGNANCY AND CHILDBIRTH.

Emetic is a substance that induces vomiting. Emetics are of two kinds. One type works by irritating the stomach, for example, common salt and ipecac (ipecacuanha). The other type stimulates a reflex center in the brain, for example, the drug apomorphine.

See also First Aid, p.568.

EMG. *See* ELECTROMYOGRAM.

Emphysema is air in the body tissues. Pulmonary emphysema is a chronic lung disease in which the normal lung structure breaks down. Surgical emphysema is air introduced into tissues as a result of injury or a surgical procedure. The air is gradually absorbed by the body; usually, surgical emphysema requires no treatment, and no permanent damage is caused.

Q: *What are the symptoms of pulmonary emphysema?*

A: There is gradually increasing breathlessness during exercise, and the chest moves less easily than normal, producing a constricted feeling. There may also be frequent bouts of coughing, and production of sputum. The patient feels generally unwell.

Q: *What causes pulmonary emphysema?*

A: Emphysema is often seen at an advanced stage of chronic bronchitis. It is also associated with other factors such as smoking, asthma, and various respiratory and occupational diseases. Heavily polluted air aggravates lung disorders that lead to emphysema. The alveoli rupture and they join together to form larger sacs (*see* ALVEOLUS). This decreases the surface area of the lungs available for the exchange of the gases oxygen and carbon dioxide, and makes the lungs less elastic.

Q: *How is pulmonary emphysema treated?*

A: The only effective way of dealing with the condition is to treat the preceding disease before emphysema develops. If emphysema is already present, treatment is directed toward preventing further lung damage. Affected persons should stop smoking, make sure that all respiratory infections receive medical treatment immediately, and perform breathing exercises to clear any mucus from the lungs. Persons with severe emphysema may require oxygen for physical exertion or sleep.

See also BRONCHITIS.

Empirin with codeine (Trademark) is a preparation of aspirin, phenacetin, caffeine, and codeine. It is primarily used as an analgesic but, because it contains aspirin, the preparation also has fever-reducing and anti-inflammatory properties.

Q: *Does Empirin with codeine produce any adverse effects?*

A: Yes. It may cause nausea, vomiting, pain, and bleeding from the stomach. For this reason, Empirin with codeine should not be taken by those with any stomach disorder. It may produce an allergic reaction, such as a skin rash, in those sensitive to either aspirin or codeine. Empirin with codeine may increase blood clotting time, so it should not be used by hemophiliacs or by those taking anti-

coagulant drugs. It may also cause sweating; dizziness; swelling of the throat; hives; and inflammation of the heart muscle (myocarditis). Large doses may produce ringing in the ears (tinnitus) and mental confusion. Prolonged use may cause kidney and liver damage, anemia, and drug dependence. Empirin with codeine should not be used by those with impaired kidney or liver functioning; those with respiratory disorders, such as bronchitis; or by those suffering from anemia. Some persons prefer to use an alternative preparation that combines codeine and aspirin.

Empyema is the accumulation of pus in a body cavity, usually the pleural cavity between the lung and the chest wall. It generally occurs because of a secondary bacterial infection that accompanies a lung disorder, for example, pneumonia or pleurisy. Infection may also come from the outside, for example, as the result of a stab wound. The symptoms of empyema include fever and sweating, other serious illness, chest pain, and cough.

Q: *How is empyema treated?*

A: The pus must be removed. This can be done either by sucking it out through a hollow needle (aspiration), or by a surgical operation to remove part of a rib and drain the pus away through a tube. Antibiotic drugs are prescribed to combat the infection, and the underlying cause is treated at the same time.

Enamel. *See* TEETH.

Encephalitis is inflammation of the brain. It

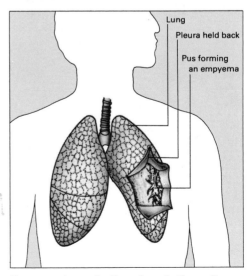

Empyema is a collection of pus in the cavity between the pleura and the lung tissue.

Encephalitis lethargica

is a serious disorder, usually caused by one of several viruses, but it can occasionally be caused by bacteria. Encephalitis viruses may be transmitted by various carriers such as ticks and mosquitoes. This form of the disease is more common in tropical countries. Rarely, encephalitis occurs as a complication of virus infections such as mumps, measles, cold sores (herpes simplex), shingles (herpes zoster), chickenpox, rabies, and some of the Coxsackie viruses. A smallpox or antirabies vaccination may lead to encephalitis.

Q: *What are the symptoms of encephalitis?*
A: Headache, high fever, vomiting, and stiffness of the neck are early symptoms. The patient's mental state varies from irritability and lethargy to confusion, delirium, convulsions, and coma in severe cases. The severity of the symptoms depends on the type of virus infection.

Q: *How is encephalitis treated?*
A: There is no specific treatment for encephalitis caused by a virus, but if the condition is traced to bacterial infection, antibiotic drugs are effective. Particular attention is paid to supportive care: an operation to make a hole in the windpipe (tracheotomy) may be performed if the patient has difficulty in breathing due to coma; fluids are given intravenously if the patient is unable to drink. If encephalitis is the result of a tumor or abscess in the brain, surgery is necessary to treat it.

Encephalitis lethargica is a particular form of brain inflammation. It is sometimes called sleeping sickness.

See also ENCEPHALITIS.

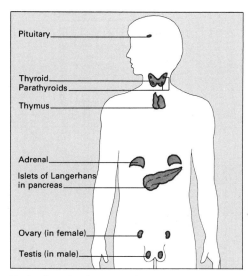

Endocrine glands secrete hormones directly into the bloodstream.

Endemic refers to any disease that is always present in a region or population.

See also EPIDEMIC; PANDEMIC.

Endocarditis is inflammation of the endocardium, the inner lining membrane of the heart. The area most commonly affected is the lining of the heart valves, and sometimes the membrane lining the heart's chambers. The cause of the inflammation is usually microorganisms in the bloodstream that lodge in a deformed heart valve. Therefore, the risk of bacterial endocarditis is greatly increased if there is a congenital deformity of the heart, and also if the valves have been damaged by rheumatic fever.

Q: *How does infection enter the bloodstream?*
A: The most common point of entry for bacteria is following minor surgery, or the extraction of an infected tooth. Bacteria may also be released into the bloodstream following a tonsillectomy, or via the womb of a woman shortly after delivery of a baby. Persons with a history of rheumatic or congenital heart disease should take antibiotic drugs several hours before visiting a dentist or before any surgical procedure, and the dentist or surgeon should be informed. A course of antibiotics may be prescribed afterward.

Q: *What are the symptoms of endocarditis?*
A: Symptoms begin gradually with fatigue, chills, and intermittent fever. If the condition is not diagnosed at this stage, increasing pallor due to progressive anemia and loss of appetite follow. Small blood spots may appear on the skin and under the nails, caused by infected clots (emboli) that have broken away from the site of the heart infection.

Q: *How is endocarditis treated?*
A: If endocarditis is suspected, hospitalization is necessary, and treatment with large doses of antibiotics is continued for at least six weeks. Penicillin is the antibiotic most commonly used, until a more specific one is selected after tests. Bed rest is an essential part of treatment. The patient may be given a blood transfusion if anemia is severe. Medical care should continue for several years.

Endocrine gland, also called a ductless gland, is a gland that produces chemicals (hormones) and secretes them directly into the blood for circulation to all parts of the body. Many endocrine glands do not act independently of each other: the balance of the body's hormones is maintained by a "feedback" system between the stimulus to produce a hormone and the ability of the hormone to regulate the strength of that stimulus.

Q: What are the main endocrine glands?

A: The main endocrine glands are: (1) PITUITARY GLAND; (2) THYROID GLAND; (3) PARATHYROID GLANDS; and (4) ADRENAL GLANDS (adrenal cortex and adrenal medulla).

These glands are purely endocrine. But (5) the GONADS (ovaries and testes) also have an endocrine function, producing sex hormones. Similarly, (6) the PANCREAS secretes insulin directly into the blood (an endocrine function) and conveys digestive juices along a duct to the duodenum.

See also HORMONE DISORDERS.

Endocrinology is the study of the endocrine glands. *See* ENDOCRINE GLAND.

Endometriosis is the presence of fragments of the lining of the womb (endometrium) in other places, such as the muscle of the womb or in the ovaries. The causes of this condition are not known.

Q: What are the symptoms of endometriosis?

A: Often there are no definite symptoms and the condition is found only during a surgical operation for some other disorder. When present, symptoms include heavy periods, often more frequent than usual, accompanied by pain (dysmenorrhea); pain during sexual intercourse (dyspareunia); and sometimes pain on defecation during a period.

The abnormally placed fragments of endometrium pass through the same monthly cycle as does the normal endometrium: they swell before a period and then bleed. Because there is no outlet for the blood, cysts form. These occasionally rupture, causing severe abdominal pain. The symptoms disappear during pregnancy, which may cure the condition, and after the menopause.

Q: How is endometriosis treated?

A: In mild cases, painkilling drugs may lessen the symptoms. Rarely, the fragments of endometrium can be found and removed surgically. All of the symptoms are relieved by artificially inducing menopause by irradiation or surgical removal of the ovaries, so that the womb and the abnormal tissue cease to be stimulated by ovarian hormones. The hormone pills used for contraception may also help, and these work without sterilizing the patient. A woman with the symptoms should consult a gynecologist.

Endometritis is inflammation of the lining of the womb (endometrium) caused by bacterial infection, which may spread to the rest of the womb and other tissues. The infection may follow gonorrhea, infection of the cervix, or any gynecological operation. Endometritis may occur after the menopause, due to lowered resistance to infection.

Q: What are the symptoms of endometritis?

A: The symptoms include fever, low backache, abdominal pain, foul-smelling vaginal discharge, and painful periods. Another symptom of senile endometritis is a watery, sometimes bloodstained discharge.

Q: How is endometritis treated?

A: The usual treatment is with antibiotic drugs to combat the infection.

Endometrium is the mucous membrane that lines the inner surface of the womb. The endometrium is under hormonal influence and undergoes various changes during the menstrual cycle. During the cycle the endometrium becomes thicker and develops a copious blood supply. If an egg is fertilized, it implants in the endometrium, part of which develops into the placenta. If fertilization does not occur, the endometrium is shed each month, causing the menstrual flow.

See also MENSTRUATION.

Endoscopy is the examination of the interior of the body using a lighted and pliable fibrous glass tube, usually with a system of lenses.

Endotracheal tube is a tube that is passed down the throat and into the windpipe (trachea). It is used to provide an airway and to prevent the inhalation of foreign material during a surgical procedure.

Enema is the introduction of a liquid into the rectum and colon through the anus. Soap and water is used to wash out constipated feces; oil to lubricate the large intestine. A barium

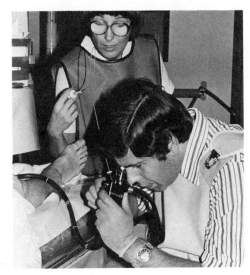

Endoscopy enables a physician to examine the internal organs without the need for surgery.

enema (a suspension of barium sulfate in water) is used in X-ray examinations to diagnose disorders of the large intestine such as diverticulitis, ulcerative colitis, and cancer.

Q: Are there any dangers from the regular use of enemas?

A: Constant home use of enemas as a treatment for chronic constipation is dangerous, because (1) the bowels' natural ability to expel feces is weakened; and (2) there is a possibility that an underlying disorder of the intestine is masked. Enemas should be given only under medical guidance.

See also COLONIC IRRIGATION.

ENT is an abbreviation for ear, nose, and throat, the medical specialty called OTORHINO-LARYNGOLOGY.

Entamoeba histolytica is a species of ameba that infects the intestine of human beings. It is the cause of amebic dysentery and amebic abscess. *See* DYSENTERY.

Enteric fevers are intestinal infections of the typhoid and paratyphoid group. *See* PARA-TYPHOID; TYPHOID FEVER.

Enteritis is inflammation of the intestine, particularly the small intestine. If the stomach is also inflamed, the condition is known as GAS-TROENTERITIS; if the colon is involved, it is called COLITIS.

Enteritis may be due to infection by a virus or bacteria; food poisoning; or chemical irritation. Symptoms of the condition are diarrhea, abdominal pain, and vomiting. Treatment is directed at the cause, and antispasmodic drugs may also be prescribed.

See also CROHN'S DISEASE.

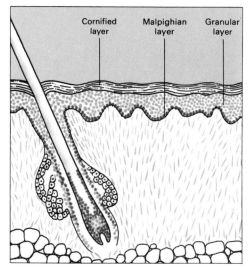

Cornified layer   Malpighian layer   Granular layer

Epidermis is continuously renewed with cells from the Malpighian layer.

Enterobiasis is infestation of the intestines by the parasitic worm *Enterobius vermicularis*. It is commonly known as pinworm or threadworm. *See* WORMS.

Enterostomy is a surgical opening in the abdominal wall to form an artificial anus. The term is also used to describe an artificial opening between two parts of the intestine.

See also COLOSTOMY; ILEOSTOMY.

Entropion is the turning inward of an edge or margin. It occurs most commonly on the edge of the lower eyelid following infection or as a condition of old age. An entropion can be treated by a special method of cautery or by plastic surgery.

See also ECTROPION.

Enuresis is involuntary urination. Nocturnal enuresis, or BED-WETTING, is common in children.

Enzymes are chemical substances, produced by living cells, that act as catalysts and speed up the rates of chemical changes in other substances. All enzymes are complicated proteins.

Q: What kinds of enzymes are there?

A: Enzymes that bring about the breakdown of complex substances into simpler compounds are found particularly in the digestive juices. Invertase (sucrase) is one of the enzymes responsible for the digestion of carbohydrates: ordinary table sugar, sucrose, is broken down into smaller compounds (fructose and glucose), which the body can digest. Other digestive enzymes break down proteins into amino acids, and fats into fatty acids.

Q: Can deficiency of an enzyme cause disease?

A: Yes. The absence of a particular enzyme is often inherited. The disorder known as phenylketonuria is caused by the absence of an enzyme that normally prevents the build-up of the amino acid phenylalamine by converting it to tyrosine.

Epidemic is an outbreak of an infectious disease or condition that afflicts many persons at the same time and in the same geographical area.

See also ENDEMIC; IMMUNIZATION; PANDEMIC; QUARANTINE.

Epidemic pleurodynia is a disease most common in children, caused by the Group B coxsackie-viruses. It is characterized by pain in the lower chest, fever, sore throat, and frequent headaches. Symptoms usually clear up in 2 to 4 days, although relapse may occur within a few days or weeks. In uncomplicated cases, epidemic pleurodynia is not serious.

Epidermis is the surface layer of the skin. *See* SKIN.

Epididymis is an oblong structure at the side

of the testicle (testis), consisting of a tightly coiled tube eighteen to twenty feet (five and a half to six meters) long. Connected with the epididymis are about twenty small tubes through which the sperm flow from the testis. The sperm gradually mature in the epididymis, before traveling along the spermatic cord to the seminal vesicles.

Epididymitis is inflammation of the EPIDIDYMIS. The inflammation causes the epididymis to become swollen and painful. The person may need to urinate more frequently, and urination may be painful. In some cases fever may occur.

The condition may be caused by the spread of the bladder infection cystitis or urethritis, or it may be a complication of gonorrhea, prostate disorders, or tuberculosis. Epididymitis can be effectively treated with antibiotic drugs and bed rest with support for the scrotum. Painkilling drugs may be prescribed until the pain subsides.

Epidural anesthetic is a local anesthetic injected into the space in the dura mater of the meninges, the tough fibrous membrane that covers the spinal cord.

See also ANESTHETICS.

Epiglottis is a leaf-shaped structure in the throat that lies in front of the base of the tongue and over the opening of the larynx and windpipe (trachea) that prevents food and liquids from passing into the trachea.

A talk about Epilepsy

Epilepsy (for EMERGENCY treatment, *see* First Aid p.534) is a symptom of brain dysfunction characterized by periodic, recurrent seizures. Seizures occur in various forms, ranging from brief periods of impaired awareness to severe convulsions with loss of consciousness. Some persons with epilepsy experience an aura, a physical sensation such as a smell, at the beginning of a seizure.

Seizures used to be described as grand mal, petit mal, psychomotor, and focal. But the new International Seizure Classification groups and describes seizures according to the area of the brain involved. The two major classes are partial seizures, which involve only a portion of the brain, and generalized seizures, which involve all of the brain.

Q: What are partial seizures?
A: Partial seizures involve only a part of the brain. Therefore only a specific area of the body or a particular level of consciousness is affected. Partial seizures with simple symptoms (traditionally called focal seizures) produce brief twitching movements of specific muscle groups, such as those controlling an arm or leg. If the area of the brain affected controls sight, hearing, or another of the senses, brief visual, auditory, or other hallucinations are experienced. The person usually retains consciousness with simple partial seizures. Partial seizures with complex symptoms (traditionally called psychomotor seizures) involve impairment of consciousness and involuntary complicated acts. During a typical complex partial seizure, the person appears to be conscious but is unresponsive, or inappropriately responsive, to his or her surroundings. He or she may perform purposeless activities, such as lip-smacking, picking at his or her clothing, or aimless wandering. This type of seizure may be brief, last for several hours, or progress to a generalized seizure.

Q: What are generalized seizures?
A: Generalized seizures affect all of the brain. The two most common forms are absence seizures (traditionally called petit mal), and tonic-clonic seizures (traditionally called grand mal). Absence seizures consist of brief lapses of consciousness lasting usually five to thirty seconds. The person may stare blankly and appear to be daydreaming or experience slight movements of the facial muscles, head, or arms. When the seizure ends, the person resumes his or her previous activity and has no awareness of the seizure. Absence seizures commonly begin in childhood and may be as frequent as 50 to 100 a

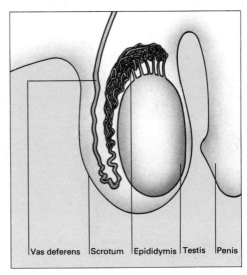

| Vas deferens | Scrotum | Epididymis | Testis | Penis |

Epididymis is a twisted tube about twenty feet long leading from testis to vas deferens.

Epilepsy

day or may occur only a few times a month.

Generalized tonic-clonic seizures are what most people think of as epilepsy. The seizure begins with a sudden loss of consciousness. The person falls and the muscles become rigid (the tonic phase). The person may also give a sharp cry, which is caused by the sudden contraction of the abdominal muscles forcing air from the lungs through the larynx. Because there is a brief cessation of breathing, the skin may turn blue. The clonic phase then follows, consisting of jerking contractual movements of the major muscle groups. Breathing resumes but is heavy and irregular, causing frothing of saliva. The person may bite his or her tongue or lose bladder control. Following the seizure, the person may have a headache, be confused, and want to sleep. Generalized tonic-clonic seizures usually last from three to five minutes.

Q: *What are some of the rarer forms of epilepsy?*

A: Rare forms of epilepsy include Jacksonian seizures in which motor activity begins in the distal portion of a limb, such as a toe or thumb, and "marches" or progresses up the limb to involve major portions of the whole body. Autonomic seizures are partial seizures involving the part of the brain that controls the autonomic nervous system. Seizure activity includes headaches, stomachaches, nausea, vomiting, fever, or similar symptoms that recur without apparent cause. In

Epilepsy produces changes in the brain patterns picked up by electrodes on the head.

atonic seizures, the person experiences a loss of muscle tone and falls with no convulsive activity. In myoclonic seizures, the individual experiences brief muscle jerks, sometimes violent enough to throw him or her to the ground. In unilateral seizures, only one hemisphere, or half, of the brain is involved and consequently seizure activity is limited to one side of the body.

Q: *What are the causes of epilepsy?*

A: Seizures are caused by the uncontrolled discharge of electrical energy by brain cells. An electroencephalograph (EEG) is used to record the electrical activity of the brain to help in the diagnosis of epilepsy. In about half of epilepsy patients, no cause can be found for the uncontrolled electrical activity, and in these persons, epilepsy is termed idiopathic. For the remaining 50 percent, an underlying cause can be identified and the epilepsy is called symptomatic.

Anyone can experience an injury to the brain or central nervous system which can result in epilepsy. Some of the more common causes are prenatal damage, injury during birth, brain tumors, head injury, cerebrovascular disease, and serious infections during childhood.

Q: *Can epilepsy be an inherited condition?*

A: A number of genetic disorders, usually rare, include recurrent seizures in their symptomology. In such cases, it is the genetic disorder and not a predilection toward seizures which is inherited.

In a low percentage of cases, an abnormal EEG pattern may be inherited. Such a condition may increase the chances that epilepsy may develop.

Q: *Does epilepsy develop only in childhood?*

A: No. Epilepsy may develop at any age, but because most cases are diagnosed in patients younger than aged eighteen, epilepsy is often mistakenly regarded as a childhood condition. Persons over the age of 55, because of the increased incidence of cerebrovascular disease, are the second most susceptible age group. Because epilepsy is not cured, but controlled by currently available treatment, it is usually a lifelong disorder.

Q: *Are there other disorders with symptoms similar to epilepsy?*

A: Yes. Breath-holding spells in children may resemble convulsive seizures. Fainting in adults may be mistaken for epilepsy. Heart disease causing rapid changes in the pulse rate may cause symptoms similar to those of epilepsy. High fever in young children can cause convulsions called febrile seizures. In otherwise normal children, febrile seizures do not usually have any serious consequences, but a physician should be consulted. In children with a family history of epilepsy or other neurological disorders, an increased chance of developing epilepsy may be present and preventive treatment may be prescribed.

Q: *How is epilepsy treated?*

A: There are sixteen anticonvulsant or antiepileptic drugs approved for use in the United States. Not all are effective for every type of seizure. A physician will begin by prescribing a single drug and increase the dosage until seizures are controlled. If side effects appear, the dosage will be reduced until a balance between a minimum of side effects and a maximum of satisfactory control is achieved. If a single drug is not satisfactory, a second drug is usually added.

A large percentage of epilepsy patients experience several different types of seizures. Sometimes the type of seizure experienced by a person may change as he or she grows older. Epilepsy patients should be regularly checked by their physician.

Because the individual's body chemistry causes him or her to absorb anticonvulsant drugs in an individual way, the physician periodically takes blood samples to determine the level of drug present in the patient's system. Blood level monitoring allows the physician to accurately tailor the drug dosage to each individual to achieve maximum seizure control with a minimum of drug side effects. Some of the most commonly used antiepileptic drugs are phenobarbital and phenytoin for generalized tonic-clonic seizures; tri-methodione, valproic acid, or ethosuximide for absence seizures; and primidone or carbamazepine for complex partial seizures.

Surgery may be used to treat epilepsy when the condition does not respond to medication or when its cause can be traced to such things as a scar on the brain or a tumor. But surgery will only be used if it can be determined that the scar or tumor is located where it can be safely removed.

Other forms of treatment are currently being researched. Biofeedback is being used to teach patients to control the brain's electrical activity. This may someday help patients to prevent seizures. Another experimental technique involves the permanent implanting of electrodes in an epilepsy patient's brain.

These electrodes can be periodically activated. The hope is that this periodic electrical activity will help to stabilize the brain's uncontrolled electrical activity and thus prevent seizures. However, it must be emphasized that both techniques are only experimental and will require more research before they can be evaluated.

Q: *What complications can result from seizures?*

A: Sometimes one seizure will immediately follow another and result in continuous seizure activity. This condition (called status epilepticus) can be life-threatening in the case of generalized tonic-clonic seizures and requires emergency medical treatment to prevent cardiac arrest or respiratory failure.

In generalized tonic-clonic, myoclonic, and atonic seizures, the person may injure himself or herself by falling against hard or sharp objects. In other seizure forms, such as absence or complex partial seizures, status epilepticus results in prolonged periods of impaired consciousness which prevent the person from behaving normally.

Untreated seizures prevent the patient from carrying out a normal life. With current treatment, more than 50 percent of persons with epilepsy can achieve complete seizure control and lead a normal life. Another 30 percent can achieve partial control over their seizures and engage in most activities.

Q: *Is epilepsy a permanent condition?*

A: In most cases, epilepsy is chronic.

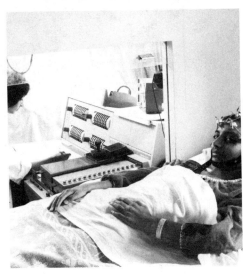

Electroencephalograph recordings of brain-waves may detect epileptic tendencies.

However, with consistent treatment, seizures may decrease in frequency after a number of years, and drugs can be gradually reduced or withdrawn. Physicians will usually begin reduction if a patient remains seizure-free for several years, but seizures often recur. A patient should never reduce medication without the advice of a physician. Abrupt withdrawal of antiepileptic drugs may result in an increase in the number and severity of seizures. Such withdrawal has also been known to trigger incidents of status epilepticus.

Q: *What precautions should a person with epilepsy take?*

A: Persons with epilepsy whose seizures are controlled can lead normal lives. However, they should be aware that excessive use of alcohol, poor eating habits, and lack of rest may precipitate seizures. All states permit a person with epilepsy to drive if he or she has been seizure-free for a specific period. The person whose seizures are less well controlled or are triggered by a specific stimulus should limit activities accordingly so as not to endanger himself or herself. The epilepsy patient should always take his or her medication exactly as prescribed and report any changes in seizure activity or drug side effects to a physician so that dosage can be adjusted.

Q: *Should a woman with epilepsy consider bearing a child?*

A: A woman with epilepsy should consult a physician before becoming pregnant.

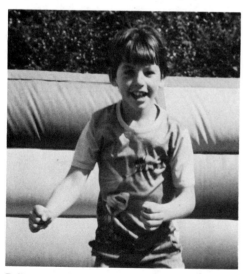

Epilepsy can be medically controlled and need not stop a child from enjoying life.

Pregnancy has been known to increase both the number and severity of seizures. Further, some anticonvulsant drugs have been shown to have a relationship to an increase in the incidence of certain birth defects, primarily cleft palate.

Episiotomy is a cut that is made into the edge of the birth canal, at the ending of the second stage of labor. It may be made to prevent tearing or to help the delivery. *See* PREGNANCY AND CHILDBIRTH.

Epsom salts. *See* MAGNESIUM SULFATE.

Epulis is any swelling or growth on the gums caused by infection or irritation. *See* GINGIVITIS; GUMBOIL.

Ergosterol is a steroid substance that is now obtained mainly from yeast, but was originally obtained from ERGOT. Ergosterol is exposed to ultraviolet rays to yield vitamin D_2, which is sometimes used in the treatment of rickets. *See* RICKETS.

Ergot is a fungus (*Claviceps purpurea*) that grows as a parasite on rye. It is extremely poisonous, but its alkaloid chemicals are the source of many drugs.

Ergot poisoning can occur by eating rye bread made from contaminated grain or by taking an overdose of an ergot drug. The poison causes blood vessels to contract. This gives rise to symptoms such as vomiting, diarrhea, tingling in the limbs, and, occasionally, convulsions. The victim needs emergency medical attention. If the patient survives, cataracts and gangrene may develop as secondary complications.

Two of the many drugs derived from ergot are ergonovine and ergotamine. Ergonovine causes the womb to contract, and may be prescribed after childbirth to stop bleeding. Ergotamine acts on the blood vessels in the head, and is used to treat migraine.

See also ERGOSTEROL.

Erosion is the breaking down of the body tissues. *See* CERVICAL EROSION.

Erysipelas is an acute, streptococcal skin infection. It tends to spread rapidly causing inflammation, fever, nausea, vomiting, and, occasionally, red lines stretching along the limbs. Erysipelas is treated with penicillin and sulfonamide drugs. A physician should be consulted if erysipelas is suspected.

Erysipeloid is an unusual bacterial skin infection resembling erysipelas. Erysipeloid produces red swellings on the skin, with tingling and itching. It is usually confined to the hands and seldom makes the patient ill. The symptoms last for several days before spontaneous recovery occurs, leaving a brown stain on the skin. Erysipeloid is generally acquired by handling fish or meat products, and it is more common in the summer. Although no treatment is necessary, antibiotics can shorten the time taken for recovery.

Erythema nodosum is a condition in which red, oval nodules appear on the skin. Over a period of several weeks, the nodules change from red to a brown color. Erythema nodosum often occurs on the shins and may be accompanied by fever, aches, and fatigue. It usually follows a streptococcal throat infection. In children, the condition can be associated with rheumatic fever. In adults, it may occur with sarcoidosis, tuberculosis, or ulcerative colitis. Certain drugs, such as the sulfonamides, may also produce erythema nodosum. The treatment consists of bed rest and aspirin until the condition improves. If the cause of the condition is a streptococcal infection, penicillin should be taken for at least one year.

Erythredema. *See* PINK DISEASE.

Erythroblastosis fetalis. *See* HEMOLYTIC DISEASE OF THE NEWBORN.

Erythrocyte. *See* RED BLOOD CELL.

Erythromycin is a preparation of an antibiotic drug derived from the mold *Streptomyces erythreus*. Like penicillin, erythromycin is a broad-range antibiotic. It produces few side effects; there may be some abdominal pain with nausea, vomiting, and diarrhea, but these usually clear up spontaneously within a few days. Because resistant bacterial strains develop rapidly to this drug, erythromycin is usually only given to patients who are allergic to penicillin.

Esophageal speech is a method of producing understandable speech, after the surgical removal of the voice box (larynx), by vibrating air in the esophagus instead.

Esophagus, also known as the gullet, is a muscular tube about ten inches (25cm) long that extends from the pharynx at the back of the throat to the stomach. In the neck, the esophagus lies behind the trachea, and enters the thorax behind the aorta and heart to join the top of the stomach.

The esophagus conveys food and drink from the pharynx to the stomach. This is achieved partly by gravity and partly by peristalsis (rhythmical waves of muscular contractions). When a person breathes in, air is directed to the larynx and the trachea. At the same time, however, saliva is able to run down the esophagus. Where the esophagus and the stomach join, there is a ring of muscle (the cardiac sphincter) that prevents the stomach contents from passing back up the esophagus.

See also ACHALASIA; DYSPHAGIA; HEARTBURN; HIATUS HERNIA.

ESR is an abbreviation of erythrocyte sedimentation rate, the rate at which red blood cells settle when an anticoagulant is added to them. *See* SEDIMENTATION RATE.

Estrogen is the collective name for several female sex hormones produced mainly by the ovaries but also by the adrenal glands.

At the onset of puberty, estrogens stimulate the development of pubic hair and of secondary female sex characteristics, such as rounded hips and breasts. Estrogens also play an essential part in the hormonal control of menstruation, being partly responsible (with progesterone) for the cyclical changes in the lining of the womb.

Estrogens have a number of medical uses. For example, synthetic estrogens are a component of most types of contraceptive pill, and are also used in the treatment of menstrual disorders and in estrogen replacement therapy (ERT) at menopause.

In men, synthetic estrogens are used in the treatment of cancer of the prostate gland.

See also HORMONES.

Ether is the general name for a class of organic chemical compounds derived from alcohols. Ether is used as a cleansing agent, and was once widely used as an anesthetic (*see* ANESTHETICS).

Eustachian tube is the narrow tube about 1.5 inches (4cm) long that connects the back of the nasal passages with the cavity of the middle ear. The Eustachian tube has two functions: it allows the natural secretions from the ear to drain into the throat; and it equalizes the pressures on each side of the eardrum. During swallowing, the lower end

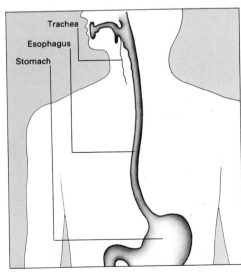

Trachea

Esophagus

Stomach

Esophagus conveys food and drink from the pharynx to the stomach.

195

Exanthem

of the Eustachian tube opens momentarily. Blockage of the Eustachian tube, with swollen tissue as in infection (otitis media), can lead to temporary deafness. If the tube is blocked and sudden pressure changes occur, as may happen during flying or diving, there may be pain and it is possible that the eardrum may rupture (*see* BAROTRAUMA).

See also EAR; EARACHE.

Exanthem. *See* RASH.

Exhaustion is a state of extreme fatigue, often accompanied by a reduced ability to respond to external stimuli.

See also FATIGUE; HEATSTROKE.

Exophthalmos is abnormal protrusion of the eyeballs. It is usually a symptom of HYPERTHYROIDISM, but may have other causes, such as a tumor behind the eye. A physician should be consulted so that the underlying cause can be treated; otherwise permanent eye damage may result. If only one eyeball is involved, the condition is called proptosis.

See also THYROTOXICOSIS.

Expectorant is a substance that helps the loosening and the discharge of phlegm.

Exploratory operation is a surgical procedure that is performed to aid the precise diagnosis of a disorder; when the urgency is such that there is no time for conventional diagnostic testing; or when conventional diagnostic methods have failed to reveal a disorder.

Exposure is a debilitated body state that results from being subjected to extremes of hot, cold, or windy weather without adequate protection. Lack of treatment may lead to loss of consciousness and further complications. Prolonged exposure may lead to death.

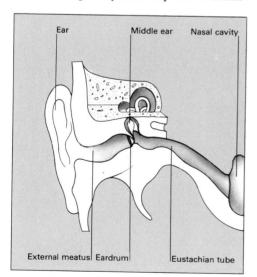

Eustachian tube connects with the nasal cavity and equalizes air pressure in the middle ear.

See First Aid, pp.560, 573.

Extradural hematoma is bleeding between the dura mater (the tough fibrous membrane that covers the brain) and the skull. The blood comes from a ruptured artery that supplies the internal surface of the skull. Extradural hematoma usually follows a head injury involving a skull fracture.

Q: *What are the symptoms of an extradural hematoma?*

A: The first sign may be a temporary loss of consciousness, followed by a period of apparently normal behavior. Other symptoms may begin hours or sometimes days after the injury. The patient's speech becomes slurred, and he or she walks unsteadily. The patient may suffer a headache, followed by unconsciousness caused by the pressure of the clotted blood on the brain.

Q: *How is an extradural hematoma treated?*

A: The patient needs urgent hospitalization. Special X rays are taken to diagnose the condition. A surgeon then performs an operation to remove the clot. The patient generally recovers immediately.

Extrasystole is a disturbance of the natural rhythm of the heart. An extra heartbeat occurs, as a premature and weak beat. When the next heartbeat is due, the heart muscles are still recovering from the extrasystole and do not respond: the heart misses a beat.

The sensation of a missed beat is usually felt in the chest, or throat, and may cause anxiety, but in an otherwise normal heart extrasystoles are no cause for alarm. They are common in many healthy persons while resting, especially in those who smoke or who drink a lot of coffee. If the extrasystoles disappear on taking exercise, they can safely be ignored. But if extrasystoles continue after exercise or occur with some regularity, a physician should be consulted.

Extrauterine pregnancy is another name for ectopic pregnancy. *See* ECTOPIC PREGNANCY.

Extravasation is the escape of a body fluid from its normal containing vessel into the surrounding tissue.

Extrovert is a psychological term that describes a person whose interests center on external objects and actions.

See also INTROVERT.

Exudate is a fluid that penetrates the walls of blood vessels and seeps into adjoining tissues. The process happens as a body defense mechanism associated with inflammation caused by infection: blood vessels dilate and become more permeable, so allowing a fluid rich in serum protein containing antibodies and white blood cells to escape. Pus and nasal mucus are also termed exudates.

A talk about the Eye

Eye is the organ of sight. It is an almost perfect sphere about one inch (2.5cm) in diameter. The eye is filled with jellylike fluid (*see* HUMOR) that helps to maintain its shape. The inside of the lids and the white of the eye are covered with the CONJUNCTIVA.

The eye's outer surface is covered with the sclera, except for a transparent area in the front, the CORNEA. Lining the sclera is the CHOROID. The front edge of the choroid is called the ciliary body. The IRIS is the colored disk in front of the LENS. The RETINA is a layer of millions of light-sensitive nerve cells that overlies the choroid. There are two types of nerve cells in the retina: rods and cones. The individual nerve fibers from these cells join to form the optic nerve.

Q: How is the amount of light entering the eye controlled?

A: This is controlled by the iris, which contains circular muscles and radial muscles. When the circular muscles contract, the pupil gets smaller. When the radial muscles contract, the pupil gets larger. These muscles are controlled by the AUTONOMIC NERVOUS SYSTEM.

Q: How is light focused on the retina?

A: Light is focused by the cornea and the lens. The cornea is the major focusing component; the lens performs fine focusing. The lens can change its shape so that near and far objects can be focused; this is called ACCOMMODATION.

Q: What happens when light hits the retina?

A: Light is focused mainly on one area of the retina called the macula lutea. In the center of the macula lutea is the FOVEA, the region that gives the greatest visual acuity. Visual acuity depends upon the number and density of the rods and cones, since each cell can record only the presence of light and, in cones, its color. There are about ten million cones and one hundred million rods in each eye.

When light falls on a rod or cone, the cell sends impulses along the optic nerve to the brain, which interprets them into a representation of the image.

Q: How do cones detect color?

A: The mechanism of color vision is not fully understood, but some specialists claim that there are three types of cone cell. Each type of cone cell is sensitive to either red, green, or blue light. These colors stimulate particular cone cells so that color is perceived.

Eye disorders. The following table lists some of the disorders that affect the eye and the basic characteristics of each condition. Sometimes an eye disorder is symptomatic of some other disorder (for example, diabetes, nephritis, or stroke). Each disorder has a separate article in the A-Z section of this book. For eye injuries, *see* First Aid, p.558.

See also BLINDNESS.

Disorder	Basic characteristics
ADENOMA (of pituitary gland)	Loss of vision due to pressure on optic nerve by a tumor
AMAUROSIS	Progressive loss of sight, leading to blindness
AMBLYOPIA	Dimness of vision
APHAKIA	Absence of the lens of the eye, causing blurred vision
ASTIGMATISM	Distorted and blurred vision
BLEPHARITIS	Inflammation of the eyelid
CATARACT	Blurred vision and loss of sight
CHALAZION	Lump on the eyelid
COLOBOMA	Cleft in the iris, the choroid, or other part of the eye
COLOR BLINDNESS	Inability to identify one or more primary colors
DACRYOCYSTITIS	Inflammation of tear sac
DETACHED RETINA	Flashes of light, followed later by sensation of curtain drawn over the eye

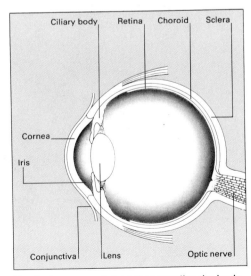

Eye is the organ of sight that supplies the body with thirty percent of sensory perception.

Eyeglasses

Disorder	Basic characteristics
DIABETES	Dimness of vision, loss of sight
ECTROPION	Inside of eyelid is turned outward
ENTROPION	Edge of eyelid is turned inward toward the eyeball
EXOPHTHALMOS	Bulging eye or eyes
FARSIGHTEDNESS	Hyperopia, diminished ability to see things at close range
GLAUCOMA	Increased pressure within eye, resulting in gradual loss of vision
GLIOMA (optic)	Tumor of optic nerve, with loss of vision
HEMIANOPIA	Defective vision or blindness in half the visual field
HYPERTENSION	Degeneration of retina as result of high blood pressure
IRITIS	Inflamation of iris with sensitivity to light
KERATITIS	Blurred vision due to inflammation of cornea
MIGRAINE	Blurred vision and flashes of light due to intense headache
MYOPIA	Nearsightedness, objects can be seen distinctly only when close to eyes
NEPHRITIS (chronic)	Deterioration of retina as result of kidney disease

Disorder	Basic characteristics
NIGHT BLINDNESS	Absence of or defective vision in the dark
OPHTHALMIA (and sympathetic ophthalmia)	Inflammation of the eye or the conjunctiva
PANOPHTHALMITIS	Infection of the whole of the eye
PAPILLEDEMA	Swelling of the optic nerve and sudden blindness
PRESBYOPIA	Diminished ability to see things at close range, due to aging
RETINITIS	Inflammation of retina
RETINITIS PIGMENTOSA	Degeneration of retina, leading eventually to blindness
RETROBULBAR NEURITIS	Inflammation of optic nerve and sudden blindness
SARCOMA	Tumor, causing pain and blurred vision
SCOTOMA	A blind or partly blind area in the visual field, surrounded by area of normal vision
STROKE	Blind spots, actual blindness, or temporary loss of vision due to interruption of blood supply to brain
STYE	Infection of one or more of the small glands of the eyelid
TAY-SACHS DISEASE	Impairment of sight, resulting in blindness

Eyeglasses are prescribed to correct certain visual defects. Recently, CONTACT LENSES have become an alternative to eyeglasses for many visual defects.

Q: What visual defects can eyeglasses help to correct?

A: Eyeglasses are commonly used to correct ASTIGMATISM (distortion of the cornea); HYPEROPIA (farsightedness); MYOPIA (nearsightedness); and PRESBYOPIA (defective vision due to hardening of the lens with age). As well as these disorders, eyeglasses may be required by young children to correct a congenital disorder.

Q: Are there special eyeglasses for particular conditions?

A: Yes. With increasing age many people need eyeglasses with divided lenses for each eye, called bifocals. These correct vision for both near and far objects. Trifocals correct vision for the middle distance as well as for near and far vision. Eyeglasses may have permanently tinted lenses, or they may be of variable

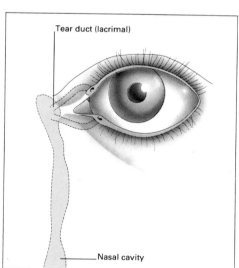

Tear duct (lacrimal)

Nasal cavity

Dacryocystitis is inflammation of the lacrimal duct and sac causing pain and swelling.

darkness according to the light intensity. Dark lenses are used by albinos; those with certain chronic eye disorders, such as IRITIS and PHOTOPHOBIA; and in conditions of extremely bright light to prevent blindness. Eyeglasses may be made with plastic or unbreakable glass lenses to prevent injury to the eyes.

Eyeglasses do not make the eyes lazy nor worsen a person's eyesight. But, because some vision defects worsen with age, this may seem to be the case. The eyes should be tested yearly.

Q: *Is there any difference between eyeglasses and contact lenses?*

A: The choice between contact lenses and conventional eyeglasses is, in most cases, a matter of personal preference. An ophthalmologist may advise the use of contact lenses in severe forms of astigmatism or myopia.

Eye injuries. *See* EYE DISORDERS; First Aid, p.558.

Eyelid is one of two movable folds of skin that protect the front of each eyeball. When closed, the eyelids cover the visible area of the eye. The upper lid is larger and capable of more movement than is the lower one. It contains a fibrous plate of tissue that gives additional protection to the eyeball. Each eyelid has on its undersurface a mucous membrane, called the conjunctiva. The conjunctiva is lubricated by tears produced by the lacrimal apparatus.

Q: *Which disorders affect the eyelids?*

A: Eyelid disorders include BLACK EYE, BLEPHARITIS, CHALAZION, CONJUNCTIVITIS, ECTROPION, ENTROPION, PTOSIS, and STYE. The eyelids are also susceptible to general skin disorders such as ECZEMA and RODENT ULCER.

See also EYE.

F

Face-lift. *See* COSMETIC SURGERY.

Face presentation describes a baby emerging face first from the vagina. *See* PREGNANCY AND CHILDBIRTH.

Facial paralysis is disablement of the muscles of the face, caused by damage to, or infection of, the nerve that supplies them.

See also BELL'S PALSY.

Fahrenheit is a temperature scale on which the freezing point of water is 32° and the boiling point of water is 212°. The normal human body temperature is 98.6°F.

See also CENTIGRADE.

Fainting, or syncope, is a momentary loss of consciousness. It is caused by a temporary deficiency in the blood supply to the brain, usually following a sudden drop in blood pressure. *See* First Aid, p.550.

Fallopian tube (oviduct) is a muscular tube that extends from the womb (uterus) to an ovary. It is about four inches (10cm) long. There are two fallopian tubes, one for each ovary.

After ovulation, the egg (ovum) passes from an ovary along the fallopian tube to the womb. Finger-like tissue at the end of the tube nearest the ovary helps to direct the egg into the tube, and hair-like cells inside the tube propel the egg along it. Sperm swim up the tube from the womb and meet the egg. If the egg becomes fertilized, fertilization usually takes place while the egg is in the fallopian tube. If for any reason the fertilized egg then moves too slowly, it may implant in the fallopian tube instead of in the lining of the womb, resulting in an ectopic pregnancy. *See* ECTOPIC PREGNANCY.

See also PREGNANCY AND CHILDBIRTH.

Q: *Can a disorder of the fallopian tubes cause sterility?*

A: Yes. After inflammation (salpingitis), any scar that remains may block the tube, or damage the finger-like tissue at its opening, or damage the hair-like cells. If the inflammation and scarring occur in both tubes, the woman is in danger of being unable to conceive. (*See* SALPINGITIS.)

Q: *Does artificial sterilization of a woman involve the fallopian tubes?*

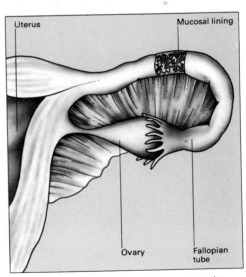

Fallopian tube extends from the ovary to the uterus and is lined with mucous membrane.

Fallot's tetralogy

A: Yes. The surgical cutting and tying of both fallopian tubes is the usual method of sterilization.

See also STERILIZATION.

Fallot's tetralogy is a congenital heart malformation that comprises four separate problems. These are: (1) a hole in the wall between the left and right ventricles; (2) narrowing of the artery that leads to the lungs (pulmonary artery); (3) blood reaching the aorta from the right ventricle as well as from the left ventricle; and (4) an increase in the thickness of the muscle of the right ventricle.

Q: What are the symptoms of Fallot's tetralogy?

A: The main symptom is a bluish tinge to the skin (cyanosis), caused by the presence in the arteries of blood that has not been properly oxygenated. Fainting sometimes occurs and a child with the disorder is often breathless.

Q: How is the condition treated?

A: Cardiac surgery during childhood may correct the condition.

False labor pains are abdominal pains that make a pregnant woman think that labor is beginning when in fact it is not. The womb contracts and relaxes slightly throughout pregnancy. A contraction may be strong enough to cause mild cramplike pain.

See also PREGNANCY AND CHILDBIRTH.

False pregnancy (pseudocyesis) is a condition in which a patient shows most of the outward, physical signs and symptoms of pregnancy, but is not pregnant. Among these signs are an enlarged abdomen, absence of menstruation, morning sickness, and weight gain. False pregnancy is thought to have an emotional origin, which causes the pituitary gland to be affected in the same way as during a real pregnancy. It occurs in women with a strong desire to have a child or in those who are anxious not to conceive. The condition has also been reported in men.

Q: Is there any treatment for a false pregnancy?

A: Psychiatric help may be useful. When the patient is asleep or under hypnosis, the enlargement of the abdomen disappears.

False teeth. *See* DENTURES.

Family planning is the control by couples of when they have children, and how many. It is achieved by practicing some form of birth control and then stopping the practice when conception is desired. *See* CONTRACEPTION.

Farsightedness (hyperopia, or hypermetropia) is a disorder of vision. Distant objects are seen clearly, but close objects appear blurred. This occurs because light rays from nearby objects are not focused normally on the back of the eye (retina). This may be because the refractive power of the eye lens is too strong, or (more commonly) because the eyeball is not long enough from front to back. Farsightedness may be inherited or it may develop after the age of 40 as the lens of the eye becomes less elastic (presbyopia). Corrective eyeglasses or contact lenses are prescribed to restore normal vision. *See* EYEGLASSES.

Fascia is a sheet of tough fibrous tissue that covers, supports, and separates muscles, or unites skin with the tissues beneath it.

Fasting is deliberate abstinence from food over a period of time. It is a medical requirement for some X-ray examinations (for example, a barium meal test), blood tests (for example, a glucose tolerance test), and before a general anesthetic.

Fasting is a requirement in some religious rites; it is also used as a means of political or social protest. Some people fast as a means of losing weight rapidly, but this method is not recommended.

Q: What happens to the body's metabolism during fasting?

A: In the absence of food, the body's energy requirements are supplied first by the body's sugar, then by reserves of fat. The "burning up" of fat is incomplete, resulting in mild KETOSIS, due to the production of by-products of fat metabolism.

Pangs of hunger occur during the first few days of a fast, but then become less noticeable.

Q: What precautions should be taken by a person who is fasting?

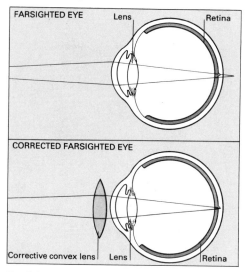

Farsightedness occurs when the lens fails to focus light rays at one point on the retina.

A: A person who intends to fast for more than two days should seek the advice of a physician. Vitamin supplements are recommended. When a fast is broken, a normal diet should be resumed gradually, beginning with light, easily digested foods.

See also WEIGHT PROBLEMS.

Fat embolus is a globule of oil, fat, or bone marrow that obstructs an artery. Such an obstruction can occur after the fracture of a large bone or after some forms of orthopedic surgery. *See* EMBOLISM.

Fatigue is a feeling of tiredness or weariness. Fatigue may be caused by many factors. Physical exertion, inadequate sleep, mental strain, boredom, or poor posture may all cause fatigue. Chronic (persistent) fatigue often occurs as a symptom of infection, deficient diet, depression, or an underlying disorder such as anemia, diabetes, tuberculosis, or cancer.

Q: *Does fatigue require medical treatment?*

A: Persistent fatigue should be brought to the attention of a physician.

A talk about Fats

Fats are one of the three kinds of energy-giving foods in the diet. They are an extremely rich source of energy, with a calorie content of about 255 calories per ounce (9 calories per gram). This is twice as much as provided by the other foods (proteins and carbohydrates). The most common fat-containing foods are butter, cream, eggs, fat meats, margarine, oily fish, and vegetable oils.

Q: *What are the functions of fats in the body's metabolism?*

A: Most fats are burned up (oxidized) to produce energy (in addition to carbon dioxide and water). Other fats become an essential part of cells. Fats that are not required immediately as a source of energy are stored in layers of fatty (adipose) tissue under the skin. They are available as fuel for energy at any time. The stored fats surround and protect internal organs such as the kidneys, and act as insulation that prevents heat loss. Fats also provide an environment in which vitamins A, D, E and K can dissolve. Some fat is stored in the liver.

Q: *What is the difference between saturated and unsaturated fats?*

A: Saturated and unsaturated fats differ chemically in the way their carbon and hydrogen atoms are arranged. Basically, unsaturated fats can absorb hydrogen, whereas saturated fats cannot. Most animal fats are saturated fats; saturated vegetable fats include coconut oil. Unsaturated fats include cottonseed oil, safflower oil, corn oil (all polyunsaturated fats that may be constituents of margarine), and olive oil.

Q: *What is the significance of this distinction?*

A: Research suggests that large amounts of saturated fats in the diet may be associated with vascular disease (arteriosclerosis). Surveys have shown that countries with high living standards, such as the U.S., have a high incidence of arteriosclerosis. But whether or not this is directly caused by staple "rich man's food" such as meat, eggs, cream, and so on (the saturated fats) is still under investigation.

Q: *Can fats be eliminated from the diet?*

A: A fat-free diet must be extremely bulky to provide enough calories because proteins and carbohydrates are only half as rich in calories as fats. Dieticians usually advise that about thirty to forty percent of the diet should consist of fats.

Fatty degeneration is a disorder involving the accumulation of fat in cells, especially of the liver and the heart. It occurs because the cells are deprived of oxygen or certain foods that make the disposal of fat possible. Poor circulation, anemia, or poisoning by alcohol or industrial chemicals, such as dry cleaning fluids, may cause fatty degeneration.

Favism is a form of acute hemolytic anemia

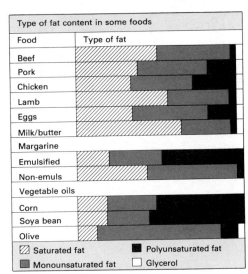

Type of fat content in some foods	
Food	Type of fat
Beef	
Pork	
Chicken	
Lamb	
Eggs	
Milk/butter	
Margarine	
Emulsified	
Non-emuls	
Vegetable oils	
Corn	
Soya bean	
Olive	

▨ Saturated fat   ■ Polyunsaturated fat
■ Monounsaturated fat   ☐ Glycerol

Fats of the saturated variety are high in animal meat, and are linked with some disorders.

Favus

caused by inhaling or swallowing fava pollen or the fava bean. It is caused by an inherited metabolic sensitivity of the red blood cells. The symptoms are fever, vomiting, diarrhea, and sometimes coma. Favism is common in the eastern Mediterranean.

Favus is a form of ringworm affecting the scalp, caused by a fungus (*Trichophyton schoenleinlii*). *See* RINGWORM.

Febrile. *See* FEVER.

Fecal analysis is the medical examination of a patient's feces to aid in the diagnosis of various disorders. *See* FECES.

Feces are the waste or end products of digestion that accumulate in the bowel (large intestine) and are expelled through the anus during defecation. The expelled product is commonly called a stool or a bowel movement. Feces are composed of: undigested or indigestible food, especially vegetable fiber such as cellulose; water; mucus and other secretions from the glands that supply the intestinal tract; bacteria; enzymes that have assisted digestion; inorganic salts; and, occasionally, foreign substances.

Q: What is the normal appearance of feces?

A: Feces are normally brown or dark brown in color, soft, and firm. Bile pigments give feces their characteristic color. The typical odor is caused by nitrogen compounds that are produced by the action of bacteria. Medical examination of the feces for abnormalities is important in the diagnosis of disorders of the intestinal tract.

Q: What disorders affect the color of feces?

A: Black feces may result from taking drugs,

such as iron tablets, or drinking red wine. The presence of blood in the feces may make them either black or bright red in color. This can occur because of infection; ulceration of the intestines; diverticular disease; malignant or non-malignant tumors; abrasive foreign bodies; or hemorrhoids. Pale yellow or white feces suggest a disorder of bile production, usually an obstruction of the bile ducts. In children, greenish feces indicate that food has passed quickly through the digestive tract.

Q: What disorders affect the consistency of feces?

A: Hard, nodular feces are associated with constipation, which may be a symptom of some other disorder. Diarrhea produces excessively watery feces. Feces that are flat and ribbonlike may be caused by an obstruction in the rectum. With jaundice, the feces may be pale and greasy.

Q: What disorders can be revealed by an analysis of feces?

A: Worms and amebic DYSENTERY are detected by inspecting the patient's feces. Chemical and microscopic analysis of a stool may show up abnormal amounts of fats, proteins, or sugars, which may indicate a disorder of digestion or malabsorption of food.

Felon is an infection of the fingertip. *See* PARONYCHIA.

Feet. *See* FOOT.

Femur is the thighbone, the bone that extends from the hip to the knee. It is the longest and strongest bone in the body; some of the most powerful muscles in the body are attached to the femur.

Fenestration is an operation in which an artificial opening is made into the labyrinth of the inner ear.

Fertility is the ability to reproduce. In a woman, fertility is the capability of an egg (ovum) to be fertilized. In a man, it is the capability of sperm to fertilize an ovum.

Fertilization is the union of an egg (ovum) and a sperm to produce a single cell (zygote) that then develops into an embryo. Fertilization usually takes place in a fallopian tube. *See* PREGNANCY AND CHILDBIRTH.

Fester is to become inflamed and produce pus. *See* INFLAMMATION; PUS.

Fetish is a person's finding sexual significance in an object rather than a person. A degree of fetishism can be involved in normal sexual stimulation, but in isolation it requires psychiatric consultation.

Fetus is an unborn baby from three months after conception to the time of birth. *See also* PREGNANCY AND CHILDBIRTH.

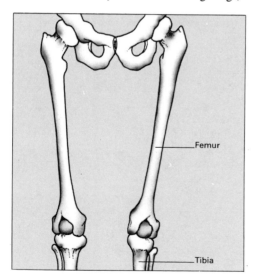

Femur

Tibia

Femur is the longest bone in the body, and can bear more weight than any other bone.

A talk about Fever

Fever is an abnormally high body temperature. In adults the normal temperature, taken orally, is up to 98.6°F (37°C). When the temperature is taken under the armpit, it is about 1°F lower than the oral temperature. The rectal temperature is about 1°F higher than the oral temperature. Children have a greater range of body temperature than adults so a moderate temperature increase in children is of less significance than the same increase in an adult. For practical purposes, fever may be defined as a temperature that is at least 0.5°F above normal on two recordings taken at least two hours apart.

For EMERGENCY treatment, *see* First Aid, p.590.

Q: What are the symptoms that commonly accompany a fever?

A: The accompanying symptoms depend on the underlying cause of the fever.

Q: What causes a fever?

A: Fever is usually caused by infection. The infecting microbes produce poisons that disturb the normal functioning of the hypothalamus, the heat-regulating center in the brain. Poisoning, drug overdose, and certain illnesses also have this effect, as does damage to the hypothalamus. Fever may also occur with certain blood disorders, breathing problems, and psychological or emotional disorders.

Q: When is a fever considered to be serious?

A: Any fever that is accompanied by mental confusion or disorientation is serious and requires expert medical attention. If the temperature rises above 103°F (39.4°C); if a continued fever has no obvious cause; or if a fever is accompanied by vomiting or diarrhea, consult a physician.

Fever sore, or fever blister, is a sore that occurs on the lips, often during a fever. *See* COLD SORE.

Fiberscope is a flexible instrument used for inspecting the body's internal organs and tissues (see ENDOSCOPY). A fiberscope is made of glass or plastic fibers that conduct light.

Fibrillation is rapid, irregular twitching of muscle fibers. Any muscle can fibrillate, and the fibrillation sometimes accompanies degenerative disorders such as motor neuron disease. It may also occur in skeletal muscle that has recently been deprived of its nerve supply. But the most serious site of fibrillation is the heart, in which the condition affects either of the two pairs of chambers, the atria (auricles) or the ventricles.

Q: What is atrial fibrillation?

A: Atrial (or auricular) fibrillation is extremely rapid twitching of the muscle of the upper chambers of each half of the heart (atria). The atria no longer contract rhythmically, causing inefficient pumping of the blood. The pulse at the wrist is irregular because the main chambers (ventricles) of the heart are not receiving a regular stimulus from the atria.

Atrial fibrillation may be caused by any kind of heart disease, such as coronary artery disease due to arteriosclerosis, following rheumatic fever with valve disease, or as a result of hyperactivity of the thyroid gland (thyrotoxicosis). In some cases, however, the cause cannot be identified.

Q: What is ventricular fibrillation?

A: This condition resembles atrial fibrillation in its action but affects the lower chambers in each half of the heart (ventricles). The disorder is rapidly fatal, because the weak, rapid heartbeats pump little or no blood into the circulation. Ventricular fibrillation may be caused by coronary thrombosis, the effect of drugs such as digitalis or chloroform, or an electric shock.

Q: How is fibrillation in the heart treated?

A: Atrial fibrillation is effectively treated either with digitalis or with other drugs used to bring the rhythm of the heart under control. All such drugs are used under medical supervision. If fibrillation is associated with a thyroid disorder, thyroid treatment is necessary.

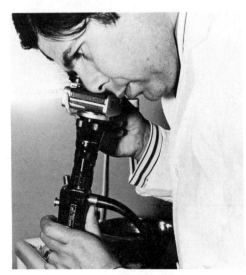

Fiberscope is used to study internal organs, and can be used to photograph them.

Fibrin

Ventricular fibrillation is an emergency treated as a cardiac arrest, and regular heart rhythm is restored using a special machine that causes defibrillation.

Fibrin is an insoluble web of protein that forms the framework of a blood clot. Synthetic fibrin, made from gelatin (fibrin foam), is sometimes used as a surgical dressing to stop a hemorrhage.

See also FIBRINOGEN.

Fibrinogen is a soluble protein in the blood plasma. It is essential for the clotting of blood: through the action of the enzyme thrombin, fibrinogen is converted into the insoluble protein FIBRIN.

Fibroadenosis is a condition that occurs in the breasts of women: the many milk-secreting ducts become enlarged and are surrounded by fibrous tissue, and the breast feels tender and lumpy to the touch, usually due to hormonal changes.

Fibrocystic disease. *See* CYSTIC FIBROSIS.

A talk about Fibroids

Fibroid is a benign (noncancerous) tumor that consists mainly of fibrous tissue. It forms in the muscle of the womb (uterus), and is also known medically as leiomyoma uteri. One or several fibroids may be present. They are of various shapes, firm, and slow-growing. They may range in size from less than an inch (2.5cm) to more than a foot (30cm) across.

Q: *What are the symptoms of a fibroid?*
A: Often a fibroid produces no symptoms

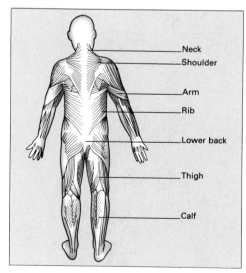

and is discovered only in a gynecological examination. Possible symptoms include heavy menstrual bleeding (menorrhagia), occasionally with pain (dysmenorrhea); if a fibroid causes pressure on the bladder, urination is more frequent. A large fibroid can sometimes be felt through the abdominal wall.

Q: *What causes a fibroid?*
A: Each month the womb increases in size, in response to the sex hormones, and then decreases at the time of menstruation. It is likely that an area of muscle in the womb fails to shrink with the rest of the womb. Each month, the area grows slightly larger under the stimulus of hormones and, as the bulk increases, a fibroid is formed. After menopause, fibroids decrease in size as the uterus becomes smaller.

Q: *Can fibroids affect fertility?*
A: Sometimes fibroids cause STERILITY. They may also be a factor in producing a miscarriage.

Q: *How are fibroids treated?*
A: Fibroids need treatment only if they produce symptoms.

Q: *Are fibroids a common condition?*
A: Yes. It is estimated that twenty percent of women have fibroids by the time menopause begins.

Fibroma is a benign (noncancerous) tumor of connective tissue. It may occur anywhere in the body, for example, in the fibrous covering of bone (periosteum) or nerve. It has a firm consistency, is irregular in shape, and grows slowly. A fibroma is not painful unless it causes pressure.

Fibrosarcoma is a rare malignant tumor formed from fibroblasts, the cells of connective fibrous tissue. A fibrosarcoma is treated by surgical removal.

See also TUMOR.

Fibrosis is the formation of fibrous scar tissue. It is a normal reaction to infection or injury, and may occur in the lungs, following pneumonia, or form adhesions in the peritoneum following peritonitis.

Fibrositis is inflammation of fibrous connective tissue anywhere in the body. The term is used imprecisely in popular usage for pain in and around muscles, either without apparent reason or caused by minor disorders such as muscle strain. Muscular aches and pains are best treated with mild painkilling drugs, heat applied locally, and massage.

Fibrous tissue is tissue containing or composed of fibers that holds organs and other structures in place.

Fibrositis is inflammation of white connective tissue, and commonly affects sites shown.

Fibula is the long, slender bone on the outside of the lower leg, extending from just below the knee to the ankle. Its lower end forms the outer side of the ankle joint. Unlike the shinbone (tibia), the fibula does not bear weight but serves as an attachment for some of the leg muscles.

Filariasis is a general term for infection by any of several tropical WORMS of the family Filarioidea. *See* ELEPHANTIASIS; LOIASIS; ONCHOCERCIASIS.

Filling, in dentistry, is the process of repairing a tooth cavity.

Finger is any of the digits of the hand. A finger consists of three bones (phalanges), except for the thumb, which has only two. The phalanges are connected by hinge joints. Tendons along the upper and lower surfaces of the fingers move the joints. These are controlled by muscles in the forearm. Other muscles in the hand help with fine finger movements. *See* DUPUYTREN'S CONTRACTURE; FROSTBITE; HEBERDEN'S NODE; RAYNAUD'S PHENOMENON.

Fingernail. *See* NAIL.

First Aid is assistance administered in an emergency to a person who has been injured or otherwise suddenly disabled. *See* First Aid, pp.503-599.

Fissure is a medical term for a crack or groove. It can be a natural division in a structure such as the brain, liver, and spinal cord, or it can refer to a cracklike sore. An anal fissure (fissure-in-ano), the most common example, is a tear in the skin of the anus. It is usually caused by passing hard, constipated feces. Pain from the fissure is sharp, and there may be bleeding during defecation. In small children, the pain may prevent defecation.

Q: How is an anal fissure treated?
A: Anal fissures often heal on their own after several days or when the constipation ceases (*see* CONSTIPATION). An anesthetic ointment may be applied to the area to prevent pain. If the condition does not improve, the anus may have to be stretched surgically under general anesthetic, to provide a wider opening; any scars are removed.

Fistula is an abnormal channel from a hollow body cavity to the surface (for example, from the rectum to the skin), or between two cavities (for example, from the vagina to the bladder). A fistula may be congenital (for example, bladder to navel), the result of a penetrating wound (for example, skin to lung), or formed from an ulcer to abscess (for example, appendix abscess to vagina or tooth socket to sinus). Fistulas arise from an abscess or wound that is unable to heal because it receives the fluid contents of some body cavity. A fistula-in-ano, for example, begins with the infection of the mucous lining of the rectum, perhaps by tuberculosis or Crohn's disease. The area becomes an abscess as it is constantly reinfected by the feces, and eventually a fistula breaks through to the skin near the anus.

Q: How is a fistula treated?
A: A fistula from a wound kept free from infection normally closes spontaneously. If a fistula is allowed to develop beyond the early stages, an operation to close it is the usual treatment.
    See also COLOSTOMY.

Fit. *See* CONVULSION.

Flatfoot is a common disorder in which the entire sole of the foot, instead of being arched, is in contact with the ground when the person stands. Normally, the bones of the foot form three arches to raise the sole; support is provided by strong ligaments in the sole and by the muscles, especially those of the big toe. Flatfoot occurs when the larger, inner arch of the bone collapses.

All children have flat feet for at least two years after they start walking. A slight outward twist of the foot (called a valgus deformity) can cause flatfoot to become a permanent condition, because it forces the inner arch of the foot downward. If the arch appears when a person with flatfoot stands on tiptoe, it is an indication that the foot is still supple enough to form a normal arch with corrective treatment.

Q: Are there any other causes of flatfoot?
A: Occasionally, flatfoot may be associated with muscular disorders or paralysis.

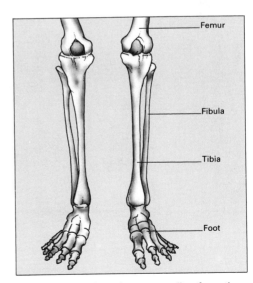

Fibula is a thin, long bone extending from the knee downward to the ankle.

Flatulence

Q: What is the treatment for flatfoot?

A: For a child, a podiatrist may suggest wedging the heels of the shoes on the inner side of the foot, and remedial exercises. But for an adult, there is no medical need to correct flat feet unless they disturb the patient.

Flatulence results from excessive gas in the stomach and intestines. A person may belch, and pass "gas" (flatus). Some gas is normally produced from fermentation in the large intestine. Flatulence often accompanies indigestion; it may also result from the nervous habit of swallowing air (aerophagia). Commercial products for the relief of indigestion help to reduce flatulence. When the condition is caused by aerophagia, it may be best treated after discussion with a physician or psychotherapist.

Flatus is gas in the intestines. Excess flatus causes FLATULENCE.

Fleas are wingless, jumping, bloodsucking insects that belong to the order *Siphonaptera*. Most fleas are parasitic on one specific species of animal, including human beings. *Pulex irritans* injects its saliva into the skin of human beings as an irritating bite.

Q: Can animal fleas afflict people as well?

A: Yes. Fleas from cats and dogs (*Ctenocephalides felis* and *C. canis*) may bite human beings, but this is unusual. One of the rat fleas, *Xenopsylla cheopis*, carries bubonic plague if the rat it lived on was infected. This flea can pass on the disease in its bite. The same rat flea may carry a form of typhus.

See also LICE.

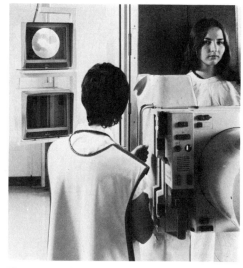

Fluoroscope is a type of X-ray device that projects the image onto a screen instead of film.

Flexibilitas cerea is a condition in which the limbs remain in any position in which they are placed. It is a rare symptom of catalepsy, a phase of schizophrenia.

Flies are winged insects that belong to the order *Diptera*. The housefly, like other flies, feeds on decomposing organic matter and can pick up disease germs on its feet and legs. A fly that settles on food contaminates it by shedding germs from its feet, in its droppings, and through its mouth while it is feeding. Illnesses that may be spread by flies include bacillary dysentery and other intestinal disorders, cholera, conjunctivitis, poliomyelitis, sandfly fever, and typhoid.

Flu. *See* INFLUENZA.

Flukes are flatworms of the class *Trematoda*. They can cause various parasitic infections in human beings. The life cycle of a fluke is complex: a small organism (miracidium) hatches from an egg, invades a snail, and develops there. When it changes into a small cystlike structure (cercaria), it is excreted by the snail and finds its home in plants, crabs, or fish. If human beings or animals drink water containing the cysts, flukes that evolve from the cysts invade the tissues and, in human beings, produce clinical symptoms. Flukes mate in the intestines of their hosts, and eggs excreted in the feces or droppings begin the life cycle again.

See also WORMS; SCHISTOSOMIASIS.

Fluorescein is a dye that is used to detect damage to the cornea of the eye, either from foreign bodies or from lesions.

Fluoridation is the addition of fluoride to the water supply. Many water supplies naturally contain an adequate amount of fluoride, and the addition of more is controversial.

Fluoride is a chemical compound of fluorine. Fluoride, in the form of calcium fluoride, occurs naturally in the soil, and in the water supply in some regions. It helps in the formation of bones and teeth. Fluoride helps to prevent tooth decay in children, but authorities are not agreed on whether or not it has the same effect in adults.

A prolonged deficiency of fluoride may lead to osteoporosis, a disorder in which the bones become brittle. A prolonged high intake of fluoride in adults may cause yellowing of the teeth; weakening of the tooth enamel; and, rarely, bone disorders, such as osteosclerosis.

Fluoroscope is a machine that aids in diagnosis. It projects onto a screen X-ray pictures of what is happening inside a person's body. The screen, which looks like a television screen, is activated when X rays strike it. By using a fluoroscope, a physician can study the movements of internal organs.

Flush is sudden redness of the skin, particularly of the face and neck. The cheeks may be flushed with a fever, or flushing may be part of such illnesses as chronic pulmonary tuberculosis. A hot flush, or flash, is accompanied by a sudden feeling of heat caused by an oversensitivity of the surface blood vessels to minor changes of temperature or emotion. This often occurs in women at time of menopause. A hot flush is also sometimes symptomatic of various neuroses.

Flutter is a state of extremely rapid, regular, vibration or pulsations. It usually occurs in the upper chambers (atria) of the heart, where the number of contractions can rise to between 200 and 400 per minute. The lower chambers (ventricles) cannot contract at such a rapid speed; instead they contract on every third or fourth atrial beat, causing irregular pulsations.

Atrial flutter may be caused by heart disease, particularly rheumatic valve disease, or by poisoning from an overactive thyroid THYROTOXICOSIS. Sometimes no cause can be found.

See also FIBRILLATION.

Folic acid is a vitamin of the B group. *See* VITAMINS.

Folk medicine is any nonorthodox but traditional way of treating illnesses and injuries. It may use herbal mixtures, physical manipulations, religious rituals, or a combination of these. It differs from orthodox medicine in that the treatments are not the products of scientific medical research. Folk medicine was the starting point from which the science of medicine developed, but it has not become a simple alternative. Some old remedies have now been incorporated into standard medical practice because their effectiveness has been scientifically proven.

Many folk remedies that do not work are useless rather than harmful. But harm might occur indirectly if a person uses such remedies instead of consulting a physician.

Follicle is a small, roughly spherical cavity or a small secretory gland.

Follicle-stimulating hormone (FSH) is a hormone that stimulates the growth of an ovarian follicle in the first half of each menstrual cycle. It also affects sperm formation in men. The hormone is produced by the frontal lobe of the pituitary gland. When the ovarian follicle has matured, the membrane surrounding it bursts, and a single egg cell (ovum) is released. *See* OVULATION.

Folliculitis is an inflammation of the hair follicles on the skin. It first appears as scattered pimples that later dry out and form crusts around the follicles. The affected area is itchy and nearby lymph glands may become swollen. In most cases, folliculitis is caused by streptococcus or staphylococcus bacteria. Sycosis barbae on the face and neck of males is a form of folliculitis.

Q: How is folliculitis treated?

A: The application of antiseptic creams or lotions to the infected area reduces the infection. A physician may prescribe antibiotic drugs.

Fomentation. *See* POULTICE.

Fontanel (or fontanelle) is a gap between the bones of the skull of a newborn baby. At birth there are six fontanels in a baby's skull. The two main ones lie along the centerline of the scalp; one towards the front of the skull just above the forehead, and the other at the base of the skull near the nape of the neck. The bones of a baby's skull are still unjoined at birth. The fontanels allow the bones to overlap and the skull to change shape during birth to fit the birth canal.

Q: Is it possible to see any of the fontanels on a baby's head?

A: Yes. The fontanel at the front of the skull, sometimes known as the "soft spot," can usually be seen and felt. It bulges when the baby cries, and may form a hollow if the baby needs fluids.

Q: Is it possible to harm the fontanel?

A: No, not through normal handling. A tough membrane covers the gap and protects the brain. The area can be touched and washed without harming the baby.

Q: When does the fontanel disappear?

A: It is usually completely closed when the child is eighteen months old.

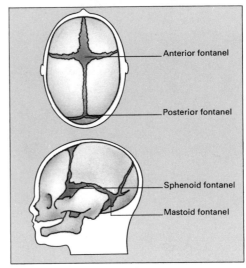

Fontanels are the spaces between the unjoined bones of the baby's skull.

Food poisoning

Food poisoning (for EMERGENCY treatment, *see* First Aid, p.568), is an acute illness caused by eating contaminated or poisonous food. The usual symptoms are vomiting, diarrhea, and sharp abdominal pain. Cramps, headache, and sweating may be additional symptoms. The patient may collapse with weakness and exhaustion. Food poisoning is rarely fatal and recovery usually takes place after about six hours.

Q: *What are the causes of food poisoning?*

A: There are several possible causes of food poisoning, the most common of which involve bacteria. (1) Bacteria in contaminated food may grow in the food and produce their own toxin. The germs usually enter the food from a staphylococcal infection (such as a boil, abscess, or other skin infection) in a person who has handled the food during processing. Although cooking kills the germs, it does not destroy the toxin that has been produced. Poisoning from the toxin takes place within two hours of eating contaminated food. Toxins produced in foods from other kinds of bacteria are rare, but BOTULISM (from the bacteria *Clostridium botulinum*) is one example.

(2) Another type of poisoning occurs when bacteria contained in food develop in the intestines of the patient (for example, salmonella or typhoid fever). Salmonella bacteria are found in many animals and the foods most likely to contain them are meats (especially chicken and processed frozen meat) and duck's eggs. The bacteria need time to grow in the intestines, and so symptoms may not appear for one or two days.

(3) Water and foods such as unwashed fruit and vegetables may be contaminated by chemicals such as pesticides, or by lead from automobile emissions.

(4) Many plants and some animals are naturally poisonous to human beings. These include some types of fungi and some shellfish. Food poisoning results with varying severity if these substances are eaten.

(5) Certain foods that are wholesome to most people may cause food poisoning as an allergic reaction in others.

Q: *What is ptomaine poisoning?*

A: Ptomaines are evil-smelling products of bacteria present in putrefying food. They were once believed to cause food poisoning, but it is now known that so-called ptomaine poisoning is bacterial infection of the intestines.

Q: *How is food poisoning treated?*

A: A physician normally concentrates on treating the symptoms by giving antinauseant drugs. The physician may also treat any water and salt deficiency, the consequence of the vomiting and diarrhea.

Q: *What measures can be taken to avoid food poisoning?*

A: Persons involved in the processing or preparation of food should be checked for skin infections. All fresh fruit and raw vegetables should be washed thoroughly before being eaten. Cooked food should be covered, cooled quickly, and stored in a refrigerator to prevent the growth of bacteria. Food that is reheated should be eaten at once and not kept warm, because this encourages the growth of bacteria.

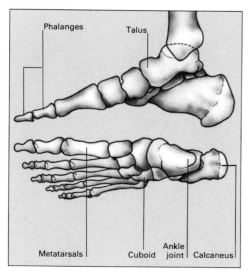

Foot is formed from thirty-eight bones and a complex set of muscles that balance the body.

Foot is joined at the ankle to the lower end of the leg. The calcaneus, which is the largest bone in the foot, forms the HEEL. Above the calcaneus, and resting on the front part of it, is the talus bone, from which extend three long narrow bones (metatarsals) that connect to the first three TOES. The cuboid bone is also in front of the calcaneus, and from it the fourth and fifth metatarsal bones connect with the fourth and fifth toes. The arch of the foot is raised higher on the instep because the talus projects farther forward than does the cuboid bone. The weight of the body is taken by the calcaneus and transmitted to the heads of the metatarsal bones.

See also FLATFOOT.

Foot disorders. The following table lists some of the disorders that affect the feet, and the basic characteristics of each condition. Each disorder has a separate article in the A-Z section of this book.

Disorder	Basic characteristics
ATHLETE'S FOOT	Skin eruptions, usually between the toes
BLISTER	Collection of fluid under the skin causing top layer to puff out
BUNION	Thickening of the skin over the joint at the base of the big toe and extension of metatarsal bone
BURSITIS	Inflammation of joint
CALLUS	Hard, thickened areas of skin on the foot
CELLULITIS	Inflammation of cellular tissue
CHILBLAIN	Itching, swelling, and painful reddening of skin
CLAW TOE (hammer toe)	Second toe is bent at its two joints, with corns over the bends
CLUBFOOT (talipes)	Forepart of the foot is twisted out of direction
CORN	Hard, cone-shaped, thickened areas of the skin on the toes
FLATFOOT	Arch of foot sinks down and the inner edge of the foot rests upon ground
FOOT DROP	Difficulty in lifting front part of foot
FROSTBITE	Reddened or whitened skin with swelling, blistering, and numbness
GANGLION	Cystic tumor on a tendon
GANGRENE	Dead tissue
GOUT	Inflammation of joint of big toe usually, but also of instep or heel
HALLUX VALGUS	Large bump on inner border of big toe joint, inclining big toe inward
IMMERSION FOOT	Blueness of skin
INGROWING TOENAIL	Edges of nail overgrown with tissue, causing pain and possible infection
MADURA FOOT	Swollen feet with ulcers
METATARSALGIA	Pain in the metatarsal region

Disorder	Basic characteristics
OSTEOARTHRITIS	Inflammation and degeneration of bone and cartilage that form joints
PES CAVUS	Abnormally high arch
POLYDACTYLISM	Extra toes
RHEUMATOID ARTHRITIS	Inflammation and degeneration of joints
WART, PLANTAR	Epidermal tumor on the sole of foot

Foot drop is a condition in which the toes drag and the foot hangs, caused by weakness or paralysis of the muscles on the side of the shinbone. It may occur as a result of damage to the nerves supplying the muscles, poliomyelitis, polyneuritis, or a muscle disorder such as myasthenia gravis or one of the muscular dystrophies.

The treatment of foot drop depends on the underlying cause. If foot drop remains after the treatment, the patient may wear a special splint or a spring on the shoe to prevent stumbling. Occasionally a physician recommends an operation called an arthrodesis, which stops ankle movement, so that the ankle is fixed with the foot at right angles to the leg. Alternatively, the base of a tendon may be transplanted from one side of the foot to the other, to strengthen the movement of the foot.

Forceps are pincers that are used in surgery for holding, seizing, or extracting.

Foreign body is an alien particle or small object that has lodged in the skin, in surface organs (for example, the eyes, ears, or nose), or internally.

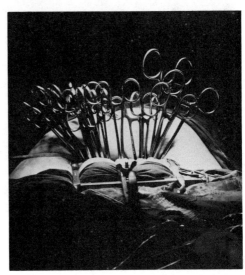

Forceps are used, during an operation, to splice blood vessels, and expose tissues and organs.

209

Forensic medicine

Forensic medicine is the branch of medical science that is related to the law and legal processes. It applies medical knowledge to legal (especially criminal) problems.

Foreskin (or prepuce) is the fold of skin that covers the end of the penis (glans penis). Before the age of eighteen months, it is held down by fine strands of tissue; after this age, it can be pulled back. Because the foreskin is subject to irritation and inflammation (balanitis), it should be pulled back and the penis washed regularly as a standard part of male hygiene.

See also CIRCUMCISION.

Formaldehyde is a pungent, poisonous gas. It is a component of formalin, a solution used in medicine as a disinfectant and preservative.

See also FORMALIN.

Formalin is a watery (aqueous) solution of the organic chemical formaldehyde, with some added methanol (methyl alcohol). It is used in medicine as a disinfectant and preservative. As a disinfectant, formalin is a component of soaps for hospital use. Clothing and towels, and samples of feces and sputum, may be sterilized in formalin. Body tissues soaked in formalin become hard, and the solution is used to preserve biological specimens for examination by a pathologist. Formalin is also sometimes used in the treatment of warts.

Formic acid (or methansic acid) is an organic chemical. It is probably the cause of the pain from certain insect bites and nettle stings. It is a clear, pungent liquid that is chemically related to formaldehyde and methanol (methyl alcohol). Formic acid is occasionally used in medicine for the relief of deep-seated inflammation.

Formication is the sensation of insects crawling over the skin. It is a form of parasthesia (an abnormal sensation without cause). Formication is sometimes a symptom of DELIRIUM TREMENS, and it is a common side effect of alcohol and cocaine withdrawal.

Fovea is any small cup-shaped depression that occurs naturally on many structures of the body; an example is the pit in the head of the thigh bone (femur). The term most commonly refers to the fovea centralis retinae, the depression on the retina of the EYE onto which light is naturally focused, and which contains only cones and no blood vessels.

A talk about Fractures

Fractures are broken bones. (For EMERGENCY treatment, *see* First Aid, pp.552–559.) Any bone in the body can accidentally be broken (fractured). But some bones, because of their awkward shapes or vulnerable positions (for example, the long bones of the arms and legs), tend to fracture more often than others. Chunky bones such as the carpals in the wrist and the tarsals in the ankle are less liable to fracture.

Q: What can cause a bone fracture?

A: Most fractures occur as the result of injury or accident. Sometimes a bone breaks following repeated minor strains. Some bones have a tendency to fracture easily because they are weak from disease.

Q: Do bones always fracture in the same way?

A: No. Physicians recognize five main kinds of fractures. (1) A transverse fracture is a straight break in a bone from side to side. (2) An oblique fracture is an angled break in a bone (for example, diagonally). (3) A spiral fracture is one in which the bone breaks as a result of a twisting action. (4) A comminuted fracture is one in which the bone is broken and splintered into more than two pieces at the fracture site. (5) A greenstick fracture usually occurs in children: because the bones are pliable, a break occurs on one side of a bone and the other side bends but, like a green twig, remains intact.

Q: Can fractures damage tissues other than bone?

A: Yes. A medical description usually classifies a fracture in terms of the effect that it has on surrounding tissues. (1) A simple (or closed) fracture does not pierce the surface of the skin. (2) A

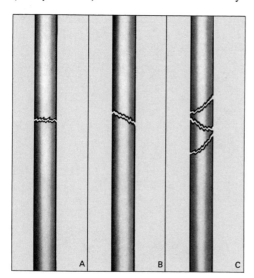

Fractures of bones are known medically as (A) transverse; (B) oblique; or (C) spiral planes.

compound fracture causes a surface wound, either leading to the site of the fracture, or caused by a broken bone piercing the skin. (3) A complicated fracture is one that damages a nearby structure such as a blood vessel, nerve, or body organ. (4) An impacted fracture is a type of fracture where one end of the broken bone becomes wedged or compressed into another bone.

Q: *What is the standard treatment for fractures?*

A: The basis of treatment for all fractures is to relocate the bone in its normal anatomical position and to hold it there until new bone has had time to heal the break.

Q: *How are unstable fractures treated?*

A: Unstable fractures may be held together with screws, metal plates, thick pins (for the hip), or wires.

Q: *How is a complicated fracture treated?*

A: A complicated fracture is treated in the same way as other fractures except that repair of the internal damage is given priority.

Q: *Is a fractured bone always displaced?*

A: No. With some fractures, particularly those of the hand, foot, or skull, the bone breaks but does not change position.

Q: *How long does a fracture take to heal?*

A: In general, an arm fracture is kept immobilized for about six weeks, but it takes at least three months for a leg fracture to heal sufficiently for the patient to be able to walk unaided.

Q: *Are there complications that can prolong the healing time?*

A: Fractures in elderly persons often take a long time to heal (called delayed union), especially when there is an underlying bone disease. With some bone diseases, the bone fails to repair itself at all (called nonunion). Sometimes not enough blood reaches the site of the fracture; this is common in fractures of the neck of the femur (thighbone) in old people.

Q: *Are there any other possible complications of fractures?*

A: Yes. If the bone has not been set in its correct position, shortening of the limb may result. A poor joining of the fractured bone (called malunion) results if one end is allowed to rotate slightly so that its contour does not lock smoothly with the other piece of bone. This problem is most common with multiple fractures, in which it is not always possible to set all the bones in their exact, original positions. If infection occurs, it is usually associated with a compound fracture, but it may also occur with simple fractures as a post-operative complication.

Q: *Can nearby muscles be exercised while the bone is healing?*

A: Yes. It is essential that the patient exercises the muscles while a limb is in a cast. Physiotherapists teach muscle contraction exercises that can be done while the limb is immobile (isometric exercises). After the cast or splint has been removed, the nearby joint is usually stiff and therapy is necessary to restore the full range of movement. Swimming is an excellent means of restoring muscle power. A high protein diet with additional vitamins is another measure that speeds the return of normal use to a fractured bone.

Fragilitas ossium is a congenital condition in which the bones are abnormally brittle. *See* OSTEOGENESIS IMPERFECTA.

Frambesia. *See* YAWS.

Fraternal twins are twin babies that result from two separate eggs (ova) that were fertilized at the same time. Unlike identical twins, fraternal twins are not necessarily of the same sex. *See* TWINS.

Freckles are small brown or yellowish-brown patches of pigment on the skin. They appear in response to sunlight: the body's cells produce more of the dark pigment MELANIN as a protection against further harmful action by sunlight's ultraviolet rays. These collections

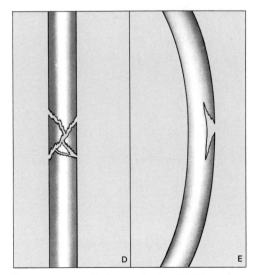

Fractures are called comminuted (D) if bone is crushed; or greenstick (E) if bone is split.

Friedreich's ataxia

of pigment tend to fade in the absence of sunlight.

Friedreich's ataxia is a serious, rare, inherited disorder of the central nervous system. It is caused by the imperfect development of some nerve fibers in the spinal cord. The first symptom of Friedreich's ataxia is poor coordination of muscles in the legs, usually beginning in childhood or early adolescence. The feet later become deformed (claw feet), the gait becomes shambling, and muscular uncoordination spreads throughout the body. Commonly, the spine curves to one side, and the patient becomes increasingly hunched. Sputtering, hesitating speech is another symptom.

Q: What are the complications of Friedreich's ataxia?

A: Friedreich's ataxia is a cause of para-plegia in children and young persons. If the heart becomes involved, heart failure may result. Diabetes is a frequent complication, and the patient is also more liable to get pneumonia.

Q: How is Friedreich's ataxia treated?

A: No effective treatment is known. But attempts can be made with physiotherapy to slow down the tightening process of the muscles. Death usually occurs within ten to twenty years, although this results from secondary infection.

Frigidity is the lack of sexual desire, and a consequent inability to reach orgasm, in a sexually mature person in good health. Frigidity is usually attributed to women only. The cause of frigidity is almost always psychological: for example, it may be a fear

of becoming pregnant. Emotional problems may prevent vaginal secretions during sexual arousal, resulting in a dry genital area and painful intercourse (DYSPAREUNIA). A physi-cian or psychiatrist can usually determine the reasons for a woman's frigidity once her sexual history is known; appropriate treat-ment can then begin. Sympathetic and careful counseling is necessary.

Only rarely is the condition caused by a physical abnormality: for example, vaginal infection or a tight hymen.

Fröhlich's syndrome is a rare glandular dis-order of childhood, more common in boys than in girls. It is caused by a disturbance in the hypothalamus, the part of the brain that regulates the supply of hormones from the pituitary gland. Essential pituitary hormones are not produced, so that the sex organs remain underdeveloped. Excess fatty tissue is distributed in areas normal for the female build: thighs, hips, and breasts. If the condi-tion begins in early childhood the patient may be a dwarf; if it occurs just before puberty, the child is fat and sluggish. The skin of an adult man with Fröhlich's syn-drome remains soft, and he has effeminate features due to the distribution of fat throughout the body. Fröhlich's syndrome in a girl causes extreme obesity.

Q: What is the treatment for Fröhlich's syndrome?

A: Provided treatment is started early enough, Fröhlich's syndrome can be most effectively treated with modern hormone therapy, such as the admin-istration of pituitary extract. This reduces the excess weight, and restores development to the sex organs.

Frostbite is an acute skin reaction to extreme cold. Particularly vulnerable areas of the body include the toes, fingers, ears, and the tip of the nose. Superficial frostbite may only damage the skin, but severe frostbite affects the deep tissues and gangrene can set in.

Q: What are the symptoms of frostbite?

A: The affected area turns unnaturally white. The victim is unaware of the condition because there is no sensation of pain at this stage. Within a few hours blood seeps back into the tissues turning them purple or black. The area becomes red, swollen, and painful. The skin may blister, and the blisters break down into ulcers. In severe cases the circulation does not return on warming, and the damage leads to gangrene.

Q: What causes frostbite?

A: In extreme weather conditions of cold and wind, the blood and tissue moisture in the affected area freezes. In severe

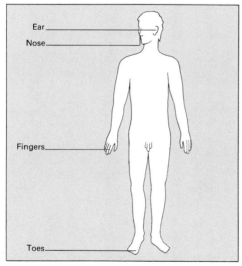

Ear

Nose

Fingers

Toes

Frostbite is most likely to affect a person's fingers, toes, nose, and ears.

cases, the blood vessels supplying the area shut down, preventing normal circulation even when gently warmed.

Q: How is frostbite treated?

A: The affected area must be warmed gradually, preferably at the same time as the rest of the body, or by immersing the area in warm, running water. Rubbing increases the damage to the already injured tissues. If the area remains white after warming, a physician must be consulted immediately. If gangrene sets in, amputation may be necessary.

Q: How can a person avoid frostbite?

A: During extremely cold weather, clothing must be well-fitting, warm, and wind-resistant. Tight shoes, socks, or gloves cut down the circulation and endanger the specific area. People with diabetes or any form of circulatory disorder are more likely to develop frostbite.

Frozen section is a technique in which an area of tissue (from a biopsy) is frozen and a thin slice cut off for examination under a microscope. The technique is useful for the immediate detection of cancer.

See also CRYOSURGERY.

Frozen shoulder is pain and stiffness in the shoulder. It is caused by inflammation of the joint capsule. This usually follows a minor injury or strain, although sometimes the cause may not be known. The inflammation restricts normal movement in the shoulder. Usually the stiffness and pain become gradually worse over a period of weeks. The pain then disappears, but the stiffness remains, with slow improvement over the next six to twelve months.

Q: What is the treatment for frozen shoulder?

A: The arm may have to be kept in a sling to reduce the pain, but some movement should be maintained. Painkilling drugs and physiotherapy help to ease the symptoms. Shortwave diathermy and the injection of a corticosteroid drug into the joint may produce some improvement. When only the stiffness remains, a physician may consider manipulation of the shoulder under a general anesthetic. This often brings about a faster recovery than does physiotherapy alone.

FSH. *See* FOLLICLE-STIMULATING HORMONE.

Fugue is a temporary disturbance of consciousness in which a person nevertheless behaves as though conscious. On "waking" from a state of fugue, a person suddenly realizes that he or she cannot account for, nor remember in any way, the time during which the fugue lasted. Because the condition usually represents a hysterical state of repressed emotions concerning some unfaceable

crisis, a person in a fugue state commonly acts a completely different role in society (*see* HYSTERIA). The condition may also be associated with epilepsy or concussion caused by a head injury.

A fugue differs from AMNESIA, in which state a person acts consciously but without memory of previous events.

Fulguration is the destruction of living tissue using an electric current. It is sometimes used to treat skin tumors.

See also DIATHERMY.

Fumigation is a method of disinfecting an area using poisonous fumes.

Functional describes a disorder in which the workings of an organ are affected, but no organic or structural cause is evident.

Fungal disorders may be caused by microscopic fungi or their spores. Many of these disorders are difficult to treat because the fungi resist most bactericidal agents. The following table lists some of the common fungal disorders and the basic characteristics of each condition. Each disorder has a separate entry in the A-Z section of this book.

Disorder	Basic characteristics
ACTINOMYCOSIS	Fibrous masses about the mouth or tongue that burst and become sinuses or ulcers; also abscesses in the lungs
ASPERGILLOSIS	Lumps in the skin, ears, sinuses and, especially, the lungs
ATHLETE'S FOOT	Skin eruptions on the foot, usually between the toes

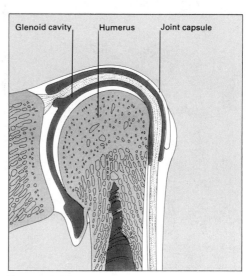

Glenoid cavity   Humerus   Joint capsule

Frozen shoulder is inflammation of the shoulder joint capsule that causes stiffness.

Funny bone

Disorder	Basic characteristics
BLASTOMYCOSIS	Lesions all over the body but, especially, infection of the lungs
HISTOPLASMOSIS	Infection of the lungs, ulcers in the gastro-intestinal tract, and possible skin lesions
MADURA FOOT	Swollen feet with ulcers
MONILIASIS (thrush)	White patches inside the mouth that later become shallow ulcers; may also occur in the vagina
RINGWORM	Raised, round sores of the skin, scalp, or nails

Funny bone is at the inner, lower end of the HUMERUS (upper arm bone). The ulnar nerve lies over this section of the humerus, close to the surface of the skin at the back of the ELBOW. A blow on the ulnar nerve is painful and often accompanied by tingling or numbness in the fingers of the affected hand.

Furred tongue is a condition in which the tongue is coated with a furry substance. It occurs during most fevers, but is an inconclusive diagnostic aid, because thirst or reduced appetite may also cause a furred tongue.

Q: What causes furring of the tongue?

A: Dead cells from the tongue are constantly being shed and are normally removed with the saliva. When the flow of saliva is reduced, this debris, together with food particles and dried mucus, accumulates on the surface of the tongue.

A furred tongue is also a symptom of chronic indigestion, poor oral hygiene, or

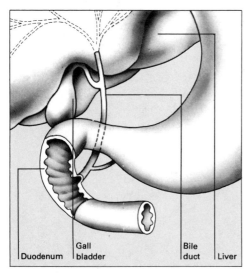

Gall bladder, situated underneath the right lobe of the liver, secretes bile into the duodenum.

Duodenum | Gall bladder | Bile duct | Liver

a throat infection such as tonsillitis.

Heavy smoking stains the tongue dark brown, and this is sometimes mistakenly thought to be a furred tongue.

Furuncle (or furunculus). *See* BOILS.

G

Gall is another name for bile. *See* BILE.

Gall bladder is a pear-shaped organ beneath the right side of the liver. It is about three to four inches (7.6–10.2cm) long, and about one inch (2.5cm) wide. The function of the gall bladder is to store BILE, a digestive liquid continually secreted by the liver. The bile emulsifies fats and neutralizes acids in partly digested food. A muscular valve in the common bile duct opens and the bile flows from the gall bladder into the cystic duct, along the common bile duct, and into the duodenum (part of the small intestine).

See also CHOLANGITIS; JAUNDICE.

Gallstone, a type of CALCULUS, is usually a mixture of cholesterol, bilirubin (a bile pigment), and protein. Resembling a stone, the calculus forms in the gall bladder, or sometimes in the common bile duct. The size of a gallstone can vary from a tiny crystal to a lump the size of a small egg. Usually, more than one gallstone is formed. The incidence of formation increases with age and among women. *See also* CHOLELITHIASIS.

Gamma globulin is a plasma protein, a component of blood serum that contains antibodies (*see* ANTIBODY). It can be extracted from the blood of a person who is immune to a certain infection and injected into another person who has been exposed to the disease (hyperimmune globulin). These extracts can provide temporary immunity to infectious hepatitis, rubeola (measles), poliomyelitis, tetanus, yellow fever, or smallpox (*see* IMMUNIZATION). Gamma globulin injections do not seem to be of much benefit against mumps or rubella (German measles).

Q: Are gamma globulin extracts used to give immunity to any other conditions?

A: Yes. A special preparation of gamma globulin, RhO (D) immune globulin, is given to a mother who has Rh- (Rhesus negative) blood after she has given birth. *See* HEMOLYTIC DISEASE OF THE NEWBORN.

Q: How important is an adequate amount of gamma globulin in the blood?

A: There is a serious risk of infection if a person has a low level of gamma globulin. For example, in a rare inherited disorder called AGAMMAGLOBULINEMIA, there is almost no gamma globulin in the blood. Infections of all kinds occur more often, and are more serious. Decreased gamma globulin levels sometimes result from the treatment of leukemia or cancer by chemotherapy. The only treatment in such circumstances is regular doses of gamma globulin.

Ganglion is an anatomical term for a bundle of nerves within the nervous system that act as a relay station outside the brain and spinal cord. A basal ganglion, however, is located within the brain and spinal cord. Ganglions are present throughout the autonomic nervous system.

As a surgical term, a ganglion is a cystlike tumor that appears on tendons.

Gangrene is the decay and death of tissue caused by a lack of blood supply to an area. It is a complication of external or internal injury, or of damage to an artery. External causes include infected bedsores; crushing injuries; deep burns; frostbite; boils; and chemical damage of the skin. Internal causes include blood clotting (thrombosis) in a diseased artery; an embolus; severe arteriosclerosis; diabetes; a strangulated hernia; torsion of the testes; Buerger's disease (a rare disorder of the leg arteries); and Raynaud's phenomenon (spasm-like contraction of the arteries in the arms and legs).

Medically, gangrene is considered either "dry" or "moist."

Q: What is dry gangrene?

A: Dry gangrene is the withering and drying out of tissue, without infection by bacteria. This process may continue unnoticed for weeks or months, especially in elderly persons. Dry gangrene is most often a complication of advanced diabetes or arteriosclerosis.

Q: What is moist gangrene?

A: Moist gangrene occurs usually in the toes, feet, or legs after a crushing injury or some other factor that causes a sudden stoppage of blood. The gangrene spreads rapidly as invading bacteria thrive and multiply unchecked by the defenses normally carried in the blood.
See also GAS GANGRENE.

Q: What are the symptoms of gangrene?

A: Areas of both dry and moist gangrene are conspicuous by a red line on the skin that marks the border of the gangrenous tissue. Dry gangrene causes some pain in the early stages. The area becomes cold, and the skin changes in color to brown, then black. Moist gangrene begins with swollen skin that may be blistered, red, and hot. The area then becomes cold as the tissues begin to die, and the skin

appears bruised. The putrefactive bacteria produce an offensive odor.

Q: Which parts of the body are susceptible to gangrene?

A: The limbs, especially the ends of the toes and fingers, are most commonly affected. The intestine may become gangrenous if an artery supplying it is twisted (volvulus), obstructed by a hernia, or diseased by arteriosclerosis. Bone gangrene is also possible.

Q: What is the treatment for gangrene?

A: The only treatment is surgical removal, with large doses of antibiotics.

Q: Can any measures be taken to guard against gangrene?

A: Patients who have severe arteriosclerosis, or diabetes, should take particular care of their feet and hands, especially the nails, because the risk of infection even from a minor injury, for example, one caused by a ragged nail, is increased. This is because the narrowed blood vessels in their fingers and toes cannot conduct sufficient blood to combat infection. Any abrasion or infection should be treated immediately.

Gas gangrene is a type of moist GANGRENE that is usually a complication of crushing injuries. The infection is caused by the bacteria *Clostridium welchii* (*see* CLOSTRIDIUM) that thrive without oxygen and release a foul-smelling gas as well as a poisonous toxin. The bacteria breed in the damaged tissue and spread rapidly to healthy tissue. Symptoms include a high fever, putrid-smelling pus, and the formation of gas bubbles under the skin

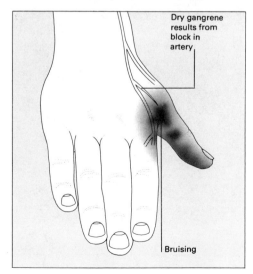

Dry gangrene results from block in artery

Bruising

Gangrene occurs when the blood supply is disrupted, causing gradual death of tissues.

Gas poisoning

Urgent hospitalization is necessary. Death occurs within about two days if the condition is not treated.

Gas poisoning (for EMERGENCY treatment, *see* First Aid, p.570). Many poisonous gases are released when solids and liquids such as mineral acids, ammonia, cyanides, and mercury are heated. Others are specially manufactured as war gases. Poisonous gases affect the body in various ways, and many are potentially fatal.

Q: What are some examples of the effects of poisonous gases?

A: Carbon monoxide and mixtures that contain it prevent the blood from carrying oxygen to tissues; hydrogen sulfide causes respiratory paralysis; carbon tetrachloride damages the liver and kidneys; carbon disulfide ultimately causes paralysis and psychoses; tear gases, such as xylyl bromide, severely irritate the eyes, nose, and throat; the various nerve gases prevent the proper functioning of nerve impulses; lung irritant gases, such as chlorine and phosgene, attack the eyes, nose, throat, and lungs; vesicant gases, such as mustard gas and lewisite gas (containing arsenic), cause blisters and ulcers on the skin; nauseant gases, such as chloropicrin, induce vomiting; nose irritant gases, such as diphenylchlorarsine, cause pain, sneezing, depression, and sometimes vomiting.

Q: How can people come in contact with such gases?

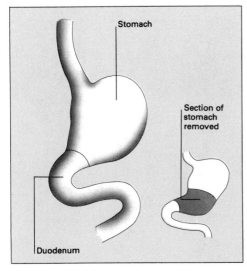

Gastrectomy of the partial type may reduce the capacity of the stomach by as much as half.

A: Carbon monoxide is the most poisonous gas likely to be present in domestic surroundings. For example, it is present in a closed garage when an automobile engine has been left running. Carbon tetrachloride is used in dry cleaning. Hydrogen sulfide is a poisonous gas produced in some chemical processes. Tear gases are used by police and military personnel. Carbon disulfide is used in the rubber industry and in making rayon.

Gastrectomy is the surgical removal of part or all of the stomach. The operation is performed to remove a perforated or bleeding stomach ulcer (partial gastrectomy), to remove scarred tissue that obstructs the passage of food, or to remove a cancerous growth. A partial gastrectomy is also one method of treatment for a peptic ulcer in the duodenum.

Q: How is the digestive process affected after a gastrectomy?

A: The small intestine is capable of maintaining the preliminary breakdown of proteins that normally takes place in the stomach. After the total removal of the stomach, however, a patient may have to make some dietary adjustments.

Q: What dietary adjustments may have to be made?

A: Supplements of vitamins and iron may be necessary. The absorption of vitamin B_{12} depends on the presence of gastric (stomach) juices; after a total gastrectomy, injections of this vitamin have to be given. Iron supplements reduce the risk of ANEMIA if a gastrectomy interferes with the amount of iron normally absorbed during digestion. After a partial gastrectomy, the patient has to adopt a routine of eating smaller amounts of food, more often.

Gastric ulcer is the ulceration of an area of the stomach lining. *See* PEPTIC ULCER.

Gastritis is inflammation of the stomach lining. The inflammation may be caused by viral infection, alcohol, smoking, certain drugs, highly spiced or poisoned food, or by stress. Gastritis may be acute or chronic.

Q: What are the symptoms of gastritis?

A: Acute gastritis causes vomiting, furred tongue, thirst, severe stomach pain, and mild fever. Chronic gastritis usually produces few symptoms although in some cases a person may experience one or more of the following discomforts: mild indigestion; slight nausea; a bloated feeling after a small meal; a bad taste in the mouth; and vague stomach pain.

Q: How is gastritis treated?

A: Acute gastritis improves of its own accord, so treatment is directed at the symptoms; antacid preparations and anti-nauseant drugs are often prescribed. Chronic gastritis can be treated only by eliminating the causative factor, for example, alcohol, smoking, or highly spiced or other foods that are difficult to digest. Sometimes antacid drugs are recommended for the relief of indigestion.

Gastroenteritis is any inflammation of the lining of the stomach and intestinal tract. The inflammation is usually caused by a bacterial infection. If it occurs in infants, there is severe liquid loss, and the patient may require hospitalization. But gastroenteritis can also be caused by alcohol, certain drugs, food allergies, contaminated food, and certain bacterial infections. The symptoms of gastroenteritis are vomiting, abdominal cramps, diarrhea, and, in severe cases, exhaustion.

Q: How is gastroenteritis treated?
A: The symptoms are treated, not the cause. The patient must stop drinking alcohol and must replace essential nutrients, especially liquids, that are lost through vomiting or diarrhea. A bland diet, such as a milk diet, is often necessary. A physician may prescribe antinauseant drugs for vomiting; antispasmodic drugs for cramps; antihistamine drugs for food allergies; or antibiotic drugs, such as penicillin or ampicillin, for bacterial infection.

Gastroenterostomy is an artificial opening that is made between the stomach and the small intestine. The operation (gastroenterotomy) is necessary if the muscle that surrounds the stomach opening is scarred and unable to pass food normally from the stomach. It is sometimes done as alternative surgical treatment for a duodenal ulcer (*see* ULCER). When removing part of the stomach (partial gastrectomy), a surgeon may perform a gastroenterotomy to connect the remaining part of the stomach to the small intestine. The lower opening is made into the jejunum beyond the duodenum. *See also* DUMPING SYNDROME.

Gastrointestinal series (GI series) is an investigation of the gastrointestinal tract in which a series of X-ray photographs are taken. This is made possible if the patient first swallows a tasteless solution of barium. X rays are taken as the radiopaque barium passes through the esophagus, stomach, and intestines. The barium is usually given to the patient early in the morning when the stomach is empty. *See* BARIUM.

Gastroscopy is the examination of the internal surface of the stomach through a special instrument (gastroscope) that is passed through the mouth and down the esophagus. The gastro-scope may be either a straight tube or flexible FIBERSCOPE. Gastroscopy is a branch of ENDOSCOPY.

Gastrostomy is an opening that is made from the outside surface of the abdomen into the stomach. The operation (called a gastrotomy) may be performed if there is some obstruction in, or damage to, the esophagus that prevents foods from passing down it (for example, cancer, or severe scarring following acid poisoning at the lower end). A gastrostomy allows the patient to be fed through the opening directly into the stomach. Gastrotomies are often performed as a temporary measure after major gastrointestinal surgery to allow stomach and abdominal tissue to heal completely.

Gaucher's disease is a rare inherited disorder caused by the absence of an enzyme that is necessary for the processing by the body of a particular group of fatty acids. The age of onset varies greatly. There is no treatment for this disease. Children generally die of the disease within one to two years of its onset, but death in adults usually results from a complication such as pneumonia.

Gene is the basic unit of HEREDITY that carries "instructions" for a particular characteristic. Within the nucleus of nearly all human cells there are twenty-three pairs of CHROMOSOMES, which contain several million pairs of genes. Exceptions are sex cells (eggs and sperm), which contain only twenty-three single chromosomes each. When an egg and a sperm fuse at fertilization, the resultant embryo carries genes from each parent cell.

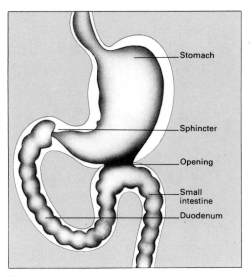

Gastroenterostomy connects stomach and small intestine to by-pass the duodenum.

Genetic abnormality

A talk about Genetic abnormality

Genetic abnormality is a disorder caused by an abnormality of a GENE, or by an incorrect number of genes.

Q: What genetic abnormalities commonly occur?

A: Conditions such as achondroplasia, hemolytic disease of the newborn, sickle cell anemia, Down's syndrome, and cleft palate are among the commonest genetic abnormalities. There are more than 2,000 genetic disorders, some of which are extremely rare, such as phenylketonuria, an inherited metabolic disorder.

Q: Are all genetic abnormalities immediately apparent?

A: No. Some genetic abnormalities, such as Tay-Sachs disease, affect the metabolism in subtle ways and may not become apparent until several months after birth. Others, such as Huntington's chorea, may not appear until the individual reaches middle age.

Q: Can normal parents have children with genetic abnormalities?

A: Yes. The effects of an abnormal gene may be masked by a normal gene in either one or both of the parents. In such a case, the parents will appear to be completely normal, but their children may be affected. Hemophilia is an example of a condition in which this situation could occur. Genetic abnormalities in children with normal parents may also occur if there is a spontaneous mutation, or change, of the parental genes, or if there is a fault in the process of egg or sperm production.

Q: Can genetic abnormalities be treated?

A: Although most genetic abnormalities are untreatable, there are a few that can be treated. Those suffering from phenylketonuria can be given a phenyl-alanine-free diet during the first few years of life while the nervous system is developing, after which they can lead a normal life. Those with celiac disease can prevent the occurrence of any symptoms by having a gluten-free diet throughout their lives. Cleft palate and spina bifida may be treated surgically, although with spina bifida, the success of the treatment depends upon the initial severity of the condition.

   See also ACHONDROPLASIA; AGAM-MAGLOBULINEMIA; ALBINO; ANKY-LOSIS; CELIAC DISEASE; CHOREA; CHRISTMAS DISEASE; CLEFT PALATE; CONGENITAL ANOMALIES; CYSTIC FIBROSIS; DOWN'S SYNDROME; DWARFISM; EPILEPSY; FAR-SIGHTEDNESS; FRIEDREICH'S ATAXIA; GAUCHER'S DISEASE; GENETIC COUNSELING; HEMOCHROMATOSIS; HEMOLYTIC DISEASE OF THE NEWBORN; HEMOPHILIA; HEREDITY; HIRSCHSPRUNG'S DISEASE; KLINEFELTER'S SYNDROME; MUTATION; MYOPIA; MYOTOMA CONGENITA; OSTEOGENESIS IMPERFECTA; PHENYLKETONURIA; POLYCYSTIC KIDNEY; PORPHYRIA; RETINITIS PIGMENTOSA; SICKLE CELL ANEMIA; TAY-SACHS DISEASE; THALASSEMIA; TURNER'S SYNDROME; VON RECKLINGHAUSEN'S DISEASE; WILSON'S DISEASE.

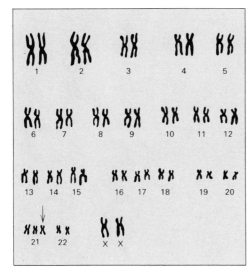

Down's syndrome occurs when an extra chromosome appears in the cell make-up.

A talk about Genetic counseling

Genetic counseling is a branch of medicine that provides and interprets information about human genetics. The main object of genetic counseling is to prevent the occurrence of CONGENITAL ANOMALIES.

Q: What types of congenital anomalies may be caused by a genetic disorder?

A: Although genetic disorders causing birth defects are comparatively rare, the range of such disorders is wide. For example, some genetic disorders, such as cleft palate, are apparent at birth; others, such as Huntington's chorea, do not appear for a number of years. For a more detailed account of genetic disorders, *see* GENETIC ABNORMALITY.

Q: What information will a genetic counselor require?

A: A counselor will need to know the ages of the couple; whether either of the couple, or any of their close relatives, has a congenital abnormality; and whether either has had children with an inherited disorder. A counselor will need as complete a family health history as possible, perhaps going back for several generations. A counselor may also perform certain tests to determine whether either of the couple has an inherited disorder of which they may be unaware.

Q: *Are there any disorders that do not affect the parents but which may occur in their children?*

A: Yes. If both parents have one recessive gene for the same disorder, neither will exhibit any abnormality. However, if a child inherits both recessive genes, one from each parent, then the disorder will manifest itself. In such a case, there is a 25 percent chance that the child will inherit both genes and so manifest the disorder.

Q: *What information does a genetic counselor give?*

A: A counselor explains about dominant and recessive genes; the kinds of chromosomal abnormalities that may occur; and why certain conditions occur. If the couple has a child with a genetic disorder, a counselor explains the chances of a second child suffering from the same disorder. Similarly, if one or both parents has an inherited disorder, a counselor tells them about the chances of a child inheriting the same disorder.

A genetic counselor's task is to provide as much information as possible. It is not for the counselor to advise on whether to have a baby or not. That decision rests with the couple. But many couples have found the decision easier to make when they have been made aware of the facts.

Q: *Can anything be done to warn a pregnant woman of an abnormal fetus?*

A: Yes. In the fourth month of pregnancy AMNIOCENTESIS, the sampling of fluid from the bag around the fetus, may be performed. This fluid can be tested for abnormal substances and for chromosomal abnormalities that may indicate an inherited disorder. For example, the abnormal substance alpha-feto protein is formed by babies with anencephaly and spina bifida. Amniocentesis may be combined with ultrasound techniques to give further information about the fetus. These techniques can detect many, but not all, abnormalities. If an abnormality is detected, the pregnancy may be terminated if the mother wishes it.

Q: *How can genetic counseling be obtained?*

A: If a couple want genetic counseling, they should consult their family physician or an obstetrician, who will refer them to a genetic counselor.

Genitourinary. *See* UROGENITAL.
Genu valgum. *See* KNOCK-KNEE.
Genu varum. *See* BOWLEGS.
Germ is any microorganism, especially one that causes disease, such as a specific bacterium, virus, fungus, or protozoan. The term also describes rudimentary living matter that has the capacity to develop into an organ, part, or organism (for example, the dental germ from which a tooth develops). Germ cell is another name for a single egg (ovum) or sperm.
German measles. *See* RUBELLA.
Gigantism is a condition of abnormal growth which occurs before puberty and results in excessive size and stature.
Gingivitis is inflammation of the gums accompanied by pain, swelling, and a tendency to bleed. If the inflammation is left untreated the teeth may become loose or fall out. The most common cause of gingivitis is poor dental hygiene. Gingivitis may also be caused by ill-fitting dentures; vitamin C deficiency disease, known as scurvy; generalized inflammation of the mouth (stomatitis); or as a complication of diabetes, leukemia, or pregnancy. In severe cases of gingivitis,

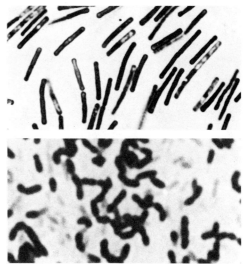

Germs of the streptococcal variety can cause septic sore throat or scarlet fever.

removal of some of the inflamed gum may be necessary.

See also DENTAL DISORDERS.

GI series. *See* GASTROINTESTINAL SERIES.

Gland is a body organ made up of specialized tissue that secretes a fluid. There are two types of glands: an exocrine gland secretes fluid into a duct or tube, and an ENDOCRINE GLAND secretes directly into the bloodstream. *See* ADRENAL GLANDS; BARTHOLIN'S GLAND; CORPUS LUTEUM; ISLETS OF LANGERHANS; OVARY; PANCREAS; PARATHYROID GLANDS; PITUITARY GLAND; PROSTATE GLAND; SALIVARY GLANDS; TESTIS; THYROID GLAND; TONSIL.

See also LACRIMATION; LACTATION.

Glandular fever is infectious mononucleosis. *See* MONONUCLEOSIS.

Glaucoma is a group of eye diseases characterized by the build-up of fluid pressure within the eyeball. The pressure severely affects the eye lens and optic nerve, resulting eventually in blindness unless the condition is detected and treated before damage becomes permanent.

Primary glaucoma usually occurs without known cause. A high incidence of glaucoma in certain families suggests that it may be an inherited tendency. It is more common in far-sighted persons.

Secondary glaucoma is a complication of other eye disorders, such as inflammation of the iris (iritis). Diabetics seem more likely to develop this condition than nondiabetics.

Q: What are the symptoms of glaucoma?

A: Acute glaucoma usually occurs suddenly with pain and a dramatic blurring of vision. The patient begins to notice

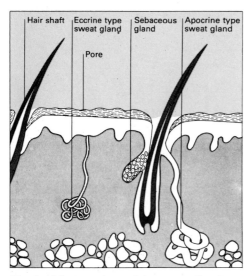

Glands of the exocrine variety secrete directly onto the epithelial surface through a duct.

rainbow-colored halos around lights and bright objects, and a loss of vision at the sides of the field of view (tunnel vision) Eyesight deteriorates, and blindness results if treatment is not obtained promptly.

Chronic glaucoma occurs slowly and without pain, so that an individual is usually unaware of the disorder until it is well advanced.

Q: How does glaucoma cause loss of vision?

A: The pressure of the fluid (aqueous humor) in the front of the lens increases the pressure in the fluid (vitreous humor) behind the lens. The resulting pressure on the retina at the back of the eye reduces the flow of blood and damages the light-sensitive rods and cones (*see* EYE). Peripheral, or side vision, is lost first, followed by total loss of vision.

Q: How is chronic glaucoma detected before eyesight deteriorates?

A: A physician measures the pressure in the eye with a special instrument called a tonometer, which is placed over the eyeball. This simple test is painless, fast, and accurate. Everyone over the age of forty should have a glaucoma check once a year.

Q: How is glaucoma treated?

A: If the condition is detected early, drug treatment prevents later damage to sight. Various eye drops can be used at regular intervals to reduce pressure within the eyeball. An ophthalmologist may prescribe pilocarpine, which increases the size of the opening through which the aqueous humor drains. Other eye drugs may also be used. Diuretic drugs, such as acetazolamide, help to decrease the amount of aqueous humor produced.

If drug treatment fails, surgery is necessary. An ophthalmic surgeon makes a small hole near the rim of the iris to create a new out-flow channel for the fluid.

Glioma is a tumor in the weblike tissue that supports nerves and the brain. A glioma may develop slowly, or grow rapidly. In many instances gliomas are malignant (cancerous). Gliomas may be treated either by surgical removal or with RADIOTHERAPY.

Globulin is one of a group of simple proteins in the blood plasma. Its main subgroups are alpha, beta, and gamma globulin. The blood clotting agents fibrinogen and prothrombin are both globulins.

Glomangioma, also known medically as a glomus tumor, is the painful but benign (noncancerous) enlargement of the glomus, a collection of tiny arteries with nerve endings. Glomera are found in the nailbeds and the pads of the fingers, toes, ears, hands, and feet. Usually located beneath a fingernail, a glomangioma causes purplish-red discoloration with slight swelling, extreme tenderness, and sometimes shooting pain. The only treatment is surgical removal.

Glomerulonephritis is a form of NEPHRITIS that involves the glomeruli, clusters of tiny blood vessels that filter the blood to extract urine in the kidneys. Glomerulonephritis may be either acute or chronic.

Q: What are the symptoms of acute glomerulonephritis?

A: Acute glomerulonephritis often follows a sore throat caused by a streptococcal infection. It is more common in children than in adults. About two weeks after the onset of infection, the patient may suddenly suffer from headaches and abdominal pain. The face swells, and the patient passes bloodstained, "smoky," or brown urine. These symptoms last for several days and the condition gradually improves within a few weeks.

Q: What causes acute glomerulonephritis?

A: In most cases, it results from a reaction to one of the types of streptococcal bacteria that cause sore throats or skin infections. The reaction damages the glomeruli, and leads to the retention of salt, water, and nitrogenous waste substances in the bloodstream, and hematuria (blood in the urine). In many cases, the cause of glomerulonephritis is not known.

Q: How is acute glomerulonephritis treated?

A: In most cases, the disease is mild enough to be treated by a restriction of salt and fluid intake, with total bed rest. If a bacterial infection is present, a physician usually prescribes antibiotic drugs. If there is high blood pressure, other drugs may be prescribed to reduce it. Occasionally, glomerulonephritis in adults causes severe kidney damage that necessitates kidney dialysis until the kidneys recover.

Q: What are the symptoms of chronic glomerulonephritis?

A: The symptoms develop slowly over a period of several months, and the condition may not be detected until it is in its final stages. The symptoms are those of kidney failure: poor appetite, fatigue, and anemia. There is also high blood pressure and the risk of heart failure. Usually, chronic glomerulonephritis is detected during a routine examination, when protein and small amounts of blood are found in the urine.

Q: How is chronic glomerulonephritis treated?

A: Treatment involves a strict diet, with restriction of salt and protein intake, and drugs to reduce high blood pressure. In severe cases, kidney dialysis and, eventually, kidney transplantation may be necessary.

Glossitis is inflammation of the tongue. Acute glossitis is often associated with other mouth disorders, such as GINGIVITIS or generalized STOMATITIS. Symptoms of acute glossitis include a painful, sometimes ulcerated tongue, thick and sticky saliva, and difficulty in swallowing. The patient may also complain of unpleasant taste and odor.

Chronic glossitis is associated with chronic ill health, DYSPEPSIA, and septic teeth. Other causes include gastritis, smoking, alcohol consumption, and sometimes the use of antibiotic drugs.

Q: How is glossitis treated?

A: Acute glossitis is treated with antiseptic mouthwashes and an anesthetic solution to reduce pain. Chronic glossitis is treated by improving the general health of the patient.

Glucose is a simple sugar that is essential to body cells for energy. It is the intermediate product in the breakdown of carbohydrates in food (sugars and starches). Glucose passes into the bloodstream from the intestines and is stored, as GLYCOGEN, in the liver. The amount of glucose in the blood is called the blood sugar content. This is carefully regulated by the pancreatic hormone INSULIN and, to a lesser extent, by other hormones such as cortisol, thyroxine, glucagon, and adrenaline. Insufficient insulin produces

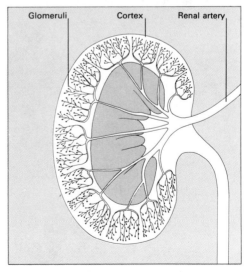

Glomerulonephritis occurs when the glomeruli within the kidney become inflamed or infected.

Glucose tolerance test

high blood sugar. *See* DIABETES MELLITUS.

Q: What other disorders are associated with abnormal blood sugar levels?

A: High blood sugar, or HYPERGLYCEMIA, is associated with acromegaly, hemochromatosis, hyperthyroidism, and hyperadrenalism. Low blood sugar, or HYPOGLYCEMIA, is associated with Addison's disease, insulin shock, hypopituitarism, and myxedema. *See* GLUCOSE TOLERANCE TEST.

Glucose tolerance test is a procedure that a physician carries out to determine whether a patient is able to use and store GLUCOSE normally. The test is most commonly carried out to diagnose DIABETES MELLITUS, but is also used to assess the functioning of the liver and the thyroid gland.

After a period of fasting, the patient's blood and urine are tested for glucose. Then, a measured quantity of glucose is administered as a drink or by injection. Further blood and urine samples are taken at regular intervals for two to four hours. A normal result shows a maximum level of glucose in the blood about an hour after the dose, followed by a gradual return to the normal level during the second hour. An abnormal result reveals an unusually high rise in the blood sugar level, an extremely slow return to normal, and sugar in the urine (glycosuria).

Glycogen is the form of carbohydrate in which GLUCOSE is stored in the liver and muscles. It acts as an energy reserve for the body because it can quickly be changed into glucose when needed.

Glycosuria is the medical term for glucose in the urine. *See* GLUCOSE TOLERANCE TEST.

Goiter is an enlargement of the thyroid gland. The resulting bulge on the neck may become extremely large, but most simple goiters are brought under control before this happens. Occasionally a simple goiter may cause some difficulty in breathing and swallowing. An overactive thyroid gland, known as HYPERTHYROIDISM, may also produce a goiter.

Q: What causes a goiter?

A: Iodine is the principal component of thyroxine, the thyroid gland's hormone. If there is not enough iodine in the diet, there is insufficient thyroxine, and the pituitary gland responds by releasing more thyroid-stimulating hormone. This causes enlargement of the thyroid gland.

However, a goiter may also be caused by overactivity of the pituitary gland or by overactivity of the thyroid gland itself. Other causes include reduced activity of the thyroid gland because of inflammation (thyroiditis), so that the gland swells in order to produce more thyroxine. Some types of drugs can produce a goiter. During adolescence or pregnancy, a goiter may appear as the thyroid gland copes with the body's need for more thyroxine. Sometimes a goiter is caused by a tumor on the thyroid gland.

Q: How is a simple goiter treated?

A: Iodized salt added to the diet is an effective treatment, as well as a preventative measure. The best drug for treating goiter caused by hypothyroidism (underactivity of the thyroid gland) is thyroxine. Such treatment prevents the pituitary gland from secreting too much thyroid-stimulating hormone. Lumps or nodules on the thyroid gland are removed surgically in case they are cancerous. Inflammation (thyroiditis) may be part of a general illness, and the goiter improves when the patient recovers. Goiters resulting from the hormone requirements of adolescence or pregnancy disappear when the demand for thyroxine is reduced naturally.

A talk about Gonorrhea

Gonorrhea is a highly contagious venereal (sexually transmitted) disease. It is common throughout the world and is widespread in the United States, where authorities estimate there are three million cases annually. If left untreated, it can lead to sterility and can be the cause of congenital blindness.

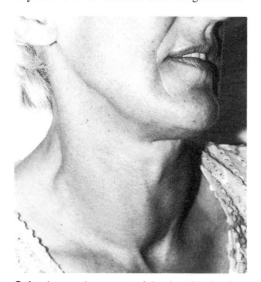

Goiter is an enlargement of the thyroid gland caused by a number of different disorders.

Gonorrhea can be treated successfully with antibiotics, if reported to a physican in time, although no immunity is given against reinfection. Any person who has a discharge from the genitals should report it to a physician at once. This consultation is important because it not only increases the chances of successful treatment, but also allows the early detection of other sexually transmitted diseases, which may also be present.

Q: What are the symptoms of gonorrhea?

A: In a male, a thick, yellow-green discharge from the penis occurs within two to ten days after infection. Inflammation and pain in the urethra (the tube through which urine is passed) are common, and urination becomes slow and difficult. If left untreated, the discharge becomes clear and sticky for several months before symptoms of fever and swollen lymph glands in the groin appear. A small number of males may develop no symptoms at all, though they are still capable of spreading the infection to a sexual partner.

In a female, the infection may produce no symptoms and so she is unaware that she may be infecting the person, or persons, with whom she comes into sexual contact. Occasionally, however, symptoms do develop slowly. These include vaginal discharge, painful or frequent urination, or pain in the lower abdomen. Gonorrhea in the rectum or throat are usually asymptomatic.

Q: What causes gonorrhea?

A: Gonorrhea is caused by the gonococcus bacterium, *Neisseria gonorrhoeae.* In most cases, the bacteria cause inflammation of the mucous membranes of the urogenital tract, but they may also affect the membranes of the throat, the conjunctiva, or the rectum.

Q: How is gonorrhea diagnosed?

A: For a male, a test (Gram's stain) of the urethral discharge produces a reliable diagnosis. In a female, this diagnosis is not as reliable, because the Gram's stain may cause confusion between the gonorrhea organism and others that resemble it but occur normally. Positive diagnosis can, however, be made from a culture.

Q: How is gonorrhea treated?

A: All cases of gonorrhea, even if only suspected, must be treated by a physician. The patient's partner must also see the physician. There is no home cure for the disease, nor will it disappear if left alone. Antibiotic treatment with penicillin is usually successful. Some strains of the bacteria are resistant to penicillin,

however, and these can be treated with other antibiotics.

Q: What are the possible complications of gonorrhea?

A: Neglected cases of gonorrhea become chronic. In a male, infection spreads from the mucous membranes into deep tissues, such as the bladder, prostate gland, and epididymis. Sometimes the urethra becomes scarred, which makes urination slow and difficult, and in some cases sterility may result.

In a female, the chronic infection may spread to the womb, fallopian tubes, and ovaries, and cause sterility. A pregnant woman with untreated gonorrhea may infect her baby's eyes during birth as the baby passes through the birth canal.

Q: How can a person avoid catching gonorrhea?

A: A person can avoid catching gonorrhea by avoiding sexual contact with an infected person. Use of the condom (sheath) offers some protection against catching the disease.

See also VENEREAL DISEASES.

Gout

Gout is a metabolic disorder characterized by inflammation and pain in affected joints. It is caused by an excess of URIC ACID in the blood and tissues. Crystals of the acid form under the skin and in the joints, causing local pain. In normal circumstances, uric acid above a certain low concentration is excreted in the urine. Gout occurs either when too little uric acid is excreted, or when there is too much of

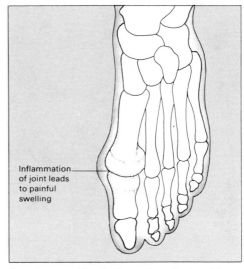

Inflammation of joint leads to painful swelling

Gout is caused by the formation of uric acid crystals that cause joint inflammation.

Graafian follicle

the acid for the kidneys to excrete. Contrary to popular belief, attacks of gout have nothing to do with diet, or alcohol intake.

Q: *What are the symptoms of gout?*

A: An attack begins suddenly with severe pain and swelling in a joint. The overlying skin becomes red and shiny. A severe attack may cause fever and nausea. Untreated, an attack of gout lasts between three and seven days. Even when the symptoms disappear, further attacks are likely.

Q: *What brings on an attack of gout?*

A: In general, the causes of acute attacks of gout are not known, but some drugs, for example, diuretics, and minor injuries, can bring on an attack.

Q: *How is gout diagnosed?*

A: A physician has to make sure that the inflamed joint is not the result of infection, osteoarthritis, or acute rheumatoid arthritis. A diagnosis of gout is made after a blood test reveals an abnormally high level of uric acid in the blood. Sometimes the fluid from an inflamed joint is examined for crystals.

Q: *How is gout treated?*

A: In an acute attack, the joint is rested until the pain subsides. The drug colchicine can bring relief within a few hours, but possible side effects make it unsuitable for the elderly and for patients with heart, liver, or kidney disorders. Other drugs prescribed for an acute attack include phenylbutazone, allopurinol, and indomethacin.

Q: *Does gout have any complications?*

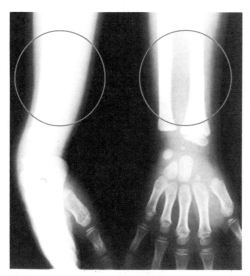

Greenstick fracture occurs when the bone splits and bends, without breaking cleanly.

A: Yes. If gout is not treated in its early stages, the condition may become chronic. Chronic gout results in deposits of uric acid (tophi) in the joints. These deposits may cause permanent arthritis. The most serious danger is that crystals may be deposited in the kidneys.

Graafian follicle is the mature follicle in an ovary that contains the ovum before OVULATION. When the follicle ruptures under the influence of luteinizing hormone (LH) the ovum is released. The CORPUS LUTEUM develops within the ruptured follicle.

Graft is healthy tissue that is transferred surgically from one place to another. Skin is the tissue most commonly grafted, although bones, tendons, and nerves can also be grafted. A cornea from the eye of a recently dead donor can be grafted to a patient's damaged cornea. The technique of skin grafting is invaluable for the treatment of deep burns and similar injuries. Healing time is reduced and the grafted skin is stronger and less disfiguring than the scarred tissue that would otherwise form.

Grand mal. *See* EPILEPSY.

Granuloma inguinale, or Donovanosis, is a venereal (sexually transmitted) disease caused by the bacterium *Calymmatobacterium granulomatis*. The first symptom is a small, painless lump in the genital area. If neglected, this rapidly breaks down and forms a deep ulcer that spreads slowly. New ulcers may develop and cover the entire genital area, buttocks, and abdomen. Effective treatment can be given with antibiotic drugs.

Graves' disease. *See* THYROTOXICOSIS.

Greenstick fracture is a type of bone fracture common among children. The fractured bone cracks only half across its width; the remaining half merely bends. *See* FRACTURES.

Grief is a normal emotion of intense sorrow expressed in response to a great loss, such as the death of a friend or relative. *See* DYING.

Q: *How may somebody be helped in the initial stages of grief?*

A: There are many ways to help a grieving person. Give practical help with the domestic tasks. Give emotional support by listening to the grieving person as he or she talks about the loss. The person may also be helped by talking to a clergyman. Encourage the person to have a rest during the day to maintain physical strength. A physician may prescribe sedatives to aid in sleeping and tranquilizers for times of acute stress, such as a funeral.

Q: *How may a grieving person be helped after the initial stages?*

A: The grieving person should be continually

invited to participate in family and social events, even if the invitations are always refused. Expert advice on any legal or financial problems may help to relieve the person's anxiety.

Despite the good will and efforts of family and friends, some people seem to cling morbidly to grief. This prolonged grief is sometimes a sign of underlying guilt and remorse and the person may require psychiatric help.

See also DYING.

Gristle. *See* CARTILAGE.

Group therapy is psychiatric treatment based on discussions among a group of people who have similar problems. *See* MENTAL ILLNESS.

Guillain-Barré syndrome is an inflammation of the nerves. Symptoms usually begin with weakness in the legs, later developing into paralysis of the muscles of the trunk, arms, and occasionally, face. The cause is unknown, but many patients have reported respiratory infections preceding the onset of Guillain-Barré syndrome. Treatment consists primarily of skilled nursing care in the early stages because of the potential risk of paralysis of the muscles of breathing. Gradual return to health generally occurs after a few weeks (or, in some cases, months).

Gullet is a common term for the esophagus. *See* ESOPHAGUS.

Gum, in medicine, is the dense fibrous tissue that surrounds the necks of the teeth. The gums are covered by a mucous membrane. It is important to keep the gums healthy by massaging them when cleaning the teeth, and by keeping the teeth free of tartar and food particles.

Fairly common gum disorders include CANKER SORE, GINGIVITIS, GUMBOIL, PERIODONTITIS, and VINCENT'S ANGINA. Spongy, ulcerated gums may be a symptom of DIABETES MELLITUS, LEUKEMIA, TUBERCULOSIS, STOMATITIS, and digestive disorders. Gums that bleed easily usually indicate gingivitis, but such a condition may also be caused by SCURVY or inflammatory illnesses such as PYORRHEA.

The color of the gums can be a useful diagnostic aid: a red line around the edge indicates gingivitis, pyorrhea, or scurvy.

Gumboil is a swelling on the gum. It is a type of abscess, usually caused by local infection at the root of a tooth. Other causes include irritation or injury to the gum, either from dentures or a toothbrush. The affected area of gum is typically red, swollen, extremely tender, and painful.

Q: How is a gumboil treated?
A: Painkilling drugs and hot mouthwashes relieve some of the symptoms. A dentist may prescribe an antibiotic drug such as penicillin. The gumboil may burst of its own accord or it may have to be cut open.

Gumma is a soft tumor of the tissues (granulation tissue). The swelling is characteristic of the third stage of SYPHILIS, but it is unusual for the disease to reach this stage untreated. A gumma may also occur as a reaction to tuberculosis or yaws. Gummata occur alone or in groups and usually affect the liver. Sometimes the heart, brain, testicles, bone, and skin are affected. On the skin, gummata may ulcerate. The ulcers are painless but heal slowly, and they may leave the skin badly scarred. Treatment with penicillin is effective.

Gut is a popular term for the INTESTINE.

Gynecological disorders. The following table lists alphabetically some of the disorders that affect the reproductive organs of women, according to their chief symptoms. Each disorder has a separate entry in the A-Z section of this book. It is important to remember that some of the symptoms are not necessarily abnormal: for example, vaginal discharge is heavier than normal at certain times during the menstrual cycle and before intercourse. Not all of the disorders listed below require medical attention, but if there is any doubt, a physician should be consulted. Breast problems are listed under BREAST DISORDERS. Similarly, problems during pregnancy are discussed under the heading PREGNANCY AND CHILDBIRTH. Other relevant sections in the A-Z section of this book are MENSTRUAL PROBLEMS and SEXUAL PROBLEMS.

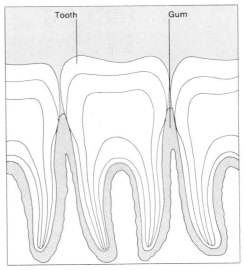

Gum is a fleshy tissue that protects teeth below the level of the hard outer enamel.

Gynecological disorders

Symptom	Related disorder	Symptom	Related disorder
Absence of, or missed period	Disorders of ADRENAL GLANDS or THYROID GLAND AMENORRHEA (medical term for lack of menstruation) Marked ANEMIA ANOREXIA NERVOSA (psychological avoidance of eating) CANCER CYST in an ovary ECTOPIC PREGNANCY (development of a fetus outside the womb) Malnutrition (*see* NUTRITIONAL DISORDERS) MENOPAUSE (cessation of periods) Pregnancy (*see* PREGNANCY AND CHILDBIRTH) TUBERCULOSIS	Difficult or painful intercourse	FRIGIDITY (psychological dislike of sexual intercourse) HEMORRHOIDS (piles) Thick or tough HYMEN (membrane across the vagina) Extreme OBESITY PROLAPSE (displacement of the womb) RECTOCELE (HERNIA of the rectum) SALPINGITIS (inflammation of a fallopian tube) VAGINISMUS (spasm in the muscles of the vagina) Atrophic VAGINITIS (inflammation of the vagina after menopause) VULVITIS (inflammation of the vulva) VULVOVAGINITIS (inflammation of the vulva and the vagina)
Aches and pains in abdomen or back	CERVICAL EROSION Chronic CERVICITIS (inflammation of the cervix) CYST in an ovary ENDOMETRITIS (inflammation of the lining of the womb) FIBROID (benign muscle tumor in the womb) Early GONORRHEA (a venereal disease) MENSTRUATION (normal) Threatened MISCARRIAGE OVULATION (normal) PREMENSTRUAL TENSION PROLAPSE (displacement of the womb) SALPINGITIS (inflammation of a fallopian tube)	Enlarged womb	CANCER FIBROID (benign muscle tumor in the womb) Pregnancy (*see* PREGNANCY AND CHILDBIRTH)
		Genital itching or soreness	ALLERGY ANXIETY DIABETES MELLITUS LEUKOPLAKIA (itchy white patches on the vulva) LICHEN PLANUS (itchy inflammation) SCABIES (itchy skin disease caused by mites) STRESS VAGINITIS (inflammation of the vagina)
Bleeding after intercourse	CERVICAL EROSION Chronic CERVICITIS (inflammation of the cervix)		
Difficult or painful intercourse	BARTHOLIN'S CYST (cyst in a gland in the vagina) DYSPAREUNIA (medical term for painful intercourse) ENDOMETRIOSIS (displacement of tissue from the lining of the womb) Fissure-in-ano (*see* FISSURE)	Headache, dizziness, moody spells	MENOPAUSE (cessation of menstruation periods in middle age) PREMENSTRUAL TENSION
		Heavy or irregular bleeding	CERVICAL EROSION ECTOPIC PREGNANCY (development of a fetus outside the womb) ENDOMETRIOSIS (displacement of tissue from the lining of the womb)

226

Gynecological disorders

Symptom	Related disorder
Heavy or irregular bleeding	ENDOMETRITIS (inflammation of the lining of the womb) FIBROID (benign muscle tumor in the womb) HEPATITIS (inflammation of the liver) Onset of MENOPAUSE MENORRHAGIA (heavy periods) METROPATHIA HEMOR-RHAGICA (abnormal bleeding from the womb) METRORRHAGIA (irregular periods) PNEUMONIA (inflammation of and liquid in the lungs) POLYP (noncancerous growth in the womb) SALPINGITIS (inflammation of a fallopian tube) TUMOR in the womb or ovary
Hot flashes	MENOPAUSE (cessation of menstrual periods in middle age)
Infertility	Extensive ENDOMETRIOSIS (displacement of tissue from the lining of the womb) FIBROID (benign muscle tumor in the womb) FRIGIDITY (psychological dislike of intercourse) Advanced GONORRHEA (a venereal disease) Endometrial HYPERPLASIA (increase in the cell structure of the womb) SALPINGITIS (inflammation of a fallopian tube)
Ovarian problems	AMENORRHEA (absence of periods) CYST in an ovary OOPHORITIS (inflammation of an ovary) TUMOR in an ovary TURNER'S SYNDROME (sex chromosome abnormality)
Painful period	DYSMENORRHEA (medical term for painful periods)

Symptom	Related disorder
Painful period	ENDOMETRIOSIS (displacement of tissue from the lining of the womb)
Postmenopausal bleeding	CANCER of the womb CYSTITIS (inflammation of the bladder) ENDOMETRITIS (inflammation of the lining of the womb) ESTROGEN drug therapy VAGINITIS (inflammation of the vagina)
Urinary problems related to genital disorders	"Honeymoon" cystitis (see CYSTITIS) NONSPECIFIC URETHRITIS (inflammation of the urethra) STRESS INCONTINENCE (involuntary urination)
Vaginal discharge	CERVICAL EROSION (bacterial destruction of the wall of the cervix) CERVICITIS (inflammation of the cervix) GONORRHEA (a venereal disease) NONSPECIFIC URETHRITIS (inflammation of the urethra) POLYP in the cervix SALPINGITIS (inflammation of a fallopian tube)

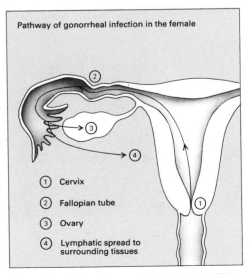

Pathway of gonorrheal infection in the female

1. Cervix
2. Fallopian tube
3. Ovary
4. Lymphatic spread to surrounding tissues

Gonorrhea in females may lead to sterility if it is not treated at an early stage.

Gynecology

Gynecology is the branch of medicine that specializes in diseases of women, particularly of the reproductive organs.

Gynecomastia is the appearance of female breasts in a boy or man. In men of fifty years or older, only one breast is affected; in children and young men, both breasts are affected. At puberty, sensitivity to female hormones produces gynecomastia in about thirty percent of boys. These hormones are produced normally by the adrenal glands before the major development of the testicles. Apart from the embarrassment that the condition may cause, there is no medical need to worry, and no need for treatment. Gynecomastia at this age disappears naturally after six to twelve months when the proper hormonal balance is established.

H

Habit spasm. *See* TIC.

Hair consists of cells of a tough protein called keratin, which grows in the hair follicle, a small pit in the outer layer of the skin (epidermis). A hair follicle produces and

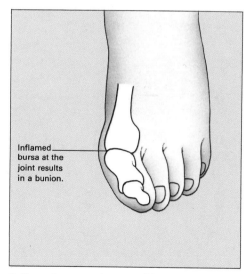

Inflamed bursa at the joint results in a bunion.

Hallux valgus may be caused by badly-fitting shoes that distort the position of the toes.

nourishes a hair. The root of the hair (hair bulb) is embedded at the base of the follicle, and it is here that growth takes place. The greasy secretions of a sebaceous gland at the side of the follicle drain into it and lubricate the hair shaft, which can be raised by a muscle attached to the follicle. There are three concentric layers of cells in a hair, and color is produced in the middle layer.

Q: Why does hair fall out?

A: Hair falls out gradually all over the body to be replaced by new hair. The follicle does not die when hair falls out; it too goes into a static period before then producing a new hair. Baldness results when hair replacement fails to keep up with hair loss (*see* BALDNESS). Abnormal hair loss (alopecia) may be caused by FOLLICULITIS or some other disorder.

Q: What factors affect the growth and condition of hair?

A: Hair growth is dependent on hormones, particularly the sex hormones. A woman's hair, for example, has a tendency to become greasier just before menstruation, because hormones then stimulate more sebaceous gland secretions, and hormonal changes during pregnancy delay the static phase of hair growth. A decreased thyroid gland or pituitary gland function makes hair become thin, dry, and brittle.

Hair, excess. *See* HIRSUTISM.

Halitosis. *See* BAD BREATH.

Hallucinations are false sensory phenomena that have no relation to reality and that may or may not be caused by external stimuli. Hallucinations are different from delusion, which is a positive belief in something unreal. In hallucinations, a person may see, hear, feel, or smell something that does not exist.

Q: What causes hallucinations?

A: Hallucinations may occur as a result of fatigue, particularly if it is accompanied by dehydration, and in an illness that produces a high fever, especially in children. Many drugs produce hallucinations, including sedatives used after a surgical operation, and in drug addiction and alcoholism, the hallucinations may be aggravated by a lack of vitamin B. In some severe forms of mental illness, hallucinations become an integral part of the condition.

Hallux rigidus is stiffness and pain in the first joint of the big toe. The condition is usually caused by repeated injury to the joint, but it may be a complication of HALLUX VALGUS.

Hallux valgus is a deformity of the big toe, usually caused by ill-fitting shoes. The toe is angled toward the other toes. The BURSA at the joint becomes inflamed, forming a BUNION. Osteoarthritis may also develop, causing HALLUX RIGIDUS. There are several surgical procedures to correct the condition. Commonly, however, the big toe is straightened, and the arthritic bone and the bunion removed.

Halothane is a gas that is used as a general anesthetic.

See also ANESTHETICS.

Hammertoe is a toe deformity in which the first joint is bent downward at a right angle.

Hamstring is any of the five tendons that connect the muscles at the back of the thigh to the lower leg.

Hand is the end part of the arm. Five long metacarpal bones form the palm of the hand; they are jointed to the bone at the base of each finger. There are three separate bones (phalanges) in each of the four fingers, and two in the thumb. The fingertips are extremely sensitive to pain, temperature, and touch, and are protected by the nails.

Q: How does the hand move?

A: The main muscles that control hand movements are in the forearm, connected to the fingers by long, strong tendons. To prevent friction, the tendons are enclosed in lubricated synovial (membrane lining) sheaths. There are also numerous small muscles in the hand.

Hand-foot-and-mouth disease is a virus infection that occurs in young children, sometimes as a minor epidemic. Small blisters appear on the palms of the hands, the soles of the feet, and in the mouth. It is a mild condition that lasts for about three or four days before recovery occurs naturally.

Hangnail is a partly detached piece of dry skin at the base of a fingernail.

Hangover is the common name for a collection of symptoms caused by drinking an excessive amount of alcohol. These symptoms often include a severe headache, nausea, vomiting, stomachache, dizziness, thirst, and fatigue.

Hansen's disease. See LEPROSY.

Hardening of the arteries. See ARTERIO-SCLEROSIS.

Harelip is a congenital cleft in the front of the upper lip. The cleft may vary in size from a notch to a fissure that extends across the whole lip. Usually it extends from the mouth up into the nostril and can be on one or on both sides of the midline. Harelip may be associated with CLEFT PALATE.

The treatment for harelip is surgery.

Hashimoto's thyroiditis is an inflammation of the THYROID GLAND caused by an increase in the fibrous tissue and an infiltration of white blood cells. It is more common in women

than in men, and usually develops during middle age. The symptoms, which develop slowly, include lethargy; loss of appetite; dry skin; underactivity of the thyroid gland; and eventually MYXEDEMA.

Hashish. See MARIJUANA.

Hay fever is an allergic condition characterized by irritation of the eyes, nose, and throat, and sometimes a rash. See ALLERGY.

Q: What causes hay fever?

A: Dust, grass, flower pollens, and mushroom spores may act as allergens, when they are inhaled, and cause the body to produce an excessive amount of HISTAMINE, a chemical that produces the symptoms of hay fever.

Q: How is hay fever treated?

A: If hay fever is seasonal and not severe, treatment with antihistamine pills may lessen the symptoms. Many cities give a daily pollen count. If the count is high, try to stay indoors, preferably in an air-conditioned room.

If hay fever is severe and long lasting, the cause of the allergy may be found by skin tests, performed by a physician, to identify the allergen. Following this, a course of desensitizing injections may be given before the hay fever season begins.

A talk about Headache

Headache is a pain or ache across the forehead or within the head itself. It is not a disorder but a symptom. Possible causes of headaches include: (1) conditions associated

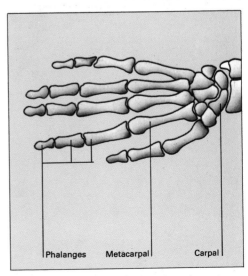

Hand consists of ten metacarpals and twenty-eight phalanges. Carpals form the wrist.

Head injury

with emotional disturbances or muscular tension; (2) disorders of the blood vessels of the brain; (3) neuralgia, caused by pressure on nerves; (4) conditions, especially infections, affecting the ears, sinuses, mouth, or the membrane that surrounds the brain; (5) head injuries; (6) conditions that affect the skull; and (7) increased pressure within the brain.

Q: *What are the commonest causes of headache?*

A: One of the commonest causes of a headache is tension in the muscles of the neck and jaw.

Another common cause is migraine, in which the headache often occurs in only one half of the head (hemicrania) and may be accompanied by nausea and vomiting.

Any generalized infection, such as influenza, may affect the blood vessels and cause a headache. Blood vessels of the brain may also be affected by external factors, such as drinking too much alcohol; smoking excessively; or inhaling or swallowing various chemicals or drugs.

Ear disorders involving inflammation, such as OTITIS and mastoiditis, may cause moderately severe headaches on the side of the head that is affected. Eye disorders, such as IRITIS, GLAUCOMA, and eye strain, may produce frontal headaches as well as pain around the eye. Sinusitis, particularly of the frontal sinuses above the eyes, may cause a severe ache at the front of the head, usually associated with a respiratory disorder such as a cold or hay fever.

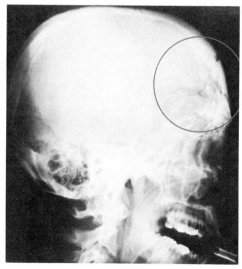

Depressed fracture of the front of the skull can be seen on the X-ray photograph.

Persistent toothache may cause headaches as well as local pain.

A head injury often causes concussion and a generalized headache of variable intensity that seems to get worse during periods of fatigue or emotional stress. It may be accompanied by dizziness, difficulty in sleeping, and loss of concentration. The injured area may also be painful and tender.

Any head injury is potentially serious, especially if there is a history of concussion. A physician should be consulted so that the skull can be X-rayed and other tests performed.

Q: *How may the common forms of headache be treated?*

A: Aspirin or preparations containing aspirin and acetaminophen are usually effective in removing the pain of a normal headache.

A talk about Head injury

Head injury (for EMERGENCY treatment, *see* First Aid, p.558) is damage to the skull or brain. It is one of the most potentially serious types of injury because it threatens the highly complex structure and functioning of the brain.

Q: *What are the various types of skull fractures?*

A: The least serious type is a hairline fracture, in which the skull cracks but the bone does not change position. If a fracture causes the bone to move, the displaced bone may press onto the tissue of the brain. This type of fracture, called a depressed fracture, causes most brain damage.

Q: *What is a brain concussion?*

A: Concussion is a severe jolting of the brain that causes microscopic damage to brain cells. Loss of consciousness may be only momentary, and the patient generally recovers completely. Symptoms of concussion include headache, difficulty in concentrating, blurred vision, feelings of depression and irritability, and, sometimes, nausea. With more serious cases there may also be loss of memory.

Q: *What is a brain contusion?*

A: Contusion of the brain is bruising that damages the nerve centers in the brain. Nerve functioning may become either depressed or accelerated.

Q: *How are head injuries treated?*

A: Although there is little that can be done to repair brain tissue already damaged, there is much that can be done to prevent further harm. Hairline fractures usually heal without complications, and an operation is seldom necessary. A depressed fracture or any type of brain hemorrhage requires an urgent surgical operation. Blood clots are normally removed as soon as possible, bringing about a rapid improvement.

For all head injuries that do not require surgery, rest is the best treatment. It may take weeks or months before the last symptoms of concussion disappear.

Q: Are there any long-term aftereffects of head injuries?

A: Yes the brain may become infected as a result of a skull fracture. Meningitis is the most serious form of infection, but preventive treatment with antibiotic drugs lessens the risk considerably.

Permanent brain damage can cause a variety of irreversible physical or mental disorders, such as weakness of the limbs (paresis), deafness, blindness, double vision, and speech-related disorders such as APHASIA, are quite common. Possible mental aftereffects include personality changes and mental impairment. Repeated minor injuries to the head can cause symptoms of disturbed coordination, memory, and concentration, and may also affect vision and hearing.

Health insurance. *See* MEDICAL EXPENSES AND INSURANCE.

Hearing is the perception of sound. For details of how this sense works, *see* EAR.

See also DEAFNESS; EAR DISORDERS.

Hearing aid. *See* DEAFNESS.

Hearing disorders. *See* DEAFNESS; EAR DISORDERS.

Heart is a strong muscular organ the size of a clenched fist, that pumps blood throughout the body. It is situated behind the breastbone (sternum) between the lungs, usually to the left side of the chest.

Q: How does the heart work?

A: There are four chambers in the heart: the right and left atria, and the right and left ventricles. The right and left sides of the heart are totally separate from each other. The atria are thin-walled upper chambers that receive blood from the veins. The ventricles are the lower chambers. The walls of both ventricles are strong, thick, and muscular, but the wall of the left ventricle is thicker and more muscular than the wall of the right ventricle, because it has to pump blood around the entire body, via the AORTA,

the main blood vessel leading from the heart.

Deoxygenated blood from the body enters the right ATRIUM from each VENA CAVA, and passes to the right VENTRICLE from which it is pumped through the PULMONARY ARTERY to the lungs. Oxygenated blood from the lungs enters the left atrium from the PULMONARY VEIN, and passes to the left ventricle.

When the atria are full of blood the ventricles relax, allowing blood from the atria to flow into them past the valves that separate the upper and lower chambers. The atria contract and force the rest of the blood into the ventricles. This is called the DIASTOLE. A split second later the ventricles contract, forcing the blood into the arteries past the semilunar valves. This is called the SYSTOLE. Backflow of blood is prevented by the opening and closing of these valves.

In an adult, at rest, the heart normally beats between 60 and 100 times per minute. The rate is usually higher in children and adolescents.

See also p.8.

Heart attack is the common term for damage to the heart muscle occurring with CORONARY HEART DISEASE. For EMERGENCY treatment, *see* First Aid, p.562.

Heartblock is a disorder in the transmission of nerve impulses between the upper chambers (atria) and lower chambers (ventricles) of the heart. A disturbance of this mechanism causes the heart beat to falter or become irregular (arrhythmia).

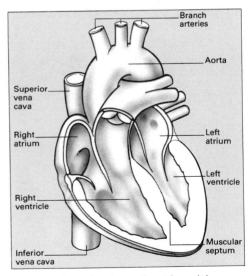

Heart has four chambers: the atria and the ventricles, separated by a muscular septum.

Heartburn

Q: *What are the symptoms of heartblock?*

A: A partial heartblock may cause no symptoms, although the irregularity of the heartbeat can be detected with a stethoscope. With a total heartblock, the contractions of the ventricles may not be fast enough to maintain an efficient blood supply. The patient may have bouts of unconsciousness (*see* STOKES-ADAMS SYNDROME). At other times, dizziness, faintness, and breathlessness may occur.

Q: *What are the causes of heartblock?*

A: Heartblock may be associated with congenital heart disease. It can be caused by infection of the heart muscle (myocarditis), damage to heart muscle from rheumatic fever, or a coronary thrombosis.

Q: *How is heartblock treated?*

A: Patients who have temporary heartblock recover spontaneously when the acute stage of the causative illness has passed. Permanent, complete heartblock may be treated with drugs but the treatment is not curative. The most effective treatment is the addition of an artificial HEART PACEMAKER.

Heartburn, also known as pyrosis, is a burning sensation in the esophagus (gullet) caused by acid rising from the stomach. It is most frequently associated with INDIGESTION.

Heart disease is the ordinary term used to describe a variety of heart disorders. All the disorders mentioned below are the subjects of individual articles in which symptoms and treatment are discussed.

The sac surrounding the heart, the pericar-dium, may become inflamed (PERICARDITIS) as a local disease or as part of a general heart inflammation, such as RHEUMATIC FEVER. The heart muscle itself may become inflamed (MYOCARDITIS) or degenerate (CARDIO-MYOPATHY) from a variety of causes.

ARTERIOSCLEROSIS can cause CORONARY HEART DISEASE which in turn may lead to coronary thrombosis. The aortic valve is frequently involved, producing narrowing and deformity and, sometimes, backflow of blood because of VALVULAR DISEASE. The distortion of the normal blood flow from valvular disease causes HEART MURMURS.

Hypertension, known commonly as HIGH BLOOD PRESSURE, produces HYPERTROPHY (increase in the size of the heart muscle) and, like other forms of heart disease, may eventually cause heart failure.

Disorders of the normal electrical impulses in the heart may produce atrial FIBRILLATION or HEARTBLOCK, and this can also occur with valvular disease, rheumatic fever, or coronary heart disease.

For further information on other conditions that may affect the heart, *see* ANGINA PECTORIS; BACTERIAL ENDOCARDITIS; BLUE BABY; DEXTROCARDIA; EMBOLISM.

Electrical disorders of the heart include BRADYCARDIA; EXTRASYSTOLE; PAROXYSMAL TACHYCARDIA; STOKES-ADAMS SYNDROME; TACHYCARDIA; VASOVAGAL SYNCOPE.

Q: *How may a physician investigate the causes of heart disease?*

A: A history of previous illness, such as rheumatic fever or muscle disorder, may help the physician to interpret any abnormal heart sounds or murmurs. But no specific cause is generally found.

There are many tests that a physician can use to assess the condition of the heart. Blood tests can detect hormone disorders such as hyperthyroidism (THYROTOXICOSIS) or HYPOTHYROIDISM. An electrocardiogram (EKG) can provide extremely useful information. This information may be supplemented by a ECHOCARDIOGRAM and PHONOCARDIOGRAM, both of which detect the effects of the heart's movement and its sounds.

Heart failure occurs when the heart's pumping ability is impaired. The heart continues to beat, but not strongly enough to maintain adequate circulation. This results in a retention of blood in the organs and tissues throughout the body. The reduction of heart function may be due to a variety of conditions including HIGH BLOOD PRESSURE, valvular heart disease, or CORONARY HEART DISEASE. For symptoms and treatment of chronic heart failure, *see* CONGESTIVE HEART FAILURE.

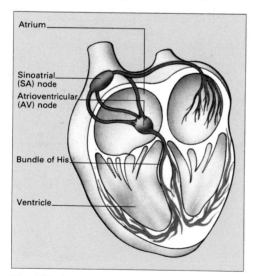

Atrium

Sinoatrial (SA) node

Atrioventricular (AV) node

Bundle of His

Ventricle

Heart block occurs when the pacemaker nerve malfunctions, disrupting the heartbeat.

Acute heart failure may follow a pulmonary embolus (a blood clot blocking an artery in a lung), or coronary thrombosis. The patient experiences shortness of breath, and coughs up bloodstained sputum. (For EMERGENCY treatment, *see* p.562.) Acute congestive heart failure may come on at night because the excess fluid moves from the legs into the circulation when the patient is lying down. This puts further strain on the heart.

Heart-lung machine is a device that permits the heart to be operated on safely. This innovation allows the surgeon to operate on a bloodless, unbeating heart. The heart-lung machine not only temporarily takes over the pumping activities of the heart, but also oxygenates the blood and removes carbon dioxide from it. Thus, the rest of the body is supplied with vital blood circulation during heart surgery. With this machine, many types of heart surgery, such as heart transplants, coronary by-passes, removal and replacement of damaged valves, and repair of other structural defects, that were previously impossible or extremely dangerous can now be done with comparative safety.

Heart massage. *See* CARDIAC MASSAGE.

Heart murmur describes the noise produced by the blood flowing through the chambers and valves of the heart.

With any abnormal murmur, a physician must be consulted. Many heart murmurs require no treatment although a few may require some form of heart surgery. A person with a serious heart murmur must inform his or her dentist of the condition who will administer drugs before treatment to prevent the possibility of bacterial endocarditis.

Heart pacemaker is a group of cells, the sinoatrial node, in the ATRIUM of the heart that regulates and generates the electrical impulses that make the heart beat.

The term also describes an artificial device that gives out electrical discharges to stimulate regular contractions of the heart muscle. The pacemaker's generator and batteries are placed under the skin, either in the armpit or in the abdominal wall, and wires are passed to the heart.

A pacemaker may be used during heart surgery, following a cardiac infarction, when an irregular heartbeat is causing episodes of dizziness or faintness, and in some forms of heart-block.

Heart stoppage, or cardiac arrest, is a temporary or permanent failure of normal heart muscle contraction (For EMERGENCY treatment, *see* First Aid, p.562). When the heart stops, blood ceases to be pumped around the body and various tissues, particularly those of the brain, become adversely affected by the lack of oxygen.

Heart stoppage may be caused by a severe electric shock; coronary thrombosis; or heart disease, particularly when it affects the heart muscle as in CARDIOMYOPATHY and MYOCARDITIS. Heart stoppage may also result from an irregular heart rhythm or Stokes-Adams syndrome. During heart surgery it is sometimes necessary to stop the heart deliberately. The heart is restarted by electrical stimulation (cardioversion).

Heart surgery is any operation on the heart. The general procedure during many operations is to connect the patient's blood circulation with a HEART-LUNG MACHINE and stop the heart beating. This enables the surgeon to operate while the heart is still and empty of blood.

Heart transplant is the replacement of an irreparably diseased heart with a healthy one. *See* TRANSPLANT SURGERY.

Heating pad is an electrical device used to relieve the pain of rheumatic disorders, or to ease stiffness after muscle damage.

Heatstroke, or sunstroke (For EMERGENCY treatment, *see* First Aid, p.573), is an acute and potentially fatal reaction to heat exposure. The onset of heatstroke may be gradual or sudden, with the symptoms of heat exhaustion (headache, weakness, and nausea) occurring in the initial stages. Then the victim ceases to sweat, causing the skin to become hot and dry, and a rapid rise in body temperature to more than 105°F (40.5°C). In the final stage, there is mental confusion, shock, and convulsions, leading to coma and sometimes death.

Hebephrenia. *See* MENTAL ILLNESS.

Heberden's nodes are small, hard lumps that sometimes form next to the joints on the ends of the fingers in persons with OSTEOARTHRITIS. There is no cure, but the discomfort of tender nodes may be lessened by wax baths and gentle heat. Disfiguring nodes can be removed surgically.

Heel is the rear part of the foot, under the ankle and behind the instep. The heel is composed of the heel bone (calcaneus), which bears the full weight of the body when standing, and a thick, firm pad of tissue beneath the calcaneus, which acts as a shock absorber when walking.

Heimlich maneuver is a first-aid procedure used to rescue a victim of choking due to an obstruction, such as food, in the windpipe. (Choking is a potentially fatal condition that requires immediate action.) The Heimlich maneuver consists of an abdominal thrust that forces the lodged material out of the windpipe. For a discussion and illustrations of this EMERGENCY maneuver, *see* First Aid, p.532.

Heliotherapy

Heliotherapy is the use of direct sunlight in the treatment of disorders such as PSORIASIS and ACNE.

Helminthiasis. *See* WORMS.

Hemachromatosis. *See* HEMOCHROMATOSIS.

Hemangioma is a tumor composed of blood vessels. It is usually benign (noncancerous) and generally affects the skin but may involve other parts of the body, such as the intestine, or the nervous system. The most common hemangiomas are types of BIRTHMARK.

Hematemesis. *See* BLOOD, VOMITING OF.

Hematocolpos is a rare condition in which menstrual blood is retained because the HYMEN completely closes the entrance to the vagina. Treatment is to make a small opening in the hymen to allow the blood to escape.

Hematology is the study of BLOOD and blood disorders.

Hematoma is a blood clot in an organ or within body tissues that forms as a result of an accident or surgery. The blood is usually reabsorbed into the body tissues and the clot disappears.

Hematuria is the presence of blood in the urine. It is always a symptom of a disorder, and a person with hematuria must consult a physician immediately.

Small amounts of blood give urine a smoky or cloudy appearance. Larger amounts make the urine dark red or dark brown. But such discoloration is not always a sign of hematuria: urine that has been standing for a while may naturally become cloudy, and reddish urine may also be caused by the pigments in certain foods, such as beets.

See also HEMOGLOBINURIA.

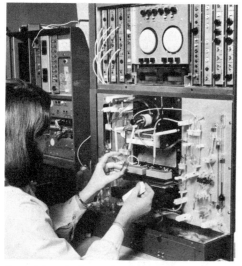

Hematology is the study of blood. Advanced machinery enables accurate blood analysis.

Hemianesthesia is the loss of sensation down one side of the body.

Hemianopia is the loss of half the normal field of vision in one or both eyes. The many types of hemianopia are classified according to which half of the vision is lost and in which eye. The most common are (1) homonymous hemianopia, in which the left (or right) half of each eye is blinded; and (2) bitemporal hemianopia, in which the outer halves of both eyes are blinded.

Hemiparesis is a type of paralysis on one side of the body only. It is commonly accompanied by loss of sensation (hemianesthesia) on the same side. *See* PARALYSIS.

Hemiplegia is total paralysis on one side of the body only. It is commonly accompanied by a loss of sensation (hemianesthesia) on the same side. Hemiplegia is generally caused by a stroke. *See* PARALYSIS.

Hemochromatosis is a disorder in which there are excessive amounts of iron absorbed by the body. It is more common in men than in women. The skin gradually darkens; diabetes mellitus usually develops because of pancreatic damage; and there may be cirrhosis of the liver.

These symptoms may be accompanied by heart failure, hypopituitarism, and loss of sex drive. Hemochromatosis may be fatal if untreated.

Q: How is hemochromatosis treated?

A: Treatment is directed toward removing the deposited iron as quickly as possible. This may be achieved by the weekly removal of a pint of blood, because hemoglobin (the red pigment in blood) contains large amounts of iron. When the patient's iron level returns to normal, removal of blood may be continued to prevent reaccumulation of iron, but at less frequent intervals; the treatment may last for up to two years.

Hemoglobin is an iron-containing protein that occurs in RED BLOOD CELLS. It consists of an iron-containing pigment called heme, and a simple protein, globin. Hemoglobin carries oxygen in the blood from the lungs to the body tissues, and also carries carbon dioxide from the tissues to the lungs.

Q: Are there different forms of hemoglobin?

A: Yes. More than a hundred types of abnormal hemoglobin have been identified, produced by rare genetic mutations. SICKLE CELL ANEMIA and THALASSEMIA, for example, are caused by different abnormal forms of hemoglobin.

Hemoglobinuria is the presence of the red blood pigment HEMOGLOBIN in the urine. It is caused by the destruction of red blood cells at a rate that releases so much hemoglobin that the liver is unable to remove it from the blood.

See also HEMATURIA; MALARIA; SICKLE CELL ANEMIA.

Hemolysis is the breakdown of RED BLOOD CELLS with the release of hemoglobin into the blood plasma. It results in a reduction in the number of red blood cells in the circulation, causing ANEMIA. Hemolysis is usually slow enough for the red blood cells to be removed by the liver and spleen. But if hemolysis occurs rapidly, it may produce shivering, fever, and JAUNDICE, and the spleen may increase in size.

Hemolytic disease of the newborn, also known medically as erythroblastosis fetalis or Rh factor incompatibility, is a serious condition affecting a baby just before, during, and just after birth. It is caused by an incompatibility between the blood of the baby and the blood of the mother.

Q: What are the symptoms of hemolytic disease of the newborn?

A: The symptoms depend on the severity of the condition. The baby may be anemic because of the destruction of the fetal blood, or have jaundice because the yellow pigment bilirubin is released when the red blood cells break down. If too much bilirubin is released, brain damage may result.

Q: How is hemolytic disease of the newborn treated?

A: Babies born with the disease are given at least one, and sometimes three, exchange transfusions of blood in which all the body's Rh+ blood is replaced by Rh−.

If necessary, after tests on both mother and child, the baby can be given a transfusion while still in the womb.

Q: What can be done to prevent hemolytic disease of the newborn?

A: Every woman should have a blood test as soon as she knows she is pregnant. If she is Rh−, the father should also be tested. If the father is Rh+, there is the possibility that the baby will develop hemolytic disease if the mother has already borne a Rh+ baby.

An injection of anti-Rh gamma globulin (Rhogam) is usually given to the mother within the first 72 hours after delivery of an Rh+ baby so that any fetal blood entering the mother's circulation is destroyed. This prevents antibodies from developing in most mothers and reduces the chances of hemolytic disease in future pregnancies. However, such treatment is effective only if the mother has had an anti-Rh gamma globulin injection during her first pregnancy.

Hemophilia is a disease caused by an inherited lack of one of the factors needed for normal blood clotting. This lack is due to a sex-linked recessive genetic defect (*see* GENE). Because the gene is sex-linked, hemophilia occurs in men, whereas women carry the abnormal gene without developing the disease.

Q: What are the symptoms of hemophilia?

A: Hemophilia is characterized by repeated episodes of spontaneous internal bleeding, and prolonged external bleeding following even minor injuries.

Q: How is hemophilia treated?

A: Injections of the missing clotting factor stop any bleeding. But for minor injuries, firm pressure over the affected area may stop the bleeding if it is maintained long enough, often an hour or more.

Q: What precautions should a hemophiliac take?

A: A hemophiliac should avoid contact sports, and any activity in which minor injuries are likely. Any operation, either surgical or dental, requires an injection of the missing clotting factor. Hemophiliacs should wear an identity disk or carry a card stating that they suffer from hemophilia.

Hemoptysis. *See* BLOOD, SPITTING OF.

Hemorrhage (for EMERGENCY treatment, *see* First Aid, p.522) is internal or external bleeding. Rapid, heavy bleeding may cause shock; slow continuous bleeding may cause anemia.

Hemorrhoidal preparations are substances that have a soothing or cleansing action on

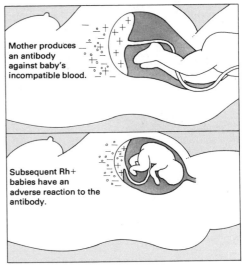

Mother produces an antibody against baby's incompatible blood.

Subsequent Rh+ babies have an adverse reaction to the antibody.

Hemolytic disease of the newborn: first (top), and subsequent pregnancies (foot).

Hemorrhoids

HEMORRHOIDS (piles), shrinking them and easing the irritation.

Hemorrhoids (for EMERGENCY treatment, *see* FIRST AID, p. 592) is the medical name for piles. A hemorrhoid is a mass of distended (varicose) veins just inside the anus. First degree hemorrhoids remain inside the anus; they may bleed from time to time. Second degree hemorrhoids also bleed and may protrude beyond the anus, being felt as a soft swelling during defecation, but spontaneously return inside. Third degree hemorrhoids, once having protruded, remain outside the anus. This type may be accompanied by slight discharge and anal itching.

Q: What is the treatment for hemorrhoids?

A: A person suffering from hemorrhoids must eat a high-roughage diet to ensure regular defecation of large, soft stools. This gently stretches the anal sphincter. Ointments, creams, and suppositories may ease the symptoms (*see* HEMORRHOIDAL PREPARATIONS). But if the hemorrhoids persist, a physician should be consulted.

Hemorrhoids can be removed surgically (hemorrhoidectomy).

Hemothorax is blood in the pleural cavity, the space between the lungs and the chest wall. The blood may be removed with a special syringe and needle, or a surgical operation (thoracotomy) may be necessary.

Heparin is an ANTICOAGULANT substance found in the liver, lungs, and other tissues. It is prepared from animal tissues for use as a drug, which is injected to prevent thrombosis in an artery or a vein, or to prevent clotting during certain heart and gynecological operations.

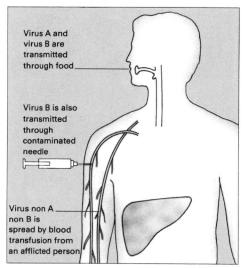

Virus A and virus B are transmitted through food

Virus B is also transmitted through contaminated needle

Virus non A non B is spread by blood transfusion from an afflicted person

Hepatitis may be caused by viral infection that can enter the body in the three ways shown.

Adverse side effects are rare.

Hepatic is the medical term for anything concerning the liver.

Hepatitis is inflammation of the liver. There are two types of hepatitis: (1) acute, caused by one of three viruses, virus A, virus B, or virus non A non B; and (2) chronic, caused by acute hepatitis, excess of alcohol, use of certain drugs, or autoimmune disease. Other infections, such as amebic dysentery and malaria, may inflame the liver.

Q: What are the symptoms of acute hepatitis?

A: Initially the patient has rapidly fluctuating fever, feels nausea, and may vomit. The patient loses his or her appetite, and a smoker finds that cigarettes taste foul. After about a week these symptoms disappear and are replaced by JAUNDICE. The skin and the whites of the eyes turn yellow, and the urine is dark colored. The patient often feels better once the jaundice appears but may still feel tired and weak.

The jaundice lasts between one and three weeks, after which the patient often becomes depressed. The depression may last for a further one or two months.

The symptoms of all forms of viral hepatitis are similar. However, the symptoms of hepatitis caused by virus B take longer to develop and tend to be more severe. It is this form of hepatitis that is sometimes fatal, with the development of ACUTE YELLOW ATROPHY of the liver.

Q: How is acute hepatitis treated?

A: In the initial stages, treatment involves bed rest. After the acute stage has passed, the patient can gradually resume normal activities. The patient need not be totally isolated, but it is essential that the feces and urine are carefully disposed of to prevent the spread of infection. Injections of GAMMA GLOBULIN may be given to persons who have come into close and prolonged contact with the patient.

Although still in the experimental stage, a vaccine offering virtually complete protection against hepatitis, type B, has been developed. Researchers expect the vaccine to be available to the public by the mid-1980's.

Q: How is acute hepatitis contracted?

A: The three viruses are transmitted in different ways. Virus A is contracted by drinking water or eating food that has been contaminated by the feces of an infected person. Virus B is usually transmitted either in saliva or in the feces of an infected person. It is also spread on contaminated hypodermic needles and is common among drug addicts.

Q: *What are the symptoms of chronic hepatitis?*

A: Chronic hepatitis means liver inflammation lasting for longer than six months. Symptoms include persistent nausea, fatigue, and jaundice. The condition may be mild, or chronic active leading to cirrhosis of the liver.

Q: *How do alcohol and drugs cause hepatitis?*

A: Alcohol leads to the accumulation of fat globules in the liver cells. If large quantities of alcohol are regularly consumed, the cells become distended with fat, burst, and die. The death of the cells produces chemical changes and causes inflammation of the surrounding liver cells. Untreated, alcoholic hepatitis leads to CIRRHOSIS and liver failure.

A talk about Heredity

Heredity is the transmission of mental and physical characteristics from parents to their children. The basic unit of heredity is a gene. Genes, which have the power to pass on hereditary characteristics, appear in strands called chromosomes in the nuclei of every cell in the body, and most importantly in the germ cells (ovum and sperm). The thousands of different genes in the body (perhaps 500 per chromosome) each carry the instructions for one specific characteristic, such as the formation of hemoglobin in the red blood cells. Sometimes the effects of several genes together determine a single characteristic: it is thought, for example, that three or four genes contribute to the determination of eye color.

Q: *What is a chromosome?*

A: A chromosome is a collection of genes in which each gene occupies a specific position in the strand. Every chromosome consists of a double strand, arranged in an helical shape, of a protein called deoxyribonucleic acid (DNA). The nucleus of every body cell contains 46 chromosomes arranged in 23 pairs. In a cell that divides to form the sex cells (ovum and sperm), the number of chromosomes is halved, so that each sex cell contains only 23 chromosomes.

At fertilization the sex cells fuse, and the 23 chromosomes from the egg unite with the 23 chromosomes from the sperm to form the embryo with 23 pairs of chromosomes. Hereditary characteristics are those contributed by the mother and by the father. One pair of chromosomes are the sex chromosomes, determining the sex of the new embryo. In males one of

these chromosomes is a shorter strand than the other. This short chromosome is called a Y chromosome and contains fewer genes; the longer chromosome is called an X chromosome. Males have XY sex chromosomes, and females XX sex chromosomes.

Q: *What is sex-linked inheritance?*

A: Sex-linked inheritance is the transmission of a characteristic that is controlled by genes on the sex chromosomes. Not all of the genes in the sex chromosomes are paired, because the X chromosome is longer than the Y chromosome. Unpaired genes on the X chromosome exert their influence, even if they are recessive, because there is no corresponding gene to modify their effects. For example, the gene for hemophilia is recessive and is carried on the X chromosome. Hemophilia occurs almost always in males because there is no corresponding gene on the Y chromosome.

Q: *Are genes always inherited in an unaltered form?*

A: No. There may be a fault in the replication of the sex cells within the parents so that one or more genes in them differ from the genes in the rest of the body. This may result in a child who has characteristics that neither parent possessed.

Q: *Can inherited disorders be predicted before birth?*

A: Prediction of some inherited disorders is possible. Through GENETIC COUNSELING,

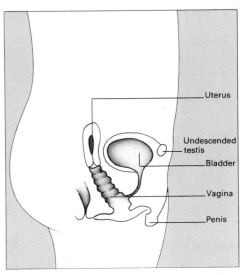

Hermaphrodite has organs of both sexes; the condition is rare in human beings.

Hermaphrodite

parents may be advised on the probability of a recurrent, inherited disorder if one has occurred in a previous child or in either of the parent's families. If a pregnancy has started, sampling of the amniotic fluid (amniocentesis) and testing the blood for alpha-feto protein may reveal any of a number of disorders.

Hermaphrodite is a person with both male and female organs. A true hermaphrodite often has sex CHROMOSOMES that are male in the testicular part of the sex glands and female in the ovarian part. This condition is rare in human beings; pseudohermaph-roditism is more common. For example, a male may have the appearance of a female, with breasts and a tiny penis, or a female may develop male characteristics. Such a condition is also termed intersex.

Q: *What may make a male appear female?*
A: This rare condition may be caused by a malfunction of the adrenal glands that makes them produce excessive amounts of certain female sex hormones. Males with this condition may appear females, with breasts, vagina, and vulva, but no womb. A male may also appear female because of an inherited disorder that makes the body fail to respond to the male sex hormone testosterone.

Q: *What condition may make a female appear male?*
A: In some girls, an adrenal gland mal-function may cause the development of male secondary sex characteristics

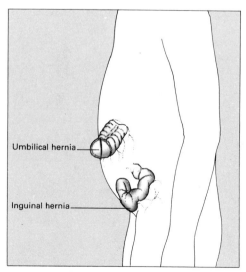

Umbilical hernia

Inguinal hernia

Hernia is more likely to protrude down the inguinal canal, or through the umbilicus.

(virilism) with hair growth in unusual places (hirsutism) and voice changes. It is more usual for females to develop male characteristics than for males to develop female ones.

Q: *If there is doubt about a baby's sex, what should be done?*
A: Sex must be determined as early as possible. The sex of a baby can be determined by examination of the chromosomes, usually in cells from inside the mouth and from blood lymphocytes, as well as by measurement of hormone levels in the urine, and special tests to examine the vagina.

Hernia, or rupture, is a lump or swelling that is formed when a tissue or organ moves out of its normal position and pushes through adjacent tissues. It may occur internally, as in a HIATUS HERNIA, when the stomach protrudes through the diaphragm muscle into the chest. Or a hernia may be external, when part of the abdominal contents, such as the intestine, protrudes through a weakness in the abdominal muscles causing a local swelling.

Q: *What are the dangers of hernias?*
A: Some hernias can be pushed back into the abdomen by a physician, and present little danger. If a hernia cannot be pushed back, it is termed irreducible. Abdominal pain, pain over the hernia, and vomiting indicate a condition called strangulation. The blood supply within the hernia is cut off and the herniated tissue dies unless an operation is performed within a few hours. A femoral hernia on the inside of the upper thigh is most likely to become strangulated because the hole is small and the ligament above the femoral artery is strong and tight.

Q: *What is the treatment for a hernia?*
A: Treatment depends on the site of the hernia. In a baby, an umbilical hernia usually disappears by the age of about four; if it does not, an operation can wait until then. In older people, an umbilical, inguinal, or femoral hernia, or one occurring in a surgical scar, is best treated with an operation called a hernia repair, which closes the weakness in the abdominal wall. Hernias in the midline of the abdomen seldom need treatment.

If the patient is too old or not well enough for an operation, a device called a truss can be worn to keep an inguinal or femoral hernia in a reduced position.

Heroin (diamorphine) is an addictive drug that is derived from the opium poppy. Heroin is illegal in the United States, but in some countries it is used medically to stop pain in the terminal stages of cancer.

Herpes genitalis is a viral infection that causes skin lesions on and around the sex organs and/or mucous membranes. Genital herpes, or Herpes simplex virus, type II, is related to COLDSORES (Herpes simplex virus, type I) and displays similar characteristics: small blisters that eventually rupture into superficial, rounded, red ulcers. Although painful, the ulcers crust over and heel in a few days, leaving scars. At this point the virus retreats to clusters of nerve cells near the spinal cord and enters a latent stage. This latent stage can last forever or for as short a span as two weeks. When a latent period is over, the virus reinfects the original site, setting off a new round of lesions.

Q: *Is genital herpes contagious?*

A: Yes, during an active period when lesions are in evidence, genital herpes is moderately contagious. It is usually contracted during intimate physical contact.

Q: *How long does it take for symptoms to appear after exposure?*

A: The incubation period is approximately four to seven days. The early symptoms include itching and soreness on or near the penis, vulva, thighs, buttocks, or mouth.

Q: *How is genital herpes diagnosed?*

A: A physician can usually diagnose herpes by examining the blisters or lesions. Diagnosis can be confirmed by taking serum from ulcerated lesions and growing tissue cultures.

Q: *Can genital herpes be cured?*

A: There is no known cure. However, for the normal, healthy adult, genital herpes is not a life-threatening condition. Herpes victims should be careful to avoid infecting other individuals, and expectant mothers should inform their physicians of the condition. Newborns, for whom the infection can be fatal, can be exposed to herpes during the passage down the birth canal.

Herpes simplex. *See* FEVER SORE.

Herpes zoster. *See* SHINGLES.

Heterograft, or xenograft, is a transplant of tissues from one species to another.

Hiatus hernia is a HERNIA that occurs when a part of the stomach protrudes upward through the sheet of muscle (diaphragm) that separates the chest cavity from the abdomen. If the hiatus hernia is small, there may be no symptoms. Sometimes, however, the condition can become serious enough to require a major operation.

Q: *What are the symptoms of a hiatus hernia?*

A: A baby with a hiatus hernia frequently regurgitates food, which may be bloodstained. The baby may appear to have difficulty in swallowing.

In an adult, a typical symptom is heartburn when bending forward or lying down. The pain may spread to the jaw and down the arms, similar to an attack of ANGINA PECTORIS. Other symptoms include hiccups, a dry cough, and an awareness of more forceful heartbeat.

Q: *How is a hiatus hernia treated?*

A: If the hernia is present at birth, the defect usually corrects itself. Until this occurs, the baby should sleep in a crib with the head raised and be given feedings that are thicker than usual.

An overweight adult patient must lose weight, and sleep propped up on a pillow. Antacid preparations can help to relieve heartburn. The patient is generally encouraged to eat a main meal at lunchtime, and have a light snack a few hours before bedtime.

If these measures fail to bring adequate relief, or if the symptoms worsen, a surgical operation may be necessary.

Hiccups are repeated involuntary spasms of the diaphragm muscle, accompanied by the closing of the vocal cords. Each spasm causes a sharp inhalation of breath and a characteristic, abrupt, coughlike noise.

Hiccups are almost always brought on by eating too fast, or swallowing stomach irritants, such as hot or cold foods, or carbonated drinks. A person suffering from a prolonged attack of hiccups should consult a physician.

A talk about High blood pressure

High blood pressure (hypertension) is a condition in which a person's blood pressure is persistently above normal. Although blood pressure varies from person to person, a pressure of approximately 120/80 is considered normal when measured while the person is at rest (*see* BLOOD PRESSURE).

High blood pressure can be caused by a variety of conditions, and if the level remains high the patient is more likely to develop heart attack, stroke, or heart and kidney failure.

Q: *What are the symptoms of high blood pressure?*

A: Symptoms are rare. High blood pressure is usually discovered during a routine examination. However, a very high blood pressure causes headaches, heart failure, and vision disturbances.

Q: *What conditions cause high blood pressure?*

A: In more than 90 percent of patients the cause of high blood pressure is unknown. Such patients are said to be suffering from

Hip

essential hypertension. Among the known causes of high blood pressure, however, are kidney disease, chronic nephritis, pyelonephritis, or polycystic kidneys tending to produce retention of salt in the body.

Q: *How is high blood pressure treated?*

A: Treatments for high blood pressure vary. Drug therapy includes the use of DIURETICS to get rid of excess salt. Sometimes, the cause of high blood pressure itself can be treated.

Q: *What is the danger if blood pressure rises during pregnancy.*

A: High blood pressure in pregnancy can indicate PREECLAMPSIA. Other symptoms are fluid retention and ALBUMINURIA (protein in the urine). If the blood pressure is not rapidly reduced to normal, there is an increased chance of the mother developing ECLAMPSIA.

Hip is the part of the body at the widest part of the pelvis, and the underlying bone. The hip joint at the top of the leg is capable of movement in many directions. It is a ball-and-socket joint in which a ball at the end of the thigh bone (femur) fits into a socket in the pelvis. The hip joint is supported by strong ligaments and is extremely secure.

Q: *What severe disorders can affect the hip?*

A: Congenital dislocation of the hip joint occurs spontaneously at, or soon after, birth. It may be caused by an inherited weakness, a breech birth, or slackening of

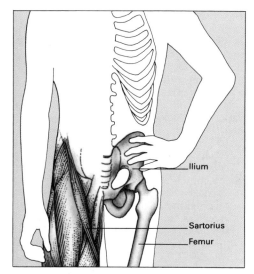

Hip is the strongest joint in the body, supported by large muscles and ligaments.

the baby's joints by hormones from the mother. If diagnosed at birth, the dislocation can be treated in a plaster-of-Paris cast.

Fractures of the neck of the femur occur commonly in the elderly. Surgical procedures either pin the bones together, or replace the head of the femur with a metal head that fits into the hip joint.

The hip may also be involved in rheumatoid ARTHRITIS or OSTEOARTHRITIS, or it may become infected, causing pyogenic arthritis.

Q: *How is severe arthritis of the hip treated?*

A: If treatment with drugs is not successful, various surgical operations can be performed. The most successful is total replacement of the joint with an artificial one made of metal or plastic and metal.

Hirschsprung's disease (megacolon) is a congenital defect of the large intestine in which there is an absence of the nerve fibers within certain segments of the intestinal muscles. As a result, the muscles in the affected area do not work and there is no peristalsis (the rhythmic movement by which the intestine moves its contents along) in the affected section. This acts as an obstruction.

Q: *What are the symptoms of Hirschsprung's disease?*

A: There is usually severe, continuous constipation, and the abdomen becomes increasingly distended as the intestine fills with feces. The affected child may vomit, and growth may be retarded.

Q: *How is Hirschsprung's disease treated?*

A: Most cases require a surgical operation in which the abnormal section of the intestine is removed, and the two normal ends joined together.

Hirsutism is the excessive growth of hair or the presence of hair in areas that are not usually hairy. Medical conditions that cause excessive hair growth are usually caused by hormonal disturbances and are much more common in females than in males. An increase in hair may occur after menopause or in patients taking corticosteroid drugs. *See also* ELECTROLYSIS.

Histamine is a chemical that is normally present in the body. Large amounts are released in response to injury or to antigen-antibody reaction, such as in an allergic reaction. Histamine is also involved in the secretion of acid by the stomach.

Histamine causes many of the involuntary smooth muscles to contract and causes the capillary blood vessels to expand. These effects account for many of the symptoms of allergic reactions and inflammation.

Q: *How may the adverse effects of histamine be prevented?*

A: The most rapidly effective antidote is epinephrine (adrenaline), which is usually given by injection. ANTIHISTAMINES are better at preventing reactions than treating them, and are useful if an allergic reaction (such as hay fever) is expected.

Histology is the study of the microscopic structure of tissues. Pathological histology is the study of diseased tissues.

Histoplasmosis is an infection caused by the fungus *Histoplasma capsulatum*. It originates in the lungs when spores of the fungus are inhaled, and may spread in the bloodstream to other parts of the body. Histoplasmosis may be mild and acute or, rarely, progressive and eventually fatal, if untreated. Mild histoplasmosis has no obvious symptoms. The only sign of infection is the presence of calcified spots on the lungs, which can be detected on a chest X ray. The primary acute form of severe histoplasmosis is characterized by a cough, breathlessness, hoarseness, coughing blood, chest pains, and a bluish tinge to the lips. There may also be fever, chills, muscle pains, weight loss, and fatigue. Occasionally, the disease spreads to other parts of the body; this is called progressive disseminated histoplasmosis.

Hives, or urticaria, is a condition characterized by red, slightly swollen eruptions or itchy lumps on the skin. The lumps are called angioneurotic edema when they occur with excessive swelling of soft tissues.

Q: *What causes hives?*

A: Hives is usually caused by an allergic reaction to an insect bite or sting; to a drug; or to certain foods, such as shell fish or eggs. Virus or streptococcus bacterial infection also cause hives in some persons; others may inherit a tendency to develop hives.

Q: *What are the symptoms of hives and how is the condition treated?*

A: Itching is usually the first symptom, followed rapidly by the formation of lumps of various sizes, which may appear anywhere on the skin.

   Hives in the mouth or throat may cause respiratory obstructions that require urgent treatment. If the throat is involved, injections of the hormone epinephrine is urgently required, followed by antihistamine drugs. In most cases, hives lasts for only a few days.

Hodgkin's disease is a maligant (cancerous) condition involving the body's lymph glands. The condition may spread throughout the body to the spleen, liver, and other organs.

   As the disease progresses, the patient experiences loss of weight, tiredness, and a general feeling of ill health.

Q: *How is Hodgkin's disease treated?*

A: Radiotherapy may be combined with CYTOTOXIC DRUGS, which may have to be taken for many months. The earlier the diagnosis is made, the more successful is the treatment.

Homeopathy is a form of medicine in which disorders are treated by giving the patient minute doses of substances that produce the same symptoms as does the disorder. Most of the substances used in homeopathy are derived from herbs that have been repeatedly diluted in a mixture of alcohol and water, sometimes with a little sugar added. The dilution of the mixture is so great that very little of the original substance remains in the final preparation.

A talk about Homosexuality

Homosexuality describes sexual orientation in which one person engages in sexual activity with another person of the same sex. A woman with this preference is called a lesbian.

Q: *What causes homosexuality?*

A: There are many theories about why homosexuality occurs but there is little real evidence of how sexual object choice is developed.

   Normal sexual development includes a transient phase, at about the time of puberty, in which a tendency toward homosexuality is normal. Sometimes, physical homosexual relations take place and sexual tension is relieved, though

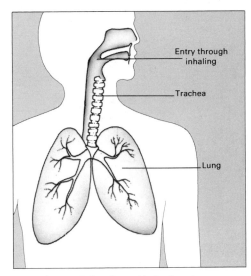

Histoplasmosis is a fungal infection that invades the lung after spores are inhaled.

such relations do not mean that the individuals concerned are permanently homosexual.

In most young people, heterosexual interest develops normally after the homosexual phase.

Q: Is it possible or desirable to treat homosexuality?

A: Many homosexual persons are perfectly happy and would not wish to change even if this were possible. Individuals who feel guilty, embarrassed, or abnormal about being homosexual can sometimes benefit from discussions with a sex counselor or psychiatrist. For homosexuals who really want to become heterosexual, psycho-analysis and psychotherapy may help.

Q: Is everyone who has ever enjoyed physical homosexuality a homosexual?

A: Not necessarily. When men or women are confined together with people of their own sex only, there is no sexual outlet other than masturbation or homo-sexuality. In such situations, homosexual activity may take place among people who are normally heterosexual. Such individuals usually revert to hetero-sexuality when they return to the mixed community.

Q: Can homosexuals lead a normal life?

A: Young homosexuals often have a period of promiscuity and then settle down with one partner in a stable relation-ship. But homosexual partnerships are more subject to turmoil than are heterosexual ones. Older homosexuals, who experience disappointment as they

become less physically attractive, may end up feeling rejected and lonely.

Q: How should parents react if they think that their child is homosexual?

A: A parent of a homosexual child should realize that love is more important than condemnation. Trying to persuade a child to change sexual interest often produces problems not solutions. Sympathy and understanding have more effect. Parents who have this concern should seek the help of a psychologist or psychiatrist.

Hookworm. *See* ANKYLOSTOMIASIS.

Hormones are powerful chemical substances produced by cells in one organ that act on other organs to regulate their activity. Several organs produce hormones. The ENDOCRINE GLANDS, such as the thyroid gland, produce hormones that are carried in the bloodstream to effect activities in other parts of the body. Other hormones are produced by the gastrointestinal tract and have a more local effect, stimulating the production of digestive juices from adjacent areas of the small intestines.

See also ADRENAL GLANDS; CORPUS LUTEUM; GONAD; GRAAFIAN FOLLICLE; OVARY; PARATHY-ROID GLAND; TESTIS; THYROID GLAND.

Horner's syndrome is a condition that affects one side of the face. The pupil of the eye constricts (myosis); the upper eyelid droops (ptosis); and the eyeball is set deeper into its socket than usual. The skin may be red and lose the ability to sweat on the affected side of the face. Horner's syndrome is caused by paralysis of the sympathetic nervous system in the neck. This condition may result from various rare nervous disorders, occasionally from SHINGLES, or as a result of nerve compression from a tumor in the upper chest.

A talk about Hospitals

Hospitals vary greatly in size, from fewer than one hundred beds to several thousand. If a physician recommends hospitalization, it is better to go to the hospital that he or she recommends, rather than requesting one that is reputed to have better facilities, but where the physicians may be strangers.

Q: How are hospitals organized?

A: The basic organization of all hospitals is similar. Within a hospital there are a number of hierarchical divisions of personnel. There are four main divisions: the Hospital Board; the medical staff; the nursing staff; and the nonmedical staff. The better the cooperation between these

Age	Muscular growth	Height spurt	Pubic hair	Penis	Testes
9					
10					
11					
12					
13					
14					
15					
16					
17					
18					

Androgens such as testosterone are essential hormones for a boy's pubescent growth.

Hormones released during puberty control gradual (gray) and fast (blue) development.

groups, the better the care received by the patients.

Q: *What is the function of the Hospital Board?*

A: The Hospital Board makes major decisions about the general running of the hospital, such as policy decisions, expansion programs, and fund-raising. The link between the Board and the rest of the hospital is usually the chief administrator.

Q: *How is the medical staff organized?*

A: The medical staff comprises not only the physicians, but also the anesthetists, pathologists, radiologists, and surgeons. The medical staff is headed by a Chief of Staff, who always holds a medical degree but whose position is administrative. Immediately below the Chief of Staff are the chiefs of various subdivisions, such as medicine, surgery, and gynecology. Should there be a complaint about a member of the medical staff, it is the responsibility of the department head and finally the Chief of Staff to take action.

The resident staff are the most junior members of the hierarchy and are in training in the various medical specialties. They deal with the patient's immediate needs at all times. If a patient needs emergency attention, it is usually a resident who gives the initial treatment. Residents have obtained their basic medical degree; a residency is an extension of their training to determine which branch of medicine they will practice. Residents are not in sole charge of a patient but are responsible to more senior and experienced physicians.

Q: *How is the nursing staff organized?*

A: The nurses are headed by the Director of Nursing, immediately below whom is the Assistant Director. Nursing Supervisors are responsible for several floors or sections. Head Nurses are responsible for individual units and organize the nurses' work on that unit.

Nurses are rated according to the length and quality of their training. An RN is a registered nurse, a rating which is at least equivalent to a college degree; an LPN is a licensed practical nurse, a slightly lower qualification than an RN; and a nursing aide is restricted to performing less skilled procedures.

Some of the nursing staff are responsible for training nurses and the revision of nursing care. This benefits both the medical staff and patients.

Q: *How is the nonmedical staff organized?*

A: The nonmedical staff supply the essential auxiliary services, such as cleaning; laundry; food; and the maintenance of complicated medical equipment. The person who is responsible for the day-to-day running of all these services is the Chief Administrator or Executive Director. There are also assistant directors and directors of various departments, who are all responsible to the Chief Administrator.

Q: *How is the government involved in the running of a hospital?*

A: There are many government regulations with which a hospital must comply. There are also periodic visits from government inspectors to ensure that a hospital maintains standards and complies with the regulations.

Hot flash, or flush, is a sensation of warmth accompanied by reddening of the skin of the face. It is a common symptom of menopause. *See* MENOPAUSE.

Housemaid's knee. *See* PREPATELLAR BURSITIS.

Humerus is the bone of the upper arm, between the shoulder and the elbow. The ulnar nerve lies behind the lower, inner end of the humerus, an area known as the FUNNY BONE.

Humor is a fluid or semifluid substance in the eyeball. There are two humors, the aqueous humor and the vitreous humor, both of which help to maintain the shape of the eyeball. The aqueous humor is a transparent liquid that fills the region between the cornea at the front of the eye and the lens. The vitreous humor is a transparent, jellylike substance

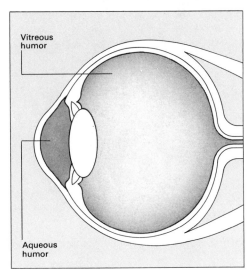

Vitreous humor

Aqueous humor

Humor of two different kinds occur in the eye—aqueous is fairly fluid, vitreous is jellylike.

that occupies the region between the lens and the retina at the back of the eye.

Q: How is the aqueous humor produced?

A: The aqueous humor is constantly secreted by the tissues within the iris, so there is a continuous flow of the humor from the rear chamber to the front chamber. The aqueous humor is kept at constant pressure by a compensating leakage in the angle between the outer rim of the iris and the back of the cornea.

Q: What is the function of the aqueous humor?

A: The aqueous humor carries nutrients and facilitates the exchange of gases (oxygen and carbon dioxide) in the cornea and other tissues of the eyeball that have no blood supply.

Q: What disorders may affect the aqueous humor?

A: Disturbances of the drainage mechanism that maintains a constant fluid pressure in the aqueous humor may cause an increase in the pressure, a condition called GLAUCOMA.

Q: How is the vitreous humor produced?

A: The vitreous humor is present from birth and remains virtually unchanged throughout an individual's life.

Q: What disorders may affect the vitreous humor?

A: Specks may occur in the vitreous humor caused by the degeneration of its cells with age. This is a normal occurrence and the presence of specks does not noticeably impair vision. Occasionally, a hemorrhage into the vitreous humor may

occur, usually caused by an injury. A hemorrhage may also occur in DIABETES MELLITUS, ARTERIOSCLEROSIS, or RETINITIS. A hemorrhage may be serious and a physician should be consulted.

Huntington's chorea is an inherited disorder of the central nervous system that is characterized by involuntary movements and progressive dementia. *See* CHOREA.

Hutchinson's teeth is a congenital anomaly in which the permanent incisor teeth are narrow and notched. It is usually a sign of congenital syphilis.

Hyaline membrane disease is a respiratory disorder of the newborn. *See* RESPIRATORY DISTRESS SYNDROME.

Hydatid cyst is a kind of CYST that forms in body tissues, especially those of the liver. It encloses the larvae of a type of tapeworm (*Echinococcus granulosus*). This parasite can infest dogs, foxes, wolves, cattle, and sheep. It is passed on to human beings in food that has been contaminated with the eggs of the tapeworm (usually from a dog).

Q: What are the symptoms of hydatid cysts?

A: Frequently, there are no symptoms, although there may be a dull ache on the right side of the abdomen and the liver may become enlarged.

Q: How is hydatid cyst disease treated?

A: When the condition has been confirmed the only treatment is to remove the cyst, or cysts, through surgery.

Hydatidiform mole is a usually benign (noncancerous) growth of the placenta (afterbirth) that may develop in early pregnancy.

There may be bleeding similar to that from a threatened MISCARRIAGE. The bleeding tends to continue and may result in the spontaneous loss of a mass of small, grapelike tissues from the womb.

Q: What is the treatment for a hydatidiform mole?

A: If the growth is not spontaneously expelled, the obstetrician induces early labor by infusion of the drug oxytocin, followed a few days later by a D AND C.

Hydrocele is an accumulation of fluid in any of the body's saclike cavities. The term is most often used to describe an excess of fluid in the scrotum, the small protective bag that surrounds each TESTIS.

Q: What causes a hydrocele?

A: The male embryo in the womb has a canal that links the abdominal cavity with the scrotum. This canal usually closes before birth but it occasionally remains open.

A less common cause of hydrocele is inflammation of a testicle or of the epididymis around it. A direct blow to

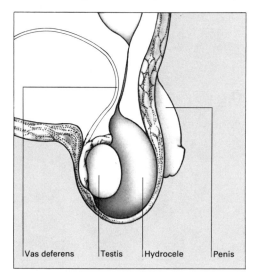

| Vas deferens | Testis | Hydrocele | Penis |

Hydrocele is an accumulation of fluid in a body cavity, especially the scrotum.

the genitals may also cause a hydrocele.

Q: How is a hydrocele treated?

A: Congenital hydrocele in children usually disappears on its own and so does not require treatment. But if it persists for more than a year, a pediatrician may advise surgery to remove the bag.

Hydrocephalus results from increased cerebrospinal fluid inside the brain. In infants this causes skull enlargement. Brain damage resulting from the excessive accumulation of cerebrospinal fluid produces mental retardation, epilepsy, and finally, in some children, death. Hydrocephalus may be associated with SPINA BIFIDA.

Q: What conditions may cause hydrocephalus?

A: In most cases, the disorder is present at birth (congenital). There is a blockage to the normal circulation and absorption of cerebrospinal fluid in the brain. Or hydrocephalus may be caused by a brain tumor that interferes with the usual circulation of the cerebrospinal fluid. This can also occur because of scarring of the membrane covering the brain following MENINGITIS.

Q: What symptoms appear with hydrocephalus?

A: The chief sign is an abnormally large head. In severe cases, the forehead bulges and the eyes appear to have receded into a face that is disproportionally smaller. The soft spots or spaces between the cranial bones of the skull (fontanels) may seem unusually tight or tense to touch.

Q: How is hydrocephalus treated?

A: In about one third of babies born with hydrocephalus, the condition does not get worse. There are various forms of brain surgery to bypass the blockage to the flow of cerebrospinal fluid. Usually a tube is run through a tunnel created under the skin to the abdominal cavity where the excess fluid is reabsorbed into the circulatory system.

Hydrocortisone. *See* CORTISOL.

Hydrogen peroxide (H_2O_2) is a colorless, nontoxic liquid used in a dilute solution in water as a disinfectant to clean wounds, ulcers, abscesses, septic tooth sockets, or inflamed mucous membranes. It may also be used to treat a sore throat, to soften hard wax in the ears, and to bleach hair.

Hydronephrosis is the swelling of a kidney caused by complete or partial obstruction of urine flow. It causes a gradual destruction of kidney tissues from the increased pressure. Often there are no symptoms, but occasionally urinary tract infection will call attention to this disorder. If both kidneys are affected, kidney failure may result.

Q: How is hydronephrosis diagnosed and treated?

A: An X ray of the kidney, called an INTRAVENOUS PYELOGRAM (IVP), shows the structure of the kidney, and blood tests may reveal uremia. It is important that any infection be treated immediately with antibiotic drugs to prevent further damage to the kidney.

Hydrophobia. *See* RABIES.

Hydrotherapy is the treatment of a disorder with water: either drinking it or bathing in it.

Hymen, or maidenhead, is a thin fold of mucous membrane surrounding the entrance to the vagina, that may initially close it.

Despite popular belief, rupture or absence of the hymen is not proof of the loss of virginity. When the hymen takes the form of an unperforated membrane, menstrual blood cannot escape (hematocolpos).

Hyoid bone is a semicircular bone that lies at the base of the tongue, just above the thyroid cartilage (Adam's apple), and partly encircles the epiglottis.

Hyperacusis is an abnormal sensitivity to sound. To a person with hyperacusis, even ordinary levels of sound may cause pain.

Hyperchlorhydria is an excessive secretion of hydrochloric acid in the gastric juices of the stomach. It may lead to the formation of a PEPTIC ULCER.

Hyperemesis is the medical term for excessive vomiting. It may be a feature of conditions such as gastric flu and intestinal obstruction. When it occurs in pregnancy it is known as hyperemesis gravidarum.

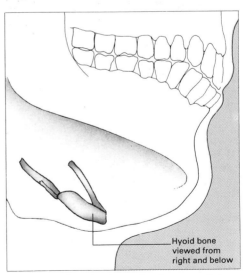

Hyoid bone is a tiny bone that is suspended within the jaw at the base of the tongue.

Hyperesthesia

Q: *What causes hyperemesis gravidarum and how is it treated?*

A: Excessive vomiting during pregnancy is a serious form of the normal, early morning sickness that affects fifty percent of pregnant women. Hyperemesis gravidarum probably develops because of an oversensitivity of the vomiting center in the brain to the hormones produced during pregnancy, but it may be of psychological origin. The vomiting causes dehydration, and should be treated in a hospital with intravenous infusions of glucose, antinauseant drugs, and sedation.

See also VOMITING.

Hyperesthesia is an increased sensitivity of a sensory organ, most commonly in the skin.

Hyperglycemia is a condition in which there is an excessive amount of glucose in the bloodstream. It results from DIABETES MELLITUS.

Hyperhidrosis is excessive perspiration. *See* PERSPIRATION.

Hyperkinesis is a disorder in which a child is physically overactive, constantly on the move, touching and feeling things but seldom remaining still enough to play with them. The condition may first be noted in early infancy when a baby cries a great deal, feeds with great difficulty, and seems to sleep less than normal for the age.

Hyperkinesis is difficult to diagnose and should be dealt with only by qualified physicians. Sometimes the child's problems are primarily emotional and treatment is directed to this area. In other cases, medications, such as AMPHETAMINES (or drugs with similar properties) are prescribed. Although amphetamines are stimulants, their effect on hyperkinetic children is paradoxically quite different—they enable these children to concentrate and think about what they are doing.

Hypermetropia. *See* FARSIGHTEDNESS.

Hypernephroma, or Grawitz's tumor, is a malignant (cancerous) tumor of the kidney. It is the most common form of kidney cancer, and is twice as common in men as women. It usually occurs after the age of forty.

Hyperopia. *See* FARSIGHTEDNESS.

Hyperplasia is an overgrowth of cells that results in an increase in the size of an organ.

Hypersensitivity is a state in which the body or part of the body overreacts to outside stimuli. All forms of hypersensitivity are similar to that occurring in an ALLERGY, such as hay fever or asthma.

See also ANAPHYLAXIS; HYPERESTHESIA.

Hypertension. *See* HIGH BLOOD PRESSURE.

Hyperthyroidism, also known as Graves' disease, or thyrotoxicosis, is overactivity of the thyroid gland, and excessive production of thyroid hormones. *See* THYROTOXICOSIS.

Hypertrophy is an increase in the size of a body tissue or organ. It may occur in the heart muscle of patients with high blood pressure, or in the remaining kidney after one has been removed. Hypertrophy can also occur as the result of changes that take place with age, such as an enlarged prostate gland.

Hyperventilation, also known as over-breathing, occurs when a person inhales much more rapidly than normal, thus disturbing the normal balance of carbon dioxide and oxygen in the bloodstream. Hyperventilation is usually caused by anxiety or emotional tension. Other causes include disorders of the central nervous system and high concentrations of certain drugs in the body.

Symptoms include faintness, dizziness, impaired consciousness, and, in prolonged episodes, muscular spasms. Immediate treatment is directed towards having the patient breathe slowly for a few minutes. Further treatment involves correcting the underlying causes that trigger the episodes.

Hypesthesia (hypoesthesia) is a reduction in the normal sensation from the skin or other sense organs. It may result from nerve damage (polyneuritis) or occur with HEMIANESTHESIA following a stroke.

Hypnosis is an artificially produced trance, similar to light sleep, which makes an individual more susceptible to suggestion. About eighty percent of all human beings can be hypnotized, but few can be put into a deep hypnotic trance. Persons in a light hypnotic trance are aware of their actions and have a distinct memory of what happens. Persons in a deep trance cannot remember details of what occurs.

Q: *What are the medical uses of hypnosis?*

A: Hypnosis can be useful in helping patients to give up habits such as smoking, and to overcome phobias such as the fear of flying. If the patient can be induced into a deeper trance, hypnosis can be used to relieve nervous tics and to reduce the awareness of pain experienced during dental operations, childbirth, or even major surgery.

Hypnotics are drugs that induce a state resembling sleep.

Hypocalcemia is a condition in which there is a lower than normal level of calcium in the blood. It may occur as a result of underactivity of the PARATHYROID GLANDS, or it may be a consequence of vitamin D deficiency (*see* RICKETS; OSTEOMALACIA).

The condition is extremely serious in newborn babies, particularly those fed on cow's milk. In babies, hypocalcemia causes vom-

Hypothyroidism

iting and breathing problems. In adults, there are often no symptoms, and diagnosis is made only after a routine blood test. In severe hypocalcemia, the patient may suffer a seizure or tetany, with muscular spasms of the hands, feet, and jaw.

Hypochondria is a condition in which a person has an undue concern about his or her physical health and well-being. It is frequently a sign of ANXIETY, although a common cause of hypochondria in elderly persons is loneliness.

Hypodermic describes anything applied or administered beneath the skin.

Hypoglycemia is a condition that occurs when the level of glucose (sugar) in the blood is abnormally low. Glucose supplies the body's cells with energy, and a low level of glucose seriously affects the brain cells.

Q: What are the symptoms and signs of hypoglycemia?

A: The patient feels anxious, may behave abnormally, has a rapid, bounding pulse, sweats, feels faint, walks unsteadily, and is confused. He or she may go into a coma.

Hypophysis. *See* PITUITARY GLAND.

Hypopituitarism is decreased function of the pituitary gland that results in an insufficient production of hormones.

Q: What are the symptoms of hypopituitarism?

A: Common symptoms of hypopituitarism include loss of weight, tiredness, lack of sex drive (libido), low blood pressure, and a feeling of faintness. Headaches and vision problems (*see* HEMIANOPIA) may also occur, if the cause of the pituitary malfunction is a tumor. Children with hypopituitarism fail to grow normally and remain small but well-proportioned (*see* DWARFISM). In men and women, the normal hair growth becomes sparse. In women, there is a failure to lactate and menstruation ceases.

Q: What is the treatment for hypopituitarism?

A: If the cause of the condition is a tumor, treatment is the destruction of the tumor using surgery or radiotherapy. If there is no tumor causing the pituitary insufficiency, or after surgery has been performed, a physician may prescribe drugs that are the hormones normally produced by the various other endocrine glands in response to the pituitary gland's stimulus.

Hypoplasia is the incomplete development of an organ or tissue.

Hypostasis is poor circulation in a part of the body, usually the legs.

Hypotension. *See* LOW BLOOD PRESSURE.

Hypothalamus is a part of the brain containing nerve centers that control appetite, thirst, body weight, fluid balance, body temperature, and sex drive (libido). It is located below the THALAMUS and above the PITUITARY GLAND, and acts as a link between the nervous system and endocrine hormone-secreting system.

Hypothermia (for EMERGENCY treatment, *see* First Aid, p.560) is a condition in which the body temperature is lower than normal. The body's normal reaction to cold is to shiver. Hypothermia may take place when the body's ability to produce heat by shivering is reduced, as may happen when the body is excessively chilled, particularly in the young (especially in sick or premature newborn babies) or in the very elderly.

Hypothyroidism is a condition that results from an inadequate supply of hormones from the THYROID GLAND in the neck. When hypothyroidism develops before birth, the infant is retarded both mentally and physically (*see* CRETINISM).

Q: What are the symptoms of hypothyroidism?

A: The symptoms of hypothyroidism include tiredness and a sensitivity to cold. The patient's skin becomes dry and puffy, especially on the face, and the hair of the scalp and the eyebrows becomes dry and brittle. The voice may become hoarse and the eyes dry (xerophthalmia). Constipation is common, and in women there are menstrual disorders, such as heavy bleeding (menorrhagia) and irregular periods.

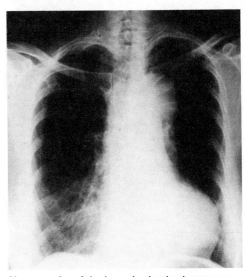

Hypertrophy of the heart is clearly shown as a white shadow in the center of the X ray.

Hypoxia

These symptoms develop gradually. Over a period of time, the individual's personality changes, with a slowing down of the thought processes, sometimes mild confusion and dementia, and occasionally symptoms that suggest paranoia. This severe form of hypothyroidism is called myxedema.

Q: *What is the treatment for hypothyroidism?*

A: A physician usually begins treatment of hypothyroidism with a small dose of one of the thyroid hormones, and then gradually increases the dose. The increase generally takes several weeks, because a sudden change may cause cardiac problems, especially in an elderly patient.

Patients who receive appropriate treatment for hypothyroidism recover completely and can expect to lead a normal life. They will, however, require treatment for the rest of their lives, with occasional blood tests to ensure that the correct amounts of hormones are given.

Hypoxia, or hypoxemia, is a condition in which there is a lack of, or low content of, oxygen in the body tissues, usually because of a reduction in the oxygen-carrying capacity of the blood.

A talk about Hysterectomy

Hysterectomy is an operation to remove the womb (uterus). In a total hysterectomy, the cervix is also removed.

Q: *Why may a physician recommend a hysterectomy?*

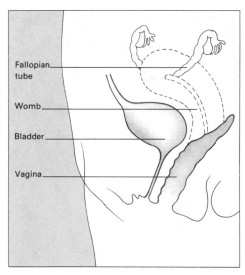

Fallopian tube

Womb

Bladder

Vagina

Hysterectomy patients keep the fallopian tubes and the vagina intact.

A: A hysterectomy is performed to treat cancer of the womb or cervix; if heavy bleeding from the womb causes anemia; or if large fibroids cause troublesome symptoms.

Q: *What is the effect of a hysterectomy?*

A: Menstruation ceases and conception is not possible.

Q: *Are the ovaries removed at the same time as the womb?*

A: In women under the age of about forty-five, the ovaries are usually left if they appear healthy at the time of the operation. In older women, the ovaries are usually removed because they will have no function within a year or two and may cause problems later in life.

Q: *How is a hysterectomy performed?*

A: The operation is usually done through an incision in the abdominal wall. The womb and the fallopian tubes are removed, and the top of the vagina closed to form a blind tube. The patient usually remains in the hospital for ten to fourteen days; the stitches or clips are removed on about the eighth day.

The patient is encouraged to get out of bed as soon as possible after the operation to prevent the risk of venous thrombosis in the legs. If the patient has varicose veins or a previous history of venous thrombosis, she may be given small doses of an anticoagulant drug for a day or two after the operation.

Q: *Does a hysterectomy affect a woman's sexual interest?*

A: There should be no effect on the woman's sexual interest. If the ovaries are removed before menopause, the physician may prescribe a course of hormones, either by implant, by injection, or by mouth. This treatment prevents the sudden onset of the symptoms that are normally associated with MENOPAUSE.

It is advisable not to resume sexual intercourse until the patient has had a postoperative check by a gynecologist about six weeks after the operation. Initially, there may be some discomfort because the top of the vagina is not as elastic as normal.

Hysteria is a form of neurotic disorder that is usually less severe than other mental illnesses. It may present itself at first as an organic disease but later prove to be entirely psychological in origin. Hysteria may be an aspect of the patient's total personality, or it may occur as a sudden (acute) event.